1 MONTH OF
FREE
READING

at

www.ForgottenBooks.com

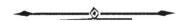

By purchasing this book you are
eligible for one month membership to
ForgottenBooks.com, giving you
unlimited access to our entire
collection of over 1,000,000 titles via
our web site and mobile apps.

To claim your free month visit:

www.forgottenbooks.com/free722398

ISBN 978-0-483-49628-6
PIBN 10722398

TRANSACTIONS

of the

American Ophthalmological Society

Fifty-Seventh Annual Meeting

SWAMPSCOTT, MASS., 1921

VOLUME XIX

Philadelphia

American Ophthalmological Society

1921

PRESS OF WM. F. FELL COMPANY
PHILADELPHIA

TABLE OF CONTENTS

4 *Table of Contents.*

OFFICERS AND COUNCIL

of the

American Ophthalmological Society

Elected at the Annual Meeting, June 14, 1921

———

President

DR. WILLIAM M. SWEET, PHILADELPHIA

Vice-President

DR. WM. H. WILMER, WASHINGTON, D. C.

Secretary-Treasurer

DR. T. B. HOLLOWAY, PHILADELPHIA

Council

DR. CASSIUS D. WESCOTT, CHICAGO, ILL.

DR. W. B. LANCASTER, BOSTON, MASS.

DR. WALTER R. PARKER, DETROIT, MICH.

DR. W. E. LAMBERT, NEW YORK

DR. HOWARD F. HANSELL, PHILADELPHIA

PRESIDENTS OF THE SOCIETY

(Since its Foundation)

1864–1868   Dr. Edward Delafield, New York.

1869–1873   Dr. Henry W. Williams, Boston, Mass.

1874–1878   Dr. C. R. Agnew, New York.

1879–1884   Dr. Henry D. Noyes, New York.

1885–1889   Dr. William F. Norris, Philadelphia.

1890–1893   Dr. Hasket Derby, Boston, Mass.

1894–1898   Dr. George C. Harlan, Philadelphia.

1899–1902   Dr. O. F. Wadsworth, Boston, Mass.

1903–1905   Dr. Charles S. Bull, New York.

1906   Dr. Arthur Mathewson, Washington, D. C.

1907   Dr. Charles J. Kipp, Newark, N. J.

1908   Dr. Samuel D. Risley, Philadelphia.

1909   Dr. S. B. St. John, Hartford, Conn.

1910   Dr. Samuel Theobald, Baltimore, Md.

1911   Dr. Emil Gruening, New York.

1912   Dr. Edward Jackson, Denver, Col.

1913   Dr. Myles Standish, Boston, Mass.

1914   Dr. Robert Sattler, Cincinnati, O.

1915   Dr. M. H. Post, St. Louis, Mo.

1916   Dr. George E. de Schweinitz, Philadelphia.

1917   Dr. Peter A. Callan, New York.

1918   Dr. William H. Wilder, Chicago, Ill.

1919   Dr. Lucien Howe, Buffalo, N. Y.

1920   Dr. Hiram Woods, Baltimore, Md.

1921   Dr. John E. Weeks, New York.

American Ophthalmological Society.

FOUNDED 1864.

LIST OF MEMBERS.

* Associate Members.   O. M. Original Members

ELECTED.	NAME.	RESIDENCE.	PLACE.
1896	DR. A. E. ADAMS,	The Inn,	Newburgh, N. Y.
1915	DR. ELLICE M. ALGER,	40 East 41st Street,	New York, N. Y.
1899	DR. A. N. ALLING,	257 Church Street,	New Haven, Conn
1883	Dr. J. A. ANDREWS,	1229 State Street,	Santa Barbara, Cal.
1913	DR. FRED. D. BAILEY,	260 Hancock Street,	Brooklyn, N. Y.
1911	DR. ARTHUR J. BEDELL,	344 State Street,	Albany, N. Y.
1908	DR. GEO. H. BELL,	40 East 41st Street,	New York, N. Y.
1905	DR. JAS. H. BELL,	Moore Building,	San Antonio, Texas.
1921	*DR. WM. L. BENEDICT,	Mayo Clinic,	Rochester, Minn.
1921	*DR. NELSON M. BLACK,	120 Wisconsin St.,	Milwaukee, Wis.
1916	DR. EUGENE M. BLAKE,	55 Trumbull Street,	New Haven, Conn.
1909	DR. JAMES BORDLEY, JR.,	Professional Building,	Baltimore, Md.
1881	DR. H. W. BRADFORD,		Wolfboro, N. H.
1918	DR. H. H. BRIGGS,	73 Haywood Street,	Asheville, N. C.
1908	DR. E. V. L. BROWN,	122 S. Michigan Blvd.,	Chicago, Ill.
1907	DR. WM. E. BRUNER,	Guardian Bldg.,	Cleveland, Ohio.
1901	DR. H. D. BRUNS,	211 Camp Street,	New Orleans, La.
1920	*DR. JOHN W. BURKE,	1740 M Street, N. W.,	Washington, D. C.
1906	DR. W. K. BUTLER,	1207 M Street, N. W.,	Washington, D. C.
1906	DR. W. GORDON M. BYERS,	346 Mountain Street,	Montreal, Canada.
1918	DR. F. PHINIZY CALHOUN,	Candler Building,	Atlanta, Ga.
1876	DR. PETER A. CALLAN,	452 Fifth Avenue,	New York, N. Y.
1885	DR. F. P. CAPRON,	118 Angell Street,	Providence, R. I.
O. M.	DR. W. H. CARMALT,	261 St. Ronan Street,	New Haven, Conn.
1898	DR. J. T. CARPENTER,	2030 Chestnut Street,	Philadelphia, Pa.
1904	DR. BURTON CHANCE,	1303 Spruce Street,	Philadelphia, Pa.
1893	DR. H. B. CHANDLER,	34½ Beacon Street,	Boston, Mass.
1904	DR. J. W. CHARLES,	509 Humboldt Bldg.,	St. Louis, Mo.
1893	DR. F. E. CHENEY,	64 Commonw'th Ave.,	Boston, Mass.
1898	DR. J. H. CLAIBORNE,	9 East 46th Street,	New York, N. Y.
1912	DR. E. W. CLAP,	390 Commonw'th Ave.,	Boston, Mass.
1891	DR. C. F. CLARK,	188 East State Street,	Columbus, Ohio.

Elected.	Name.	Residence.	Place.
1912	Dr. G. S. Crampton,	1700 Walnut Street,	Philadelphia, Pa.
1890	Dr. C. M. Culver,	36 Eagle Street,	Albany, N. Y.
1906	Dr. R. J. Curdy,	1134 Rialto Building,	Kansas City, Mo.
1902	Dr. Colman W. Cutler,	24 East 48th Street,	New York, N. Y.
1907	Dr. A. E. Davis,	47 East 57th Street,	New York, N. Y.
1878	Dr. W. S. Dennett,	36 Gramercy Park,	New York, N. Y.
1918	*Dr. David N. Dennis,	221 West 9th Street,	Erie, Pa.
1909	Dr. George S. Derby,	23 Bay State Road,	Boston, Mass.
1874	Dr. Lewis S. Dixon,	232 Clarendon Street,	Boston, Mass.
1912	Dr. Oscar Dodd,	1604 Chicago Avenue,	Evanston, Ill.
1902	Dr. Alexander Duane,	139 E. 37th Street,	New York, N. Y.
1908	Dr. J. L. Duncan,	Jenkins Bldg.,	Pittsburgh, Pa.
1912	Dr. E. C. Ellett,	Exchange Building,	Memphis, Tenn.
1887	Dr. J. B. Emerson,	40 East 41st Street,	New York, N. Y.
1890	Dr. Arthur E. Ewing,	Metropolitan Bldg.,	St. Louis, Mo.
1920	*Dr. Marcus Feingold,	4206 St. Charles Ave.,	New Orleans, La.
1896	Dr. T. H. Fenton,	1319 Spruce Street,	Philadelphia, Pa. '
1920	*Dr. William C. Finnoff,	318 Majestic Building,	Denver, Col.
1915	Dr. Carl Fisher,	1028 Pacific-Mutual Bldg.,	Los Angeles, Cal.
1893	Dr. George F. Fiske,	25 E. Washington Street,	Chicago, Ill.
1909	Dr. M. L. Foster,	106 Centre Avenue,	New Rochelle, N.Y
1904	Dr. W. H. Fox,	1826 Jefferson Place,	Washington, D. C.
1913	Dr. Lee M. Francis,	636 Delaware Avenue,	Buffalo, N. Y.
1902	Dr. Percy Fridenberg,	38 West 59th Street,	New York, N. Y.
1894	Dr. H. Friedenwald,	1029 Madison Ave.,	Baltimore, Md.
1913	Dr. H. G. Goldberg,	1925 Chestnut Street,	Philadelphia, Pa.
1895	Dr. G. M. Gould,	215 Atlantic Avenue,	Atlantic City, N. J.
1896	Dr. H. Y. Grant,	Falls View,	Ontario, Canada.
1919	*Dr. John Green, Jr.,	626 Metropolitan Bldg.,	St. Louis, Mo.
1908	Dr. L. S. Greene,	1624 I Street, N. W.,	Washington, D. C.
1905	Dr. Allen Greenwood,	101 Newbury Street,	Boston, Mass.
1914	Dr. J. Milton Griscom,	1925 Chestnut St.,	Philadelphia, Pa.
1892	Dr. G. W. Hale,	210 Hitchcock Building,	Nashville, Tenn.
1895	Dr. Wm. D. Hall,	416 Marlborough Street,	Boston, Mass.
1887	Dr. H. F. Hansell,	17th and Walnut Streets,	Philadelphia, Pa.
1918	*Dr. D. F. Harbridge,	Goodrich Building,	Phoenix, Ariz.
1918	Dr. Wm. F. Hardy,	Metropolitan Bldg.,	St. Louis, Mo.
1901	Dr. Herbert Harlan,	516 Cathedral Street,	Baltimore, Md.
1889	Dr. David Harrower,	13 Elm Street,	Worcester, Mass.
1896	Dr. N. D. Harvey,	114 Waterman Street,	Providence, R. I.
1904	Dr. H. H. Haskell,	29 Commonwealth Ave.,	Boston, Mass.
1914	Dr. Edw. B. Heckel,	Jenkins Building,	Pittsburgh, Pa.
1913	Dr. Chas. R. Heed,	1205 Spruce Street,	Philadelphia, Pa.
1920	*Dr. Emory Hill,	Professional Building,	Richmond, Va.
1896	Dr. Ward A. Holden,	8 East 54th Street,	New York, N. Y.

ELECTED.	NAME.	RESIDENCE.	PLACE.
1909	DR. T. B. HOLLOWAY,	1819 Chestnut Street,	Philadelphia, Pa.
1883	DR. E. E. HOLT,	723 Congress Street,	Portland, Me.
1921	*DR. E. E. HOLT, JR.	723 Congress Street,	Portland, Me.
1917	*DR. HARVEY J. HOWARD,	Union Medical College,	Peking, China.
1878	DR. LUCIEN HOWE,	520 Delaware Avenue,	Buffalo, N. Y.
1891	DR. D. W. HUNTER,	80 West 40th Street,	New York, N. Y.
1898	DR. J. W. INGALLS,	328 Stuyvesant Ave.,	Brooklyn, N. Y.
1895	DR. E. E. JACK,	215 Beacon Street,	Boston, Mass.
1885	DR. EDWARD JACKSON,	318 Majestic Building,	Denver, Col.
1912	DR. P. C. JAMESON,	139 Montague Street,	Brooklyn, N. Y.
1918	*DR. J. WILKINSON JERVEY,	Jervey-Jordan Bldg.,	Greenville, S. C.
1892	DR. W. B. JOHNSON,	170 Broadway,	Paterson, N. J.
1908	DR. B. R. KENNON,	Taylor Building,	Norfolk, Va.
1919	*DR. BEN WITT KEY,	180 W. 59th Street,	New York, N. Y.
1903	DR. ARNOLD KNAPP,	10 East 54th Street,	New York, N. Y.
1889	DR. CARL KOLLER,	681 Madison Avenue,	New York, N. Y.
1888	DR. CHAS. W. KOLLOCK,	86 Wentworth Street,	Charleston, S. C.
1913	DR. ROBERT S. LAMB,	Stoneleigh Court,	Washington, D. C.
1891	DR. W. E. LAMBERT,	112 East 35th Street,	New York, N. Y.
1902	DR. W. B. LANCASTER,	522 Commonw'lth Ave.,	Boston, Mass.
1919	*DR. FRANCIS LANE,	25 E. Washington Street,	Chicago, Ill.
1912	DR. H. M. LANGDON,	2014 Chestnut Street,	Philadelphia, Pa.
1903	DR. J. C. LESTER,	616 Madison Avenue,	New York, N. Y.
1907	DR. GEORGE F. LIBBY,	Majestic Bldg.,	Denver, Col.
1883	DR. J. A. LIPPINCOTT,	Jenkins Building,	Pittsburgh, Pa.
1878	DR. F. B. LORING,	1420 K Street,	Washington, D. C.
1909	DR. R. G. LORING,	140 Beacon Street,	Boston, Mass.
1899	DR. D. B. LOVELL,	340 Main Street	Worcester, Mass.
1914	DR. W. H. LOWELL,	101 Newbury Street,	Boston, Mass.
1919	*DR. W. H. LUEDDE,	311 Metropolitan Bldg.,	St. Louis, Mo.
1918	DR. HUNTER H. MCGUIRE,	105 N. Braddock Street,	Winchester, Va.
1913	DR. A. L. MACLEISH,	1101 Brockman Bldg.,	Los Angeles, Cal.
1891	DR. F. W. MARLOW,	731 University Block,	Syracuse, N. Y.
1878	DR. W. V. MARMION,	1300 Fairm'nt St., N.W.,	Washington, D. C.
1907	DR. C. H. MAY,	698 Madison Avenue,	New York, N. Y.
1874	DR. C. S. MERRILL,	27 S. Hawk Street,	Albany, N. Y.
1908	DR. H. S. MILES,	881 Lafayette Street,	Bridgeport, Conn.
1883	DR. J. LANCELOT MINOR,	Bank of Commerce Bldg.,	Memphis, Tenn.
1916	DR. JOHN H. OHLY,	22 Schermerhorn St.,	Brooklyn, N. Y.
1908	DR. W. R. PARKER,	David Whitney Bldg.,	Detroit, Mich.
1908	DR. S. McA. PAYNE,	542 Fifth Avenue,	New York, N. Y.
1920	*DR. ADOLPH O. PFINGST,	Francis Building,	Louisville, Ky.
1895	DR. R. J. PHILLIPS,	123 So. 39th Street,	Philadelphia, Pa.
1898	DR. W. CAMPBELL POSEY,	2049 Chestnut Street,	Philadelphia, Pa.
1895	DR. H. R. PRICE,	146 Remsen Street,	Brooklyn, N. Y.

ELECTED.	NAME.	RESIDENCE.	PLACE.
1906	DR. BROWN PUSEY,	7 West Madison Street,	Chicago, Ill.
1901	DR. ALEX. QUACKENBOSS,	143 Newbury Street,	Boston, Mass.
1906	DR. McCLUNEY RADCLIFFE,	1906 Chestnut Street,	Philadelphia, Pa.
1885	DR. ALEX'R RANDALL,	1717 Locust Street,	Philadelphia, Pa.
1901	DR. R. G. REESE,	50 West 52nd Street,	New York, N. Y
1899	DR. H. O. REIK,	300 E. 30th Street,	Baltimore, Md.
1912	DR. W. G. REYNOLDS,	1165 Dean Street,	Brooklyn, N. Y.
1901	DR. G. O. RING,	17th and Walnut Streets,	Philadelphia, Pa.
1895	DR. H. W. RING,	185 Church Street,	New Haven, Conn.
1908	DR. J. NORMAN RISLEY,	238 Union Street,	New Bedford, Mass.
1920	*DR. WILLIAM H. ROBERTS,	461 E. Colorado Street,	Pasadena, Cal.
1899	DR. DUNBAR ROY,	Gr. Opera House Blk.,	Atlanta, Ga.
1875	DR. JOHN D. RUSHMORE,	129 Montague Street,	Brooklyn, N. Y.
1880	DR. ROBERT SATTLER,	30, The Groton,	Cincinnati, Ohio.
1912	DR. A. C. SAUTTER,	1421 Locust Street,	Philadelphia, Pa.
1898	DR. T. B. SCHNEIDEMAN,	1831 Chestnut Street,	Philadelphia, Pa.
1919	*DR. M. J. SCHOENBERG,	103 E. 81st Street,	New York, N. Y.
1889	DR. G. E. DE SCHWEINITZ,	1705 Walnut Street,	Philadelphia, Pa.
1895	DR. P. N. K. SCHWENK,	1417 North Broad St.,	Philadelphia, Pa.
1918	*DR. WM. E. SHAHAN,	Metropolitan Bldg.,	St. Louis, Mo.
1913	DR C. E. G. SHANNON,	1633 Spruce Street,	Philadelphia, Pa.
1905	DR. JOHN R. SHANNON,	17 East 38th Street,	New York, N. Y
1916	*DR. FRANCIS W. SHINE,	33 West 52d Street,	New York, N. Y.
1911	DR. J. F. SHOEMAKER,	1006 Carleton Bldg.,	St. Louis, Mo.
1902	DR. WM. A. SHOEMAKER,	1006 Carleton Bldg.,	St. Louis, Mo.
1902	DR. WM. T. SHOEMAKER,	109 South 20th Street,	Philadelphia, Pa.
1905	DR. E. A. SHUMWAY,	2046 Chestnut Street,	Philadelphia, Pa.
1918	DR. DORLAND SMITH,	834 Myrtle Avenue,	Bridgeport, Conn.
1912	DR. E. T. SMITH,	36 Pearl Street,	Hartford, Conn.
1910	DR. ALBERT C. SNELL,	53 S. Fitzhugh St.,	Rochester, N. Y.
1909	DR. F. M. SPALDING,	128 Newbury Street,	Boston, Mass.
1911	DR. CHAS. N. SPRATT,	900 Nicollet Avenue,	Minneapolis, Minn.
1884	DR. MYLES STANDISH,	51 Hereford Street,	Boston, Mass.
1903	DR. EDW. STIEREN,	Union Arcade Bldg.,	Pittsburgh, Pa.
1887	DR. T. Y. SUTPHEN	992 Broad Street,	Newark, N. J.
1900	DR. WM. M. SWEET,	1205 Spruce Street,	Philadelphia, Pa.
1917	DR. WILLIAM TARUN,	605 Park Ave.,	Baltimore, Md.
1888	DR. LEWIS H. TAYLOR,	83 So. Franklin Street,	Wilkesbarre, Pa.
1880	DR. SAMUEL THEOBALD,	Cathedral & How'd Sts.,	Baltimore, Md.
1903	DR. EDGAR S. THOMSON,	39 East 61st Street,	New York, N. Y.
1898	DR. JAS. THORINGTON,	2031 Chestnut Street,	Philadelphia, Pa.
1911	DR. FRED. T. TOOKE,	368 Mountain Street,	Montreal, Canada.
1912	DR. E. TÖRÖK,	8 East 54th Street,	New York, N. Y.
1906	DR. H. H. TYSON,	11 East 48th Street,	New York, N. Y.

ELECTED.	NAME.	RESIDENCE.	PLACE.
1916	DR. DERRICK T. VAIL,	24 East 8th Street,	Cincinnati, Ohio.
1898	DR. C. A. VEASEY,	Paulsen Building,	Spokane, Wash.
1905	DR. F. H. VERHOEFF,	101 Newbury Street,	Boston, Mass.
1903	DR. F. L. WAITE,	68 Pratt Street,	Hartford, Conn.
1916	*DR. CLIFFORD B. WALKER,	317 Main Street,	Springfield, Mass.
1893	DR. J. E. WEEKS,	46 East 57th Street,	New York, N. Y.
1914	DR. WALTER B. WEIDLER,	137 East 60th Street,	New York, N. Y.
1900	DR. C. D. WESCOTT,	22 E. Washington St.,	Chicago, Ill.
1916	*DR. JOHN M. WHEELER,	30 West 59th Street,	New York, N. Y.
1891	DR. EDWARD WHEELOCK,	400 Cutler Building.	Rochester, N. Y.
1892	DR. J. A. WHITE,	200 E. Franklin Street,	Richmond, Va.
1919	*DR. LLOYD B. WHITHAM	514 Cathedral Street,	Baltimore, Md.
1895	DR. W. H. WILDER,	122 S. Michigan Blvd.,	Chicago, Ill.
1910	DR. CARL WILLIAMS,	School L. & Greene St.,	Philadelphia, Pa.
1912	DR. EDW. R. WILLIAMS,	1069 Boylston Street,	Boston, Mass.
1893	DR. WM. H. WILMER,	1610 I Street, N. W.,	Washington, D. C.
1906	DR. J. SCOTT WOOD,	172 Sixth Avenue,	Brooklyn, N. Y.
1900	DR. HIRAM WOODS,	842 Park Avenue,	Baltimore, Md.
1915	*DR. H. W. WOOTTON,	319 Lexington Avenue,	New York, N. Y.
1881	DR. J. P. WORRELL,	20 South 7th Street,	Terre Haute, Ind.
1905	DR. WM. ZENTMAYER,	1506 Spruce Street,	Philadelphia, Pa.
1903	DR. S. LEWIS ZIEGLER,	1625 Walnut Street,	Philadelphia, Pa.

Total   188

HONORARY MEMBERS.

1868	DR. J. S. PROUT,	Fishkill,	Dutchess Co., N.Y.
O. M.	DR. F. P. SPRAGUE,	229 Commonw'lth Ave.,	Boston, Mass.

EMERITUS MEMBERS.

1905	DR. S. C. MAXSON,	235 Genesee Street,	Utica, N. Y.
1869	DR. THOMAS R. POOLEY,	26 Trinity Street,	Newton, N. J.
1878	DR. J. A. SPALDING,	627 Congress Street,	Portland, Me.

Whole number   193

IN MEMORIAM

DR. ARTHUR MATHEWSON, elected 1868

DR. GEORGE T. STEVENS, elected 1873

DR. ADOLF ALT, elected 1882

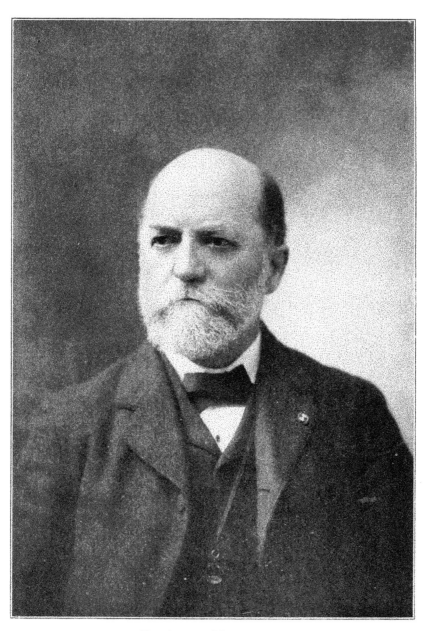

DR. ARTHUR MATHEWSON.

NECROLOGY.

ARTHUR MATHEWSON, A.M., M.D.*

JAMES W. INGALLS, M.D.,
Brooklyn, New York.

Dr. Arthur Mathewson, son of Rufus Smith and Faith (McClellan) Mathewson, was born in Brooklyn, Conn., September 11, 1837. After having suffered several years from paralysis, he died at his home in Washington, D. C., December 31, 1920. Dr. Mathewson was descended from Pilgrim ancestry. On the paternal side he was the ninth lineal descendant of John Alden. On the maternal side, the McClellans came from Scotland and were among the early settlers of Worcester, Mass. Preparation for college was received at Woodstock Academy, Woodstock, Conn. He graduated at Yale in 1858 and then spent one year as private tutor in a planter's family in McIntosh Co., Georgia. He received the degree of M.D. from the Medical Department of New York University on March 4, 1861. He passed first of 37 in a competitive examination. For a short time he was on duty at the Naval Hospital in Brooklyn and then served two years on the gunboat Winona in Farragut's squadron. In 1864 he was promoted to Passed Assistant Surgeon, passing first of 30 competitors. In March, 1865, was promoted to the position of Surgeon, and in the same year he received his M.A. degree from Yale. In May, 1867, he began practice in Brooklyn, N. Y., specializing in ophthalmic and aural surgery. In the spring of 1868. associated with Dr. Cornelius R. Agnew, of New York, and others,

* For much of the data in this memoir the writer is indebted to the courtesy of the librarian of Yale University.

Dr. Mathewson aided in establishing the Brooklyn Eye and Ear Hospital, in which institution he served as Senior Surgeon for thirty-two years. In collaboration with Dr. Homer G. Newton he translated Dr. Adam Politzers' work on diseases of the ear, which was published under the title of "Membrana Tympani, in Health and Disease, Clinical Contributions to the Diagnosis and Treatment of Diseases of the Ear." In 1868 Dr. Mathewson was elected a member of the American Ophthalmological Society. In 1869 he spent about eight months studying abroad. In 1870 he joined the New York Ophthalmological Society, and was honored on two occasions by being elected president. Upon his resignation in 1904 he was made an honorary member. Dr. Mathewson was elected a member of the American Otological Society in 1872, and of the International Otological Society in 1876. In the Transactions of the International Otological Society for 1876 Dr. Mathewson described a new operation for the removal of bony growths from the external auditory meatus.

Also in 1876 Dr. Mathewson delivered the first course of lectures on ophthalmology and otology in the Yale Medical School. In 1883 he was appointed lecturer on otology in the Long Island College Hospital. He served St. Mary's Hospital, St. John's Hospital, and Brooklyn City Hospital as ophthalmic and aural surgeon for many years. In 1885 he became a member of the American Academy of Medicine. In 1886 he was appointed Professor of Otology in the Long Island College Hospital. This position he held for ten years, and after his resignation was appointed Professor Emeritus. In 1893 he was elected vice-president of the American Otological Society and president in 1894, 1895, 1896, and 1897. In 1902 Dr. Mathewson was elected vice-president of the American Ophthalmological Society, and in 1906 he served as president. He retired from practice in 1904. After leaving Brooklyn, Dr. Mathewson took up his

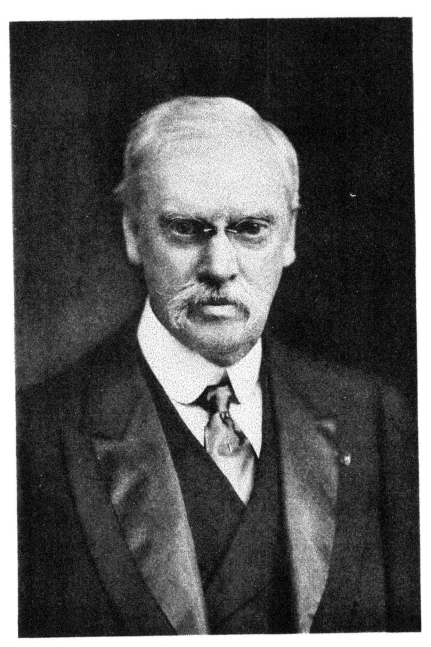

DR. GEORGE THOMAS STEVENS.

residence in Washington, D. C. For many years it was his custom to spend a part or the whole of the summer on his Woodstock estate, comprising several hundred acres of magnificent pine forest bordering on a beautiful lake. Dr. Mathewson was married in Washington, D. C., in 1870, to Harriet Silliman, daughter of Thomas and Emily (Silliman) Blagden. Mrs. Mathewson died a number of years ago. Two sons and a daughter survive.

Dr. Mathewson, while in Brooklyn, was a member of the Church of the Pilgrims (Congregationalist). Although dignified in bearing, yet he was modest and unassuming. His strong, sturdy nature always reminded me of an oak tree, and when the news of his death was received, the exclamation came to my lips, "a noble oak has fallen."

GEORGE THOMAS STEVENS, M.D., Ph.D.

ALEXANDER DUANE, M.D.,
New York.

Dr. George Thomas Stevens was the son of Rev. Chauncey Coe Stevens and Lucinda Hoadley Stevens. He was born in Jay, Essex County, New York, on July 25, 1832, and died at his residence, 350 West 88th Street, New York, on January 30, 1921.

His childhood and early youth were spent in Elizabethtown and Crownpoint, New York, where his father was a Congregational minister. He received his early education in the schools of the county and through studies with his father, who was a man of high literary attainments.

He received his medical education at the Castleton Medical College, Vermont, where he graduated in medicine in 1857. He commenced the practice of medicine in Wadhams Mills, Essex County, New York. On April 17, 1861, he married Harriet Weeks Wadhams, of Wadhams Mills, New

York. Their children were Frances Virginia Stevens, who married Professor George Tiumbull Ladd, of Yale University; Dr. Charles Wadhams Stevens, who is now practising ophthalmology in New York city; and Georgina Wadhams Stevens, who died in childhood.

At the outbreak of the Civil War in 1861 he was commissioned an assistant surgeon in the Seventy-seventh Regiment, New York State Volunteers. He was later made surgeon, and for two and one-half years was operating surgeon of his division. He served in all the campaigns of the Army of the Potomac, and for a time was Medical Inspector of the Sixth Corps.

At the close of the war he resumed the general practice of medicine in Albany, New York. Early in his career he began to devote special attention to ophthalmology, and while still in Albany had become widely known as an enthusiastic student of the subject and as an operator. In 1870 he was appointed Professor of Physiology and Diseases of the Eye in the Albany Medical College, the Medical Department of Union University. In 1877 he was given the honorary degree of Doctor of Philosophy by Union. He became a member of the American Ophthalmological Society in 1873.

Being desirous of confining his work solely to ophthalmology, he moved to New York in 1880. He continued in active practice there up to the time of his last illness. about two years before his death, and retained his steadiness of hand and ability to perform delicate eye surgery into his eighty-sixth year.

In 1881 he presented and described at the International Medical Congress in London his recording perimeter, probably the first of its kind.

In 1883 he received the highest award in a competition instituted by the Royal Academy of Medicine of Belgium for an essay on Functional Nervous Diseases.

Soon after this he performed one of the first operations done in this country for removing a foreign body from the eye with a magnet. The foreign body, visible with the ophthalmoscope, was located in the retina. The writer of this paper had the opportunity of seeing the case at least twenty-five years after the operation, and found the eye perfectly normal except for a cataract.

Dr. Stevens was, indeed, a natural operator—dexterous, careful, and cool, and with some it was a matter of regret that he did not give more attention in his later years to general ophthalmology, in which his skill would have made him preëminent. But comparatively early he turned from general ophthalmic work to the study of motor anomalies, and to this study he devoted almost exclusively the last forty years of his life. Strongly convinced of the dependence of many nervous conditions (chorea, epilepsy, migraine) on ocular conditions, and particularly on disorders of the ocular muscles, he wrote much concerning these inter-relations, and constantly exemplified his faith in his practice. It was his life work, which he pursued with the zeal of a missionary almost to the day of his death. Particularly he advocated operations on the eye muscles as a means of relieving these conditions.

Apart from his writings on these topics, presented with admirable clearness and great force, we may say that his main contributions to the subject were these: First, he propounded a nomenclature of motor anomalies, which is now firmly established and universally employed; second, he devised the phorometer, clinoscope, clinometer, and tropometer, instruments that form an important part of the armamentarium of ophthalmologists who are at all interested in the study of motor anomalies; third, he suggested and praetised a variety of new operations on the muscles, which required a delicacy and skill that his numerous imitators have not always been able to command; fourth, for conducting these operations he invented a set of instruments which are among the best that we have.

As is well known, his radical views and his uncompromising way of presenting them aroused much antagonism. He was a born fighter and, possessing strong convictions, expressed them in no uncertain tones. He had consequently many opponents as well as many adherents. Not a few regarded his views as ultra-radical, mistaken in principle and dangerous in practice. This opposition at times waxed bitter, and in conducting it many forgot the considerable services that he had rendered to ophthalmology and quite overlooked the essential sincerity and integrity of the man.

It is on this last point that the author would specially speak. It was his fortune to be associated with Dr. Stevens for some eight months in the beginning of his own work in ophthalmology. It was by such close personal contact that he learned to know Dr. Stevens as a man genial, courageous, virile, and sincere, a man of warm attachments and with a host of friends. Although engaged a good part of his life in controversies, he was the reverse of bittei in his antagonisms, and rarely, if ever, let slip an expression indicative of a personal animus. It was a characteristic trait that he was very fond of children and animals.

Dr. Stevens was a man of great industry, ingenuity, originality, and genius. His was a many-sided character. A skilful artist, he made excellent sketches of the fundus and, as one of his hobbies, made extra-illustrated books.

He was a lover of good books and had a large general library. He was also an ardent student, not only of all branches of his profession, but also of natural history in all its forms. His principal recreation was the study of botany. His extensive herbarium included plants and flowers from all parts of America and Europe. His Guide to Flowering Plants, mentioned below, was published in his seventy-eighth year. It was illustrated with hundreds of drawings made by him from nature with great accuracy and remarkable skill. Of nature, indeed, he was always a great lover and an enthusiastic student.

In politics he was a Republican; in religion, a member of the Congregational Church. Always interested in current events, always, as one ot his friends said, intensely alive and of remarkable intellectual vitality, he retained his interests and his mental vigor to the very end of his eighty-eight years.

His published works include: "Three Years in the Sixth Corps," 1866; "Flora of the Adirondacks," 1868; "Les Maladies des Centres Nerveux," 1883; "Functional Nervous Diseases," 1884; "Coaching through North Wales," 1895; "Les Muscles Moteurs de l'Oeil et l'Expression du Visage," 1892; "A Treatise on the Motor Apparatus of the Eyes," 1905; "An Illustrated Guide to Flowering Plants," 1910; "A Series of Studies of Nervous Affections," 1911; as well as numerous articles on ophthalmologic and general scientific topics.

ADOLF ALT, M.D.

WM. F. HARDY, M.D.,
St. Louis, Mo.

The death of Dr. Adolf Alt occurred June 28, 1920, after two and a half years of invalidism the result of a myocarditis. Throughout his long illness the gentleness and patience which were his characteristics in health were never absent. If he entertained doubts as to his restoration to health, he carefully concealed them from his friends and those he loved in order to spare them pain.

If simplicity, honesty, and candor are attributes of greatness, then Adolf Alt deserved that distinction. Whether in private or public life, in professional or literary activity, these qualities were ever dominant. To create a false impression by word or deed in his professional relations with patients would have been considered by him dishonesty and hypocrisy. The many little arts used by many professional men to psychologically influence their patients were considered beneath his dignity. His criticisms were ever kindly, honest, and constructive, if not always agreeable. One could always obtain a candid opinion from Dr. Alt. Dissimulation had no place in his character.

While well versed in every branch of ophthalmology, it was his literary work and knowledge of ophthalmic pathology which gave him his greatest renown. Pathology might well be called his hobby. A great deal of his preparation of specimens, sectioning, staining, and microscopic examinations, was done in his office. If not busy with patients, he was working with specimens or looking through a microscope. He always contended that if this work was left to be done at leisure time in a hospital laboratory or at home, it would not be done. He did everything himself, even to the making of microphotographs. This latter work was done at home with an apparatus of his own construction.

His mind was a veritable storehouse of information, and his memory of past events in ophthalmology was almost uncanny. It behooved one with a new idea or theory to seek out Dr. Alt and obtain his opinion as to its originality. Nine times out of ten he would unhesitatingly and unerringly state who had promulgated the same idea or theory and where it was recorded.

His own writings were voluminous, the bibliography of his articles comprising 206 numbers. Most of these dealt with pathologic subjects. One of his earliest efforts was a monograph, "The Normal and Pathological Histology of the Human Eye." For many years, from 1884 to 1918, he edited the *American Journal of Ophthalmology.* Virtually all the work of getting out this monthly publication fell on his shoulders. It was this which kept him in such intimate touch with the progress of ophthalmology throughout the world. A perfect knowledge of French and German aided much in this work.

He belonged to no clubs or lodges and to few societies. His diversions were art and music. A violinist of no mean ability, he was one of a quartet of amateur musicians who, for many years, met regularly once a week at his home. Year in and year out found him a regular subscriber to and patron of the Symphony Society. He could not resist the appeal of a good painting or a beautiful rug. He was not what is known as a "mixer," and preferred his home and family above all else. Each year six weeks of rest in the woods of northern Wisconsin in the late summer gave him renewed zest and vigor for the work of the winter.

Dr. Alt was the son of a physician and was born at Mannheim, Germany, August 13, 1851. As was not uncommon in the land of his birth, he was given a superfluity of Christian names, Gustav Adolf Fredrich Wilhelm, all of which he dropped except Adolf. His educational training included the usual gymnasium course, followed by a period at a boarding school and later his matriculation at Heidelberg. The death of his father and the breaking out of the Franco-Prussian War altered his plans temporarily. After service in the army he continued his medical studies, graduating from Heidelberg in March, 1875. On completion of his military service as Infantry Surgeon, which required but five and a half months, he departed for America, influenced in great measure by Dr. Herman Knapp, of New York City.

Becoming assistant to Dr. Knapp, he served two years as House Surgeon in the New York Ophthalmic and Aural Institute. Leaving New York, he located in Toronto, becoming a member of the College of Physicians and Surgeons of Ontario. In 1880 he removed to St. Louis, which became his permanent home and the seat of most of his ophthalmologic activities. His editorship of the *American Journal of Ophthalmology* began in 1884. From 1886 to 1901 he was

Professor of Ophthalmology in the Beaumont Hospital Medical College, and after its consolidation with the Marion Sims Medical College to form the Medical Department of St. Louis University, Dr. Alt continued in the chair of ophthalmology until 1910. He resigned then to take the appointment of Clinical Professor of Ophthalmology in the Washington University Medical School. By reason of the age limit he was retired as Professor Emeritus of Ophthalmology in 1917.

He was elected a member of the American Ophthalmological Society in 1882, and this membership he prized above all others. One of the founders of the American Academy of Ophthalmology and Oto-Laryngology, he served as its president the first two years of its existence. In 1911 he presided as chairman of the Section of Ophthalmology of the American Medical Association at its meeting in Los Angeles. Early in his career he combined otology with ophthalmology, but soon dropped it when he found men, as he stated, who knew much more about it than he did.

Dr. Alt was married in 1879 and had two children, one of whom died in childhood. He leaves a widow and son, Arnold D. Alt.

The true test of a gentleman is a consideration for others. No veneer of gentility can replace or counterfeit it. This, when coupled with simplicity, candor, honesty, and erudition, makes up a composite whole which we term gentleman and scholar. Thus was Adolf Alt.

MINUTES OF THE PROCEEDINGS.

FIFTY-SEVENTH ANNUAL MEETING.
New Ocean House,
Swampscott, Mass., June 14, 1921.

The Fifty-seventh Annual Meeting of the Society was called to order at 9 A. M. by the Vice-President, Dr. William M. Sweet, of Philadelphia.

Dr. Sweet said that he occupied the Chair in the absence of the President, Dr. John E. Weeks, who had been in the Orient, and was unable to secure steamer accommodations to return in time for the meeting. The Secretary received a letter from Dr. Weeks, which he asked to be read at the meeting:

Yokohoma, Japan, February 22, 1921.

To the Members of the American Ophthalmological Society and their Guests:

Your President sends hearty and sincere greetings and best wishes for a successful and enjoyable session. He regrets that, because of the inability to secure suitable accommodations for the return trip from Japan in time to enable him to be at the place of meeting on June 14, he will not be able to attend. However, he is consoled, and his disappointment is partly compensated for, by the knowledge that his absence will not be detrimental to the Society as, because of his long experience as Secretary, the session will be much more ably presided over by our Vice-President than it could be by him.

Your President wishes to extend his sympathy to the members of the families of those of our number who have passed from this life since our last meeting, and to acknowledge the loss to our Society of their fellowship and of their participation in our scientific proceedings.

He wishes to acknowledge to Dr. Lucien Howe the indebt-

23

edness of the Society to him for his excellent contribution to the inducements for original research on the part of the members of our Society, and to express his conviction that this feature of our endeavor should be extended.

In conclusion, he would suggest that a change be made in the manner of the selection of the personnel of the Council. The number of the members of the Council and the term of service should remain as now, but he would suggest that the personnel be constituted of the ex-presidents of the Society, they becoming automatically members of the Council on expiration of the term as President.

Respectfully,
JOHN E. WEEKS.

Before taking up the scientific business the Chair introduced Lieutenant-Colonel Henry Smith, C.I.E., of London, England, and formerly of Amritsar, India, a guest of the Society.

The following papers were read and discussed:

1. "Some Features in the Technic of Trephining the Cornea for the Relief of Glaucoma." Frederick Tooke, M.D., Montreal, Can.

Discussed by Drs. Thomson, Lambert, Wilmer, Charles, Fisher, Andrews, Koller, Verhoeff, and Tooke.

2. "Repeated Operations for Glaucoma. Report of Case." Oscar Dodd, M.D., Evanston, Ill.

3. "Friability of the Iris a Factor in Iridectomy for Hypertension." Hiram Woods, M.D., Baltimore, Md.

Papers Nos. 2 and 3 discussed by Drs. Knapp, Wilder, E. V. L. Brown, Dodd, and Lieutenant-Colonel Smith.

4. "The Action of Adrenalin on the Glaucomatous Eye." Arnold Knapp, M.D., New York.

Discussed by Drs. Charles, Verhoeff, Derby, Schoenberg, E. V. L. Brown, and Knapp.

5. "The Physiologic Mode of Action of Mydriatics and Miotics, Explaining Their Effects in Hypertension (Glaucoma)." Carl Koller, M.D., New York.

Discussed by Drs. Duane, Verhoeff, Schoenberg, Clark, and Koller.

6. "After-Cataract." Henry Smith, C.I.E., Lieutenant-Colonel, I.M.S., London, England.

Discussed by Drs. Lambert, Chance, Holloway, de Schweinitz, Jackson, Burke, Wilder, G. Oram Ring, Dorland Smith, Thomson, Parker, Woodruff, and Lieutenant-Colonel Smith.

7. "Intracapsular Cataract Extraction by Traction Alone." Allen Greenwood, M.D., Boston, Mass.

Discussed by Lieutenant-Colonel Smith, and Drs. Clark, Holloway, and Greenwood.

The following, who were present at the meeting, were invited to be guests of the Society and take part in the discussions: Lieutenant-Colonel Henry Smith, C.I.E., I.M.S., London; Drs. F. J. Arnold, Burlington, Vt.; S. Judd Beach and John W. Bowers, Portland, Me.; W. L. Benedict, Rochester, Minn.; W. H. Boiler, Iowa City, Iowa; E. F. Curran and James W. May, Kansas City, Mo.; P. DeLong, Philadelphia; L. E. Elliott, Melrose, Mass.; C. E. Ferree and G. Rand, Bryn Mawr, Pa.; Frederick Frisch, Atlantic City, N. J.; Wm. J. Holzer, Worcester, Mass.; E. W. Jones and Archibald H. Martin, Lynn, Mass.; C. L. LaRue, Boulder, Col.; F. C. Leavitt, Belmont, Mass.; Alexander L. Prince and George E. Tucker, Hartford, Conn.; Francis I. Proctor, David W. Wells and C. F. Worthen, Boston; L. V. Stegman, Battle Creek, Mich.; David A. Strickler, Denver, Col.; F. Jackle, Dunkirk, N. Y.; V. Wescott, Chicago, and H. W. Woodruff, Joliet, Ill.

TUESDAY AFTERNOON, JUNE 14TH.

8. "The Insertions of the Ocular Muscles as Seen in Text-Books and in the Dissecting Room." Lucien Howe, M.D., Buffalo, N. Y.

9. "The Action of the Obliques and the Bearing of Head-

Tilting in the Diagnosis of Paralysis." Alexander Duane, M.D., New York.

Papers 8 and 9 discussed by Drs. Duane and Howe.

10. "A Case of Intermittent Exophthalmos." W. Gordon M. Byers, M.D., Montreal, Can.

Discussed by Dr. Posey.

11. "Double Luxation of the Eyeballs in a Case of Exophthalmic Goiter." Walter R. Parker, M.D., Detroit, Mich.

Discussed by Drs. Langdon, Fisher, and Parker.

12. "Loss of Vision from Sympathetic Inflammation with Recovery Following the Use of Tuberculin." Harry Friedenwald, M.D., Baltimore, Md.

Discussed by Dr. E. V. L. Brown.

13. "Loss of Vision in One Eye Restored by Pituitary Feeding in a Case of Compensatory Pituitary Hypertrophy." Edward Stieren, M.D., Pittsburgh, Pa.

Discussed by Drs. de Schweinitz, Friedenwald, and Stieren.

14. "The Estimation of Compensation in Disability Resulting from Accidental Loss of Visual Acuity." E. Terry Smith, M.D., Hartford, Conn.

Discussed by Drs. Prince, Tucker, Holt, and E. Terry Smith.

15. "An Unusual Case of Conjunctival Irritation." H. H. Briggs, M.D., Asheville, N. C.

EXECUTIVE SESSION, JUNE 14TH.

The meeting was called to order by the Vice-President, Dr. William M. Sweet.

As the Minutes of the last meeting had appeared in full in the TRANSACTIONS, a motion was made and carried that the reading of them be dispensed with.

The Chair announced the following appointment:

Auditing Committee: Dr. R. J. Curdy.

The report of the Secretary-Treasurer was read. The

Auditing Committee certified to its correctness, and it was accepted and filed. In presenting the report the Secretary-Treasurer stated that, notwithstanding the continued high cost of paper and labor in the printing trade, the bill for the TRANSACTIONS for last year was considerably less than for the previous year. The deficit in the treasury of the Society last year had been met by a loan, which has been considerably reduced. It was felt that after the present dispute between the printers and their employees shall have been adjusted, the cost of the TRANSACTIONS this year would show a further decrease in cost. As there still remained, however, a deficit from last year, it was recommended that an assessment be made in addition to the regular annual dues.

Dr. W. H. Wilmer, Chairman of the Committee on Theses, reported that six theses had been presented, of which number five were acceptable. Of these, two were from candidates who failed to write acceptable theses last year, but after consultation with them, they submitted theses this year that were satisfactory.

Dr. C. F. Clark, Chairman of Council, presented the following recommendations:

1. That the following named candidates be elected as Associate Members of the Society:
DR. W. L. BENEDICT.
DR. NELSON M. BLACK.
DR. E. E. HOLT, JR.

2. That Section 8, Article 3, of the Constitution be so changed as to provide for a three years' term of office for members of the Committee on Theses.

3. That the Constitution be so amended as to provide for an emeritus membership as follows: Any active member on request may be transferred to the emeritus membership roll if in the judgment of the council said member is no longer able to comply with all the requirements of the Constitution and By-Laws of the Society. Emeritus members not to be required to pay dues, nor will they have a voice in the proceedings of the Society.

4. That the dues for 1921 be $10.00, and that an assessment of $10.00 additional be made on each member of the Society to apply on the deficit of the year.

5. The following named members are nominated for officers of the Society for the ensuing year:

President: Dr. William M. Sweet.

Vice-President: Dr. William H. Wilmer.

Secretary and Treasurer: Dr. Thomas B. Holloway.

Member of the American Board for Ophthalmic Examinations: Dr. William Zentmayer.

Board of Governors, American College of Surgeons: Dr. William H. Wilder, Dr. Alex. Quackenboss, and Dr. Hiram Woods.

6. Next place of meeting, Washington, D. C., at the time of the Congress of American Physicians and Surgeons, May, 1922.

The names of other candidates for membership were referred to the Council for 1922.

Upon motion the report of the Council with recommendations was adopted.

As no objection was made to the three candidates recommended, the Chair declared them elected Associate Members of the Society.

The Secretary was directed to cast a ballot for the nominees for officers, and they were declared elected.

The report of the Committee on Prize Essays for the medal for research of the American Ophthalmological Society was read by the Secretary:

At our last meeting a committee was appointed to perfect arrangements for the preparation and acceptance of the prize medal offered to the Society in 1919 by one of its members. That committee consisted of the donor, with our President and Secretary.

On inquiry it was found that the incorporation of the Ophthalmological Society, as provided by the donor, would probably prove inconvenient, as that might necessitate annual meetings in whichever State the incorporation was registered.

Therefore that point was waived by the donor.

Another formality yet to be complied with is the acceptance by resolution of the prize—that was omitted at the time, in spite of the expressions of approval and thanks which appear in the records of that meeting.

The committee has agreed on a model for the prize.

If a vote of acceptance is passed by the Society, this medal will be handed to the President now, to be awarded by the proper committee next year and the fifteen hundred dollars in liberty bonds will be deposited with the Metropolitan Trust Company of New York, or such other institution as the officers of the Society may prefer, to be used by the Society, without its incorporation, but otherwise in accord with the conditions mentioned by the donor.

(Signed)   Lucien Howe.

Dr. C. D. Wescott made the following motion, which was carried:

That the offer made by Dr. Howe when he was President of the Society of a prize medal to be awarded by the American Ophthalmological Society be hereby accepted, with the understanding, however, that the Society need not now be incorporated.

Dr. G. E. de Schweinitz, Chairman of the General Committee, presented the report of the Committee on an International Congress of Ophthalmology.

I have so recently made a report in regard to the activities of the membership of the committee appointed to take charge of an International Congress that I do not know that it is necessary to add anything to it, except to say that, through the great activity of all the various committees, the arrangements are well in advance of what we had hoped. An extensive program has been elaborated by the Committee on Scientific Business, of which Dr. Jackson is chairman. The next meeting of the committee will be in October at the meeting of the American Academy of Ophthalmology and Oto-Laryngology. It is desired that the gentlemen here present shall use their personal influence to increase the membership of the Congress. We necessarily must depend in large measure upon such membership for financial support as well as for scientific communications of value.

Dr. Myles Standish, one of the representatives of this Society on the American Board for Ophthalmic Examinations, made the following report:

The Board consolidated its gains within the year. It has had several examinations, and there has been an increasing number of applicants. What is more satisfactory, the applicants that actually come to have examination either prepare themselves better or are a better class of men, I do not know which, but the results in examinations within the past year have been much more satisfactory to the Board than those that preceded. Of course, the Board has had to feel its way to a certain extent as to what to require and expect the men to know, but the Board has been in existence now six years, and we are beginning to know what we expect the men to pass on when they come. The increasing number of applicants and the increasing number of inquiries have been very encouraging. I think that it was a step in the right direction. I think if all of you gentlemen would manage to get your names on the list the Board would be very much aided in its work in the future. The long list of licensed men who are well known will make it easier for the Board to keep up the standard.

Dr. W. H. Wilder, Secretary of the Board, made the following statement of the work of the Board:

Before the date of the last meeting of the American Medical Association the Board had certificated 219 ophthalmologists in this country, and I think that at the meeting in Boston something over 40 more were certificated. Dr. Standish has stated we would like very much for members of this Society to present their applications for the certificate of this Board. It would tend to encourage the work, would support the Board in its endeavors, and it would give a fine foundation for the superstructure of ophthalmology in this country. Many men say, "Of what use is it to me to be certificated by this Board? I do not want to go up for examination; I do not want to present case reports, and it requires an outlay of $25 in order to secure this certificate." It will mean much to the young men in the future, because we are writing into our constitution what has already been written into that of the American Academy of Ophthalmology and Oto-Laryngology, a section which states that membership can be acquired only after a certificate of this Board has been granted to the individual. This being the case, it seems to me that members of this Society should encourage the movement by making application for this certificate. We require that the application be made on a formal blank. It is not likely that any man who knows ophthalmology well enough to qualify for membership in the American Ophthalmological Society would be rejected by the Board.

The Secretary announced the following death of members during the year: Dr. Arthur Mathewson, Washington, D. C., elected 1868, President of the Society in 1906; Dr. George T. Stevens, New York, elected in 1873; Dr. A. Alt, St. Louis, Mo., elected in 1882.

The Publication Committee announced that the price of the TRANSACTIONS had been fixed at $5.00 a copy.

The following Committees were announced by the Chair:

Council: Drs. Cassius D. Wescott, Walter B. Lancaster, Walter R. Parker, Walter E. Lambert, and Howard F. Hansell.

Committee on Theses: Dr. E. V. L. Brown, to serve for three years; Dr. Lee M. Francis, to serve for two years; and Dr. George S. Derby, to serve for one year.

Committee on Program: Drs. William T. Shoemaker, E. A. Shumway, and the Secretary.

Committee on Publication: Drs. Harry Friedenwald, J. W. Charles, and the Secretary.

Committee on Prize Essays for the Medal for Research of the American Ophthalmological Society: Drs. Lucien Howe, John E. Weeks, and W. Gordon M. Byers.

Committee on an International Congress of Ophthalmology:

Drs. G. E. de Schweinitz, W. H. Wilmer, and Frederick T. Tooke.

Representatives on the American Board for Ophthalmic Examinations: Dr. Wm. Zentmayer, to serve for three years; Dr. E. C. Ellett, to serve for two years; and Dr. John E. Weeks, to serve for one year.

Committee on Arrangements for the Congress of American Physicians and Surgeons: Dr. W. H. Wilmer, Delegate, and Dr. L. S. Greene, Alternate.

Second International Eugenics Congress: Dr. Lucien Howe, Delegate.

Dr. Wm. Zentmayer presented the report of the Committee to Revise the Constitution and By-Laws. The report as sent out to each member of the Society was printed in parallel columns, the first showing the old Constitution and By-Laws, and the second the changes as proposed by the Committee.

A motion was made and carried that the report of the Committee be accepted. It was also decided that the sections be taken up seriatim and considered. After considerable discussion, the wording of the several sections was agreed upon, and the Chair put the motion of the adoption of the report of the Committee as a whole with the amendments made, the eliminations, and the substitutions, and this was carried. The Executive Session then adjourned at 10.10.

The Executive Session was called to order by the Chair at 10.20.

A motion was made to adopt the Constitution as finally passed at the previous meeting of the Executive Session of the Society. Carried. The Chair then announced that the Constitution as adopted becomes the new Constitution and By-Laws of the Society.

A motion was made and carried that the Committee on Revision of the Constitution and By-Laws be discharged with thanks.

WEDNESDAY MORNING, JUNE 15TH.

EXHIBITION OF NEW INSTRUMENTS AND APPARATUS.

The meeting was called to order at 9.30 o'clock by the Vice-President, Dr. Sweet.

16. "Illuminated Eye Spud with Magnifier." George S. Crampton, M.D., Philadelphia.

17. "Foreign-Body Spud Illuminator." W. Holbrook Lowell, M.D., Boston, Mass. Discussed by Dr. Posey.

18. "Tonometric Chart." E. C. Ellett, M.D., Memphis, Tenn.

19. "A Modified Accommodation Line and Prince's Rule." Alexander Duane, M.D., New York.

20. "Special Forceps for Tendo-Muscle Lengthening." W. Holbrook Lowell, M.D., Boston, Mass.

21. "Microscopic Sections of Coralliform Cataract, and a Specimen of Vitreous Humor from Asteroid Hyalitis." F. H. Verhoeff, M.D., Boston, Mass.

The reading of papers was then continued.

22. "A Case of Mooren's Ulcer." Arthur J. Bedell, M.D., Albany, N. Y.

Discussed by Drs. Ellett, Kollock, Feingold, and Bedell.

23. "Sarcoma of the Cornea. Case Report." George S. Derby, M.D., Boston, Mass.

24. "Melano-Sarcoma of the Choroid Occurring in Brothers." Adolph O. Pfingst, M.D., Louisville, Ky.

25. "Report of a Case of Primary Tubular Epithelioma of the Lacrimal Sac." William Campbell Posey, M.D., Philadelphia.

26. "Glioma Retinæ Treated by X-Rays, with Apparent Destruction of the Tumor and Preservation of Normal Vision." F. H. Verhoeff, M.D., Boston, Mass.

27. "The Use of Radium Plugs in the Dissolution of Orbital Gliomatous Masses Developing after Excision of the Globe." Burton Chance, M.D., Philadelphia.

3

Papers Nos. 26 and 27 discussed by Drs. E. Terry Smith and Verhoeff.

28. "Coats' Disease of the Retina.   Report of Two Cases." A. Edward Davis, M.D., New York.

Discussed by Drs. Zentmayer and Davis.

29. "Lipæmia Retinalis." Wm. F. Hardy, M.D., St. Louis, Mo.

30. "Some Impressions Derived from the Study of Recurrent Hemorrhages into the Retina and Vitreous of Young Persons." William C. Finnoff, M.D., Denver, Col.

Discussed by Drs. Holloway, Wilmer, Friedenwald, Derby, Knapp, Davis, Langdon, Hill, Benedict, Jackson, Verhoeff, Parker, and Finnoff.

31. "The Ocular Symptoms of Epidemic Encephalitis." Matthias Lanckton Foster, M.D., New Rochelle, N. Y.

Discussed by Drs. Woods, Finnoff, Friedenwald, and Foster.

32. "The Effect of Variations in Intensity of Illumination on Acuity, Speed of Discrimination, Speed of Accommodation, and Other Important Eye Functions." C. E. Ferree, Ph.D., and G. Rand, Ph.D., Bryn Mawr College, Bryn Mawr, Pa. (By invitation.)

Discussed by Drs. Clark, Foster and Ferree.

33. "Some Hitherto Unrecognized Signs in Skiascopy." J. H. Claiborne, M. D., New York.

Discussed by Drs. Tarun, Lambert, and Claiborne.

34. "The Ocular Changes in Infantile Scurvy. Report of a Case." Eugene M. Blake, M.D., New Haven, Conn.

Discussed by Dr. Jack.

35. "The Relation of Headache to Functional Monocularity." Albert C. Snell, M.D., Rochester, N. Y.

36. "Three Cases of Word-Blindness." Ellice M. Alger, M.D., New York.

Discussed by Drs. Jack, Claiborne, Chance, Stieren, Jackson, and Langdon.

The following members were present and registered at the Fifty-seventh Annual Meeting:

ALGER, ELLICE M.
ALLING, A. N.
ANDREWS, J. A.
BEDELL, ARTHUR J.
BLAKE, EUGENE M.
BORDLEY, JAMES, JR.
BRIGGS, H. H.
BROWN, E. V. L.
BURKE, JOHN W.
BYERS, W. GORDON M.
CALHOUN, F. PHINIZY
CHANCE, BURTON
CHANDLER, H. B.
CHARLES, J. W.
CLAIBORNE, J. H.
CLAP, E. W.
CLARK, C. F.
CRAMPTON, G. S.
CURDY, R. J.
CUTLER, COLMAN W.
DAVIS, A. E.
DENNIS, DAVID N.
DERBY, GEORGE S.
DODD, OSCAR
DUANE, ALEXANDER
ELLETT, E. C.
EWING, ARTHUR E.
FEINGOLD, MARCUS
FINNOFF, WILLIAM C.
FISHER, CARL
FOSTER, M. L.
FOX, W. H.
FRANCIS, LEE M.
FRIDENBERG, PERCY
FRIEDENWALD, H.
GREENE, L. S.
GREENWOOD, ALLEN
HARBRIDGE, D. F.

HARDY, WM. F.
HARLAN, HERBERT
HARROWER, DAVID
HASKELL, H. H.
HILL, EMORY
HOLLOWAY, T. B.
HOLT, E. E.
HOWE, LUCIEN
JACK, E. E.
JACKSON, EDWARD
JAMESON, P. C.
KENNON, B. R.
KEY, BEN WITT
KNAPP, ARNOLD
KOLLER, CARL
KOLLOCK, CHAS. W.
LAMB, ROBERT S.
LAMBERT, W. E.
LANCASTER, W. B.
LANGDON, H. M.
LORING, R. G.
LOVELL, D. B.
LOWELL, W. H.
LUEDDE, W. H.
McGUIRE, HUNTER H.
MARLOW, F. W.
MAY, C. H.
MILES, H. S.
OHLY, JOHN H.
PARKER, W. R.
PFINGST, ADOLPH O.
POSEY, W. CAMPBELL
PUSEY, BROWN
QUACKENBOSS, ALEXANDER
REYNOLDS, W. G.
RING, G. O.
RING, H. W.
RISLEY, J. NORMAN

SCHOENBERG, M. J.
DE SCHWEINITZ, G. E.
SHANNON, JOHN R.
SHINE, FRANCIS W.
SHOEMAKER, J. F.
SHOEMAKER, WM. T.
SMITH, DORLAND
SMITH, E. TERRY
SNELL, ALBERT C.
SPALDING, F. M.
STANDISH, MYLES
STIEREN, EDW.
SWEET, WM. M.

TARUN, WILLIAM
THOMSON, EDGAR S.
TOOKE, FRED. T.
TYSON, H. H.
VERHOEFF, F. H.
WESCOTT, C. D.
WILDER, W. H.
WILLIAMS, EDW. R.
WILMER, WM. H.
WOOD, J. SCOTT
WOODS, HIRAM
WOOTTON, H. W.
ZENTMAYER, WM.

SOME FEATURES IN THE TECHNIC OF TREPHINING THE CORNEA FOR THE RELIEF OF GLAUCOMA.

FREDERICK TOOKE, M.D.,
Montreal, Canada.

An approach to my subject cannot better be made than to quote Mr. Priestley Smith's remarks in introducing the discussion on the operative treatment of glaucoma at the Seventy-ninth Annual Meeting of the British Medical Association, held at Birmingham in 1911. He asks the pertinent question: "In operating for glaucoma, ought we to adhere to the time-honored iridectomy of von Graefe, or to adopt one or other of the substitutes lately introduced? The object of every glaucoma operation is to establish filtration from the eye; if we fail in that, we fail entirely."

Glaucoma cannot well be described by any one stereotyped definition. A series of pathologic, or rather of etiologic, features underlying the symptoms acknowledged clinically as glaucoma have been presented of recent years. These are as many as they are varied. Burgers, Wessely, Parisotti, Kummel, Hamburger, Bjerrum, Parsons, Thompson, Martin Fisher, and Priestley Smith himself are some of the contributors who have attempted to solve the riddle of our science. Almost as many have presented operative procedures designed to minimize, if not actually to eliminate, the symptoms which these pathologic features have induced. The outstanding contributors of recent years have been Lagrange, Herbert, and Elliot, the object of each being to establish a filtering scar.

The purpose of this contribution is not to bring into discussion the merits or faults of the operations designed by the authorities whom I have mentioned: it would be an impertinence on my part to attempt to do so. My brief for the time being is with the technic of trephining the cornea as advocated by the chief exponent of the operation, Colonel H. R. Elliot, as the operation with which I am most familiar.

It is quite probable that an enthusiastic support of this procedure will not go unchallenged by some, if not by many. To these I may as well at once reply by inquiring of them if they, in cases of chronic glaucoma have, through their actual operative experience, anything better to offer as an operative procedure that will more consistently, and with less risk, diminish tension, maintain vision, and retain blind eyes whose lot was formerly an enucleation. May I further be permitted to inquire if the terror of a late infection has not been one of anticipation, rather than one of actual fact n many, many cases? I feel sure that my colleagues at the Royal Victoria Hospital, Montreal, would wish to share with me in making the following assertions: That we have practised the operation of trephining the cornea for the relief of chronic glaucoma consistently since it was first introduced to this continent, and even before that time. Further, that in a series of nearly 150 cases we have had less than 2 per cent. of late infections. That there has not been one case of initial infection recorded, and that our material has, as in any large city, included all classes of society, from pauper to patrician.

As Colonel Elliot very aptly remarked in one of his contributions on this subject: "Magna est Veritas et prevalebit." The selection of my subject must not be interpreted as a presumption. The few following remarks on operative technic are the acknowledgment of an opportunity of acting as Colonel Elliot's assistant during his visit to Montreal in 1914. The enthusiastic and kindly interest which he evinced during the progress of several operations impressed us all most forcibly at the time how best the operation might be

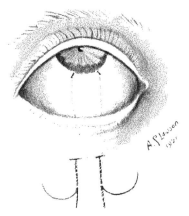

Fig. 1.

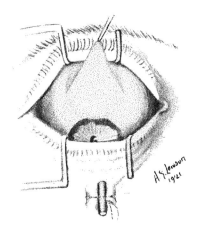

Fig. 2.

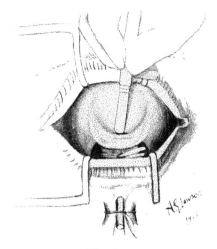

Fig. 3.

performed, and how pitfalls and possible complications might be avoided.

Since undertaking the operation on my own responsibility, or when assisting my colleagues in the department, I have always felt that one of the greatest difficulties experienced was to keep the patient looking down. Compared with a cataract extraction, or even with an iridectomy, trephining is a slow, tedious operative procedure. There is always the desire on the part of the patient to look up,—call it curiosity if you will,—and even though traction be applied by fine forceps below, or pressure by a horn spatula above, at some unguarded moment, when these are released, the patient looks up, with the result that the conjunctival flap in the process of dissection is buttonholed.

At the present time it is my practice to fix the eye downward by a double-armed suture. After anesthetizing the conjunctiva and cornea, a few drops of 2 per cent. anocain solution are injected into the lower lid. The needles, which should be moderately long and curved, should be inserted in a horizontal direction at the limbus corneæ below, and should include some of the episcleral fibrous tissue, very much as in the case of an advancement operation. The needles should then be passed downward in a vertical direction, beneath the conjunctiva bulbi, as far as the lower fornix, being brought forward through the skin surface of the lid in a line with the lower margin of the orbit. Traction is brought to bear on the two ends of the suture until the globe assumes the desired position, when the suture is secured about a small piece of rubber tubing. After the introduction of an eye speculum, the operation may be proceeded with (Figs. 1 and 2).

If there is one point more than another upon which all who support this operation are agreed, it is that the trephine must pass entirely through corneal tissue—and for this reason: The object of the trephine hole is to drain the aqueous through the cornea from the anterior chamber to the subconjunctival capillaries. It has been computed that the corneoscleral margin lies 1 mm. forward of the actual filtration angle (Priestley Smith). Should one operate with a 2 mm., or even with a 1.5 mm., trephine, the actual corneal tissue not being exposed, it would be impossible to reach the anterior chamber without wounding the ciliary body, subsequently plugging the wound with pigment and lymph exudate, the result of a complicating cyclitis. Satisfactory filtration can best be secured by a procedure known as splitting the cornea, a point emphasized by Colonel Elliot in all his writings. It is, in my humble opinion, the salient feature of the operation.

How best, then, may one approach the cornea, and how best expose that portion required to accommodate the trephine without complicating any of the underlying structures? The idea is to dissect or undermine the conjunctival flap so that its mid-portion will expose the actual corneoscleral margin. This mid-point of dissection is extended still further forward into the corneal tissue proper, toward the apparent limbus of the cornea, thus exposing a tiny crescentic or semilunar patch of actual corneal tissue. This area may measure between 1 and 2 mm. in a vertical diameter, and lies directly behind the attached or hinged end of the conjunctival flap. I have seen various instruments used in the execution of this, the most tedious, but, I claim, the most important, step of the operation, a knife-needle, a blunt keratome, the separated blade of the scissors used in dissecting the conjunctival flap, all with the same facility of buttonholing the conjunctiva.

For some time past it has been my practice to use an instrument which I have called, for want of a better name, a corneal separator. I made the original by grinding down an old Beer's knife. The blade is short, its cutting surface is 4 mm. wide, it is rounded at the end and beveled on both surfaces. When properly approximated to the cornea it is, consequently, almost impossible to buttonhole the cornea forward, on the one hand, or to completely penetrate the substantia propria backward, on the other. The instrument actually resembles a very fine mastoid chisel. A sufficient area of the substantia propria is exposed with the greatest ease, especially when the instrument is used with a lateral motion rather than vertically alone. It was made for me by Messrs. Tieman and Company, New York, to whom my thanks are due. The proper use of this very simple instrument has afforded us an opportunity of out-Ellioting Elliot at this particular and important stage of the operation (Figs. 2 and 3).

Having exposed an area of underlying corneal tissue, allow me to digress for a moment and to define very briefly the histologic features of a filtering corneal cicatrix. In an uncomplicated incision of the cornea, healing begins almost immediately. The severed ends of the corneal fibers at the mid-point of the substantia propria are the first actually to unite by primary intention. A secondary downgrowth of epithelial cells and an ingrowth of endothelium follow which successfully plug the wound. As union of the corneal fibers proceeds, these plugs are pushed forward, on the one hand, and backward, on the other, so that when fibrous union of the substantia propria is complete, there being no inclusion in the wound, there is little or no evidence of the epithelium or endothelium remaining.

When the cornea is trephined, a definite plug of corneal tissue is excised. At a circumscribed point, at least, the severed ends of the substantia propria cannot approximate. Primary union of the corneal fibers cannot take place before an ingrowth of endothelium has occurred which completely lines the trephine hole. Consequently, the apposition of the severed ends of the substantia propria is inhibited where primary union was wont to take place. A cystoid scar thus replaces a fixed scar (Plate 1).

In a recent article by Colonel Elliot appearing in the Transactions of the Ophthalmological Society of the United Kingdom, a series of histologic sections were shown which were intended to demonstrate part of the ligamentum pectinatum in the excised corneal plug. I must confess that I am distinctly dubious in my interpretation of the presence of the fibers of the ligament in some of the sections. For, after all, why should they be included? Granted that we expose the cornea sufficiently well forward, as I have already attempted to describe. If a not too large trephine be used, and it be properly approximated near the hinge of the conjunctival flap, then it should penetrate the cornea forward before Descemet's membrane breaks up to form the fibers of the ligamentum pectinatum (Plate 2).

Plate 3 shows a section through the cornea near the apparent limbus for the extraction of a senile cataract. The incision has, in fact, come out well beyond the apparent limbus of the cornea, with the inclusion of a conjunctival flap. Should such a conjunctival flap have been extended still further forward according to the procedure of Colonel Elliot, and one which I am attempting to emphasize, it is difficult to suppose that the proper apposition of a moderately sized trephine could possibly include any of the fibers of the ligamentum pectinatum. That it is done by himself on occasions is admitted: it is also acknowledged by Mr. Freeland Fergus that a fine spatula or probe is almost invariably inserted into the wound, breaking down the more underlying fibers of the ligamentum pectinatum before drainage is complete. In the operation as performed by us we practically always meet with a hernia of the iris after trephining without having to insert any instrument whatsoever into the anterior chamber.

But need we regard the ligamentum pectinatum as a factor in the operation? Indirectly yes, and directly no, depending entirely upon the underlying pathologic cause and the clinical form which the condition exhibits. Clinically we note two

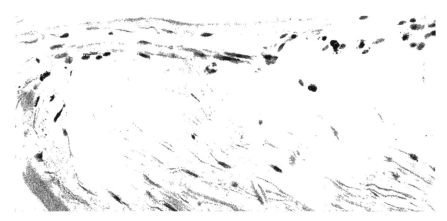

Plate 1.—A cystoid scar occurring near the limbus corneæ. This has been induced mechanically by the accidental inclusion of a portion of Descemet's membrane. The apposition or primary union of the severed ends of the corneal fibers has been inhibited not so much by the inclusion of the membrane as by the ingress of endothelium from the anterior chamber lining the walls of the incision. There is absolutely no evidence of inflammatory reaction. The eye was removed post-mortem eight days following operation.

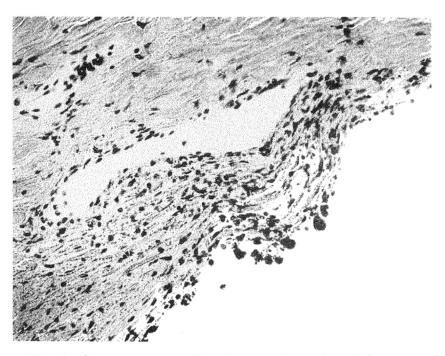

Plate 2.—Structures concerned in the normal excretion of the aqueous about the filtration angles. The splitting up of Descemet's membrane to form the fibers of the ligamentum pectinatum is particularly well shown. One may also clearly distinguish the spaces of Fontana and the canal of Schlemm.

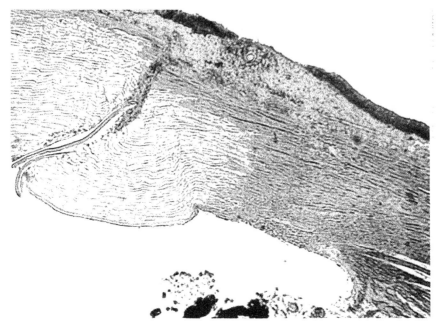

Plate 3.—A section through the cornea for the extraction of a senile cataract. The section has come out well beyond the apparent limbus, and has included a large conjunctival flap. An iridectomy has also been performed. Notwithstanding, the aperture through the cornea appears to be well forward and to be quite remote from the structures concerned in the filtration of the aqueous about the filtration angle.

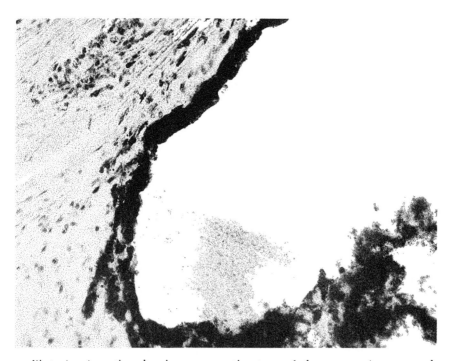

Plate 4.—A section showing a congestive type of glaucoma. An engorged anterior ciliary process with complete occlusion of the anterior chamber through the falling forward of the iris. The canal of Schlemm can still be

types of glaucoma, one with a shallow, the other with a deep anterior chamber. An excellent illustration of the first type, which might be interpreted as one of the congestive variety, shows an engorged anterior ciliary process pushing the root of the iris forward, blocking the natural egress of the aqueous through the spaces of Fontana and the canal of Schlemm (Plate 4). In such a condition the trephine operation relieves congestion, released filtration allows the iris to fall back to its former position, the normal depth of the anterior chamber is restored, the filtration angle consequently freed, and the circulation of the aqueous reëstablished, not only by the cystoid cicatrix, but also the former physiologic channels.

Take, on the other hand, the question of colloid changes occurring in the aqueous, a view advanced by Martin Fisher in his work on edema. Such a condition may manifest itself in the anterior chamber, and from an altered specific gravity the structures about the filtration angle are unable to aecommodate the aqueous. Such a condition is also shown in Plate 4, but existing in the posterior rather than in the anterior chamber. A feature such as this would be relieved, primarily, by the action of the cystoid cicatrix itself, independent of any mechanical or physiologic release on the parts concerned in the normal channel of circulation.

One practical point in conclusion: The operation with which I am dealing has been criticized as requiring a keen near vision and a steady hand. But such essentials are necessary in every branch of ophthalmic surgery. Granted that the trephine area is small, that we cannot all be myopes, and that presbyopia is the lot of man. With such problems facing us a means had to be found to afford one the best possible vision of the field of operation without disturbing the general relationship of existing conditions. My first practice was to employ a small loupe which was worn as a monocle, one which I was in the habit of carrying about with me for the detection of foreign bodies embedded in the conjunctiva or cornea. This served my purpose admirably. It had the distinct disadvantage, however, of not being worn with equal facility by every operator. Dr. Byers was one to appreciate this difficulty very early, and adopted the practice of using a Zeiss binocular. But this proved to be clumsy, and had the distinct disadvantage of closing off all but the actual field of operation. We have compromised by using the Betz Hardy binoculars, which are of inestimable assistance at every stage of the operation, but more especially in exposing the corneal lamellæ before the trephine is applied.

DISCUSSION.

DR. EDGAR S. THOMSON, New York: I would like to speak of one feature of technic, that is the position of the trephine opening. Dr. Tooke has said that it should be well forward in the cornea. I have seen a case that shows that this principle is sometimes productive of disadvantage. A gentleman was operated upon by Dr. Marple five years ago for chronic glaucoma in both eyes. The trephine opening was placed well forward in the limbus, principally in corneal tissue, as Colonel Elliot advised. The patient came into my hands after Dr. Marple's death, and he had a perfectly classic cicatrix. Two years ago he had one of these infective attacks (they have all been evanescent in my cases). The trephine opening was filled with plastic exudation which ultimately entirely absorbed, but the area around the sclera seemed to have been walled in by the infection, forcing the drainage to make unusual strain upon the cornea, so that the corneal lamella have been separated one-third down the cornea, forming a whitish bleb. This is composed of thick, indurated tissue and is probably composed of epithelium and Bowman's membrane. If it had gone on further it might have interfered with his vision. As it is it has not done so. It is a very thick, white pellicle, which is very annoying to him when he closes the eye. I mention this as a possible complication in getting the trephine opening too far forward.

DR. W. E. LAMBERT, New York: In our experience at the New York Eye and Ear Infirmary the danger of infection has not been so great as we have been told, and only in one instance has it occurred in the large number of cases operated upon in my service. I have never experienced any great difficulty in the fixation. It seems to me that sutures are unnecessary and complicate the operation. The instrument is similar to that which we have been using for many years.

DR. WILLIAM H. WILMER, Washington, D. C.: I am still doing sclerocorneal trephining, and while I am perhaps not so enthusiastic as I was at one time, still in cases of chronic glaucoma it is my operation of choice and the one I should select were it necessary to have an operative procedure upon my own eye. In nervous patients who find it very difficult to look down I meet the situation by drawing the conjunctival flap down with the suture, instead of the cotton-tipped probe of Colonel Elliot. The eye is held fast in the proper position by an assistant, who grasps with a fixation-forceps the insertion of one of the recti muscles. In some cases of chronic glaucoma the intra-ocular tension remains high and the anterior chamber very shallow, in spite of the frequent instillations of a miotic and a resulting "pin-point" pupil. In such cases I have found the so-called "splitting of the cornea" a very difficult, but necessary, procedure; I have never had to regret making the site of the trephine too far forward, but in one case I trephined too far back to obtain a good result. As a rule, the conjunctival suture to hold the flap in place seems to be a distinct advantage, but some nervous patients have seemed to find more discomfort from the removal of the suture than from the original operation. In such cases the knowledge that a catgut suture has been used eliminates the dread of suture removal and brings much peace of mind to the patient in consequence. I inject subconjunctivally at the site of the operation a solution of novocain and epinephrin.

DR. J. W. CHARLES, St. Louis, Mo.: When Colonel Elliot was in this country I think he laid stress on the fact that the dangers of late infection with the trephining operation were not much greater than those after iridectomy, providing the object of the iridectomy was obtained, viz., a filtering scar. It has seemed to me that the proportion of results from corneoscleral trephining has been so good that it offsets the dangers of late infection. I remember one case which I had, with an acute conjunctivitis, in which Colonel Elliot himself had operated. The wound had become yellow, the hole in the sclera seemed plugged with pus, and I was very fearful that the patient would not pull through again with normal vision, but under silver nitrate and general treatment, combined with the aid of the rhinologist, he recovered without ill results, and is still able to work normally, seven years after the operation.

DR. CARL FISHER, Los Angeles, Cal.: It seems to me that men are more important than methods. One hears much of the various ways of treating chronic glaucoma,—trephining, Lagrange, iridectomy,—but as one visits the standard clinics he sees excellent results obtained by various methods. I have been struck by the fact that some surgeons in their trephinings obtain such thin, friable flaps that secondary infection seems almost to be invited. I have had much comfort from the infiltration of the site of the flap with 1 per cent. cocain. It gives a thick, bloodless flap, not easily torn by even rather rough handling, and almost self-dissected. Another comfort has been the W. A. Fisher lid hook, which holds the upper lid securely out of the field of operation.

DR. J. A. ANDREWS, Santa Barbara, Cal.: Did you use any particular means to allay infections?

DR. CARL KOLLER, New York: I wish to confirm one of the minor points Dr. Tooke made—the necessity of seeing well; not only in this operation, but in most operations we do not see well enough. This has led me for many years to use strong convex glasses, adding about 5 diopters to my refraction, and besides prisms of 6 degrees base in. In order not to blur distant vision, I have added neutralizing glasses on top. These bifocal glasses have given me good service in this and other operations.

DR. F. H. VERHOEFF, Boston, Mass.: I should like to ask Dr. Tooke whether his description of the healing of the trephine hole is based on theoretic grounds or upon actual histologic examinations. His description does not agree with my findings in a case of successful trephining in which the eye later developed sarcoma and had to be removed. In this particular case, which, so far as I know, is still the only case of the kind yet reported, the endothelium had not lined the wall of the opening, but the latter was filled with very delicate connective tissue, containing openings analogous to iris crypts. In regard to Dr. Thomson's case of keratitis following trephining, it seems to me remarkable that this does not happen more often when an opening is made in the cornea. If there is much intra-ocular pressure, you would think that the fluid would get into the cornea and cause bullous keratitis. I have seen several cases in which this condition existed to a slight degree near the trephine opening. In one recent case operated on by a colleague in which the conjunctiva had been buttonholed and a large sliding conjunctival flap had to be made, a persisting condition of bullous keratitis resulted, so extreme that the whole epithelium of the cornea was loosened and could be picked up anywhere.

Dr. Tooke (closing): The case reported by Dr. Edgar Thomson was undoubtedly one of bullous keratitis. I have never met such a condition in my experience with this operation. I would reply to Dr. Lambert by saying that anything that secures confidence in the patient and relieves him from anxiety is justified. A spud has the same facility of buttonholing the cornea as the other instruments I have mentioned. I am pleased to learn that he belittles the possibility of late infection, but would refer him to the general discussion of the subject in the Transactions of 1914. Dr. Andrews has requested information regarding the use of bactericidal solutions, and I may say that such are never used by us. Dr. Verhoeff has described what he has found microscopically after trephining the cornea. Doubtless his description of a downgrowth of reticular connective tissue from the conjunctiva is quite correct. I can only refer him to Plate 1, which definitely shows the ingrowth of endothelium as the primary means of inhibiting union of the cut ends of the corneal fibers. It is quite possible that following this the process which he has described might occur, a great deal depending on the post-operative inflammatory reaction.

REPEATED OPERATIONS FOR GLAUCOMA: REPORT OF CASE.

OSCAR DODD, M.D.,
Evanston, Ill.

The subject of my paper is one that has been much discussed, but as our results from the operation for simple glaucoma are still unsuccessful in many cases, consideration of the causes of these failures seems not out of place. The case which I shall report has been interesting to me in that it illustrates many of the difficulties we may encounter, and the necessity of watching the cases carefully for a long period of time.

Family History.—My patient's mother went blind at the age of seventy-one years from glaucoma—three years before her death. Her eyes were operated upon, but it was said to have been too late to prevent blindness. One sister had an operation for glaucoma when forty-nine years of age, which preserved the sight of one eye for about six years, but she eventually became blind. Another sister had glaucoma when fifty-two years old, and in 1896, when she came under my care, had lost the sight in one eye and the vision in the other eye was 20/120. I did a simple iridectomy, using a broad keratome, which relieved the tension so her vision was improved to 20/40. This vision had been retained with normal tension when I saw her last in 1913—seventeen years. I have recently heard that her vision remains the same. The fields, which had narrowed considerably before operation, improved some upon the restoration of normal tension, and were retained. The blind eye, on which she refused to have an operation, became so severely painful that she returned in 1913 to have it removed.

History of Case.—Mrs. H., aged fifty-nine years, consulted me first in 1912. She had noticed failure of vision in her right eye the past three years, and for one year had been having electric treatments, probably high-frequency current, with no improvement. The vision of her left eye had also begun to fail, and as her physician said the trouble was not glaucoma, and that he could promise nothing from the electric treatments, she decided to consult some one else. Her vision equaled fingers at two feet with the right eye, and 6/12 in the left. The left could be improved by a +0.75 sph. to 6/7.5. There was no congestion in either eye, the media were clear, but the optic discs were deeply cupped, the right more than the left, and were pale, with narrowing of the retinal vessels. The right field was nearly normal in outline for white, but had a large crescentic scotoma below, involving the fixation-point. The left field was normal in extent, with an abnormally large blind spot. The tension was 60 mm. in the right eye and 40 mm. in the left. After the use of the miotic the tension five days later was 40 mm. right and 30 mm. left.

As I advised consultation before operating, she consulted Dr. Wilder, and we decided the best procedure would be to do the Lagrange operation, as our experience at that time with the Elliot operation had not been favorable enough to depend upon it. I did a Lagrange operation on both eyes, under general anesthesia, removing a large sector of iris and a good-sized piece of the sclera, and covering the wounds well with a conjunctival flap. The conjunctival flap healed readily, but the scleral wound did not close completely for some time, the aqueous escaping under the conjunctiva. Massage was used daily. At the end of a month the tension was normal in both eyes, the wounds were closed with the conjunctival bleb showing, and the vision was some better than before operation. Five months after operation the tension was 18 mm. in the right eye and 24 mm. in the left. The tension continued the same until nine months after operation, when I found it to be 24 mm. in the right and 40 mm. in the left. As the large iridectomy prevented doing a trephining above, I did it below with a 2 mm. trephine, removing a peripheral piece of iris. Healing took place readily with a large bleb persisting. Two months later the tension was 22 mm., and three months after operation the tension was only 10 mm.; her vision with correction was 6/10−, and the large bleb over the trephine opening remained. This vision continued until April, 1914, seven months after the second operation, when I found her vision reduced to 6/15—, and a small opacity at the posterior part of the lens. The vitreous was clear and no changes could be seen in the fundus except the cupping of the optic disc. Two months later her vision was reduced to 6/60, and there was diffuse opacification of the lens. There was no central scotoma. Dr. Wilder saw her again and was of the opinion that the opacity of the lens was the only cause of the poor vision, as the tension was as low as 5 mm. at this time. A little later a mild form of inflammation began in the eye, and upon the use of a mydriatic some adhesions of the iris to the lens were found. Whether these were caused by the low tension or were part of a low-grade iridocyclitis producing the low tension, I could not determine. It quieted down under treatment and the tension improved slightly.

In October, 1915, the opacity of the lens having become almost complete, I operated for removal of cataract. The lens was very sticky and difficult to remove, but after needling the capsule a month later, her vision was 6/10 with a correcting glass. She returned in May, 1916, complaining of pain in the eye, and I found the tension was 28 mm. By the use of pilocarpin solution the tension was kept down fairly well until June, 1917, when it went up to 40 mm., and I decided it was best to operate again. I did another trephining below, near the former trephine site, which gave good drainage, so that the vision returned to 6/10 with the correcting glass, and the tension was normal. This condition continued until October, 1918. As she lived some distance away, I did not see her again until August, 1920, when she returned complaining of failing vision. I found her sight reduced to 6/60, and there was a small scotoma involving the fixation-point. The tension varied from 27 mm. to 33 mm., being reduced somewhat by the use of miotics. There was great thickening of the bulbar conjunctiva below, but it was solid and did not show the pitting which was present when she passed from under my observation in 1918. Examination showed that she had some diseased teeth, and these were removed, but no improvement in the eye condition followed. In January of this year the tension had risen to

35 mm., and in February I operated again. I dissected up a large conjunctival flap below and found it to be very thick and fibrous for a long distance from the trephine opening, and directly over the trephine opening I found a dense, glistening membrane grown fast to the sclera, preventing drainage. This I dissected away, also considerable of the hyperplastic tissue, giving good drainage, so the tension was once more reduced to normal (22 mm.), with vision of 6/60 with her glasses. There is a good-sized bleb present, and the condition seems exactly as after the first trephining, except for the thickened conjunctiva.

The history of several cases of glaucoma in a family during two or more generations has been frequently reported. In 1908 Lawford,[1] of London, collected the histories of 24 families, including one reported by Dr. Howe[2] in 1887. Dr. Calhoun[3] also reported several cases in a family during three generations. In most of the families the onset of the glaucoma is at a younger age in each succeeding generation.

In the family of my patient the age of the mother was seventy-one years, and the daughters forty-nine, fifty-two, and fifty-six years when they were attacked. I have been unable to determine any cause for this predisposition. The two sisters who came under my care were seemingly in good health, with blood-pressure normal or slightly below. The refraction of one was slightly myopic and the other slightly hyperopic, with no deviation from the normal in the size of the corneas.

As to response to treatment, Nettleship[4] remarked that in some families the prognosis is bad, while in other families there does not seem to be any difference from the ordinary cases. In the family whose history I have given the only eye which retained good vision was the one on which I did a simple iridectomy at a time before sclerostomy came into use. I have recently been consulted by a physician with simple glaucoma of both eyes. He explained his reluctance to have an operation, as I advised, by giving the history of blindness in father, uncle, and three brothers, in spite of their having had operations by good surgeons in different parts of the country.

My experience with the first few cases of trephining was not so favorable as to make it the operation of choice. I could find no reason, in the case I am reporting, why the Lagrange operation, done as nearly alike as possible on the two eyes, should have been so successful in the poorer eye, which has retained normal tension ever since, and proved so unsatisfactory in the other eye, necessitating another operation at the end of nine months. I used massage to facilitate drainage during the period of healing, and a filtering scar was present in both eyes for some time when the bleb disappeared, as is usually the case.

When a second operation became necessary, the only choice left, on account of the broad iridectomy, was to make it below or to one side of the coloboma, where the bleb would be exposed when the eye was open. I decided to make it below, although I think the danger of secondary infection is much greater at this point than under the upper lid. The constant irritation of the lower lid undoubtedly produced the great thickening of the subconjunctival tissue, and in this way probably caused a blocking of the opening, with return of tension. This hyperplasia of the subconjunctival tissue, producing closure of the scleral opening, is reported by a number of operators with no explanation given for its occurrence. In a large number of trephinings which I have done with the flap under the upper lid I have never had this occur, and considered it due to the location. In the cases reported, however, this does not explain the condition. It is worthy of note that in animal experimentation the hyperplasia of tissue causes a closure of the opening in nearly every case.

Why there should have been hypotony after the second operation, following a period of normal tension, I could not determine. It is probable that there was good drainage with a diminished secretion of fluid in the eye as a result of the previous tension. That there was a close relation of the hypotony to the development of the cataract I have no doubt. With the lack of normal tone in the eye it seems reasonable to suppose that the lens, which depends on absorption of the fluid surrounding it for its nutrition, should not be sufficiently nourished.

E. Treacher Collins,[5] in his paper on Sequelæ of Hypotony, stated that he had watched cases of minus tension following sclerocorneal trephining for years in which apparently there had been no ill effects. Elliot, in his discussion of the paper, said that the prevalent idea that opacity of the lens would follow hypotony was due to the experience with cases due to decreased ciliary secretion. That hypotony due to operation had never been followed by this result in his experience, and he had followed cases as long as six years in which there had been no changes in the lens or diminution of the vision.

Dr. Knapp[6] does not consider the continued low tension as harmless. He reported six eyes in four patients with tension varying from 2 to 10 mm. at a period of four to five years after trephining. One was lost with phthisis bulbi, and in two the lenses became opaque.

Considering the marked changes to be found in the other structures of the eye, it would be strange if the lens escaped.

It is interesting to note that in my last operation on this patient the blocking of the trephine opening was caused by a dense membrane covering the opening. Dr. Verhoeff,[7] in his histologic examination of an eye on which a successful sclerostomy had been performed, mentioned the fine reticulated tissue which had grown down into the scleral opening, but in my case, as far as macroscopic examination could determine, there was none present. The removal of the membrane has restored the drainage, the permanency of which it is too soon to determine. I removed part of the hypertrophied subconjunctival tissue, and should have removed more of it except for the fear of secondary infection. I can find no report of cases in which this has been done, but I could see no reason for making a new opening when a former one was patent and sufficient to give the necessary drainage.

A recent report of her condition from Dr. Edgar, of Dixon, Ill., under whose observation my patient has been since the operation, says the tension of the eye was 13 mm. in April, and has remained about the same, with a rather prominent bleb always present, and there has been no change in vision.

REFERENCES.

1. Lawford, J. B.: Royal London Ophth. Hosp. Rep., 1908.
2. Howe, Lucien: Arch. Ophth., 1887.
3. Calhoun, F. Phinizy: Jour. Amer. Med. Asso., 1914.
4. Nettleship, Edw.: Trans. Ophth. Soc. U. K., 1909, vol. xxix.
5. Collins, E. Treacher: Trans. Ophth. Soc. U. K., 1917.
6. Knapp, Arnold: Jour. of Ophth., iii, 88.
7. Verhoeff, Fred'k H.: Arch. Ophth., 1915, 129.

FRIABILITY OF THE IRIS A FACTOR IN IRIDECTOMY FOR HYPERTENSION.

HIRAM WOODS, M.D.,
Baltimore, Md.

While breaking of the iris in an attempted iridectomy has been with me a rare occurrence in a fairly extensive experience with glaucoma, it is possible that others have found it more common and have considered it unworthy of record. This may account for my never having heard it discussed. We do not like to report disastrous results; but when such results seem to carry definite teaching, they may be worthy of record. I have used the term "friability" because the first sign of trouble was found when the iris tissues broke from the use of the forceps. Doubtless such cases should be classified under the more general term, "atrophy of the iris."

The subject receives comparatively little space in literature. Fuchs, in the fifth edition of his text-book, page 140, has this to say: "Either the repeated recurrences of an acute iritis or the sluggishly progressing chronic inflammations, may lead ultimately to *atrophy of the iris.* This is characterized by a bleached-out, gray or grayish-brown aspect of the iris (resembling gray felt or blotting paper): the delicate markings of the anterior surface have disappeared, and in their stead dilated vessels can often be recognized as reddish blotches upon the surface of the iris. The pupillary margin is thinned down, often looking as if it had been frayed out; the reaction of the iris is diminished or altogether lost. The great friability of the atrophic iris often renders the correct performance of iridectomy impossible.

"Atrophy of the iris may set in: (1) As a result of long-continued or frequently recurring inflammation. (2) In consequence of increase of tension. Here the main agent is the compression of the blood-vessels at the root of the iris, which is pushed away from the ciliary body and against the sclera."

Case 1.—Mrs. R., aged seventy-four years, came to the dispensary of the University Hospital on December 30, 1918. On Thanksgiving morning, nearly five weeks before, she had awakened with pain and sudden loss of sight in the left eye. There had been no treatment. She was an ignorant woman, and it was impossible, in spite of evident visual loss in both eyes, to get any history antedating what she claimed as sudden loss of sight in the left eye. V.R.E., 5/200; L.E., counts fingers at two feet.

Before coming to the dispensary she thought the right eye was free from trouble. There was left circumcorneal injection; none in the right eye; both pupils were dilated but reacted to light. Tension elevated to fingers. No tonometer record was made at this time. She refused to enter the hospital, and was given eserin to use at home. One week later the tonometer showed right eye 40, left 60, and she entered the hospital. She was given a thorough physical examination, with negative results. Vision had not changed. Blood pressure was 155; urinalysis negative for sugar and albumin; no definite arteriosclerosis could be noted; in fact, her arteries were unusually soft for her age. She was, however, poorly nourished.

Three days after admission Dr. Tarun undertook an iridectomy on her left, or worse, eye. There seems to have been no complication, but there was only transient and very slight, if any, improvement in vision. The eye became worse, apparently from progressive atrophy. She left the hospital on the sixth of February against advice. At this time, under eserin, her right central vision has improved to 20/120 from 5/200 in December. The fields were contracted; tension 35 to 45; pupil small and no pain.

February 11th (five days later) she applied for readmission, as she thought the vision of the right eye was failing. There was considerable right circumcorneal injection; tension was elevated to the fingers; no tenderness on pressure. Central vision was reduced to counting fingers at 20 feet against 20/120 five days before, when she left the hospital.

Considering the outcome of the left iridectomy, I had doubts of any operative interference doing good. From the date of her second admission, February 11th, to March 4th, her eye condition changed very little. Tension was usually moderately elevated, 35 or so, and occasionally went into the fifties. There was no pain and only moderate injection. She had the regular use of eserin while in the hospital. On March 4th I went over her eyes carefully. Vision was greatly reduced; tension was elevated to fingers (tonometer not used); anterior chamber shallow; cornea hazy, eye injected, but the iris showed no characteristics of atrophy, so far as I could judge, and the pupil was of pin-head size.

On March 5th, I attempted an iridectomy. My reasons for operating were that vision was failing, the eye was becoming more inflamed and it was impossible to secure the regular use of a miotic at her home. I felt that the worst we had to anticipate was failure to secure improvement in vision or to stop the inflammatory outbreak. I had no conception of stumbling into the troubles that followed the operation. The spade knife easily entered the anterior chamber through the sclera, 2 mm. behind the limbus. Then an attempt was made to draw out a piece of iris. The forceps cut right through.

This happened two or three times. I decided to try to make a peripheral opening only. A small bit of iris came out in the forceps. As soon as it was cut off there was a gush of semifluid vitreous. Four days later, after the wound had healed, she complained of sudden pain in the right eye, and the anterior chamber was found full of blood. The blood was slowly absorbed; but from this time on, sometimes in the hospital, and sometimes at her home, she had a succession of hemorrhages into the anterior chamber, and was finally discharged blind on June 21, 1919.

CASE 2.—Mrs. G., aged sixty-six years, consulted me first November 25, 1917. Apparently there was no particular reason for her doing so at this time—at least no reason of which she was aware, except that she had been urged to have her eyes watched. There was no pain and she was not conscious of failure in vision. While her physical history indicated no particular abnormality, there were certain things which led me to suspect the presence of degenerative nerve changes. Her physician, Dr. Louis Hamburger, an extremely careful diagnostician, told me that he had known her for years and that the conditions I found had always been present. While she appeared in good health, her eyes showed small pupils with very feeble light reaction. It was better in convergence. There was a slight ptosis on both sides, and she had to throw her head back or elevate her lids to obtain clearest possible vision. This was 20/30 each with correction of a low grade of hyperopic astigmatism. The patella reflex was almost lost, and I thought there was a suggestion of Romberg's sign. I suspected a beginning tabes, but, owing to the long duration of these symptoms, according to Dr. Hamburger, the theory was dismissed. He thought serologic study unnecessary.

Her form fields, which remained pretty constant, are illustrated in Fig. 1. In the right eye, there was contraction with some improvement after the use of pilocarpin. The left field, at first contracted, gradually widened to within 15° or 20° of normal; color fields, of any value, could not be obtained. Tension, to the fingers, was normal. She protested so against the use of the tonometer that results were unreliable. However, on December 22d, about one month after I first saw her, a fairly quiet state was obtained, and tension was found to be 70 for the right and 45 for the left eye. She had neglected the use of pilocarpin, and was persuaded, with some difficulty, to go back to it. In forty-eight hours her tension had fallen to—right, 38; left, 33. Vision, 20/40 each. Up to this time there had been no definite bending of the vessels, so far as I could see, with cocain dilatation; no pulsation. Six weeks later, however (February 4th), one could easily make out bending of the vessels in the right eye. V.R.E., 20/50; L.E., 20/30; fields unchanged. Two days later the tension of the right eye went to 75, but under the vigorous use of pilocarpin, two

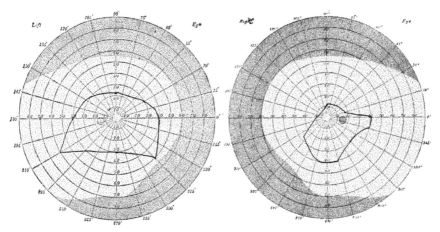

Fig. 1.—Mrs. G. Nov., 1917, and May, 1918.

grains to the ounce, and rest, it fell to 33 with 20/30 vision. It is unnecessary to record the various changes in the tension of the right eye. As long as she used pilocarpin faithfully, tension was kept in the thirties, while in the left it was normal or below. On May 29th it was—32 right; 24 left; central vision, 20/30 each. On July 18th tension was—right, 28; left, 24; central vision, 20/30 each; fields unchanged. This was nearly eight months of treatment with a miotic.

When I returned from my vacation early in September, her central vision was—right, 20/50; left, 20/20; tension—right, 33; left, 23. On September 24th there was apparently a fall of central vision in the right eye to 20/200, but there was no elevation of tension and vision of 20/40 was recorded two days later. On October 17th central vision was 20/30, each eye with tension as last recorded (33). Eleven days later (October 28th) tension suddenly went to 90, with a falling in vision to 20/200. I urged operation, which was finally accepted. The iris showed no clinical evidence of degeneration; the pupil was small from the use of the miotic; yet when, on October 31st, I attempted an iridectomy, it was simply impossible to remove a satisfactory piece of iris. My forceps did, however, extract a small bit of the periphery, with decided benefit to tension and vision. Four months later (February 17th) the vision was 20/30 and tension 24. This improvement persisted during the spring of

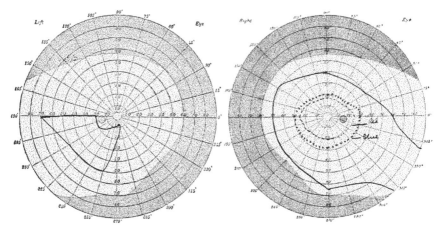

Fig. 2.—Miss T   April 7, 1921.

1919. She was kept on pilocarpin. In spite of the reduction in tension following the unsatisfactory operation the right nerve underwent atrophy and sight was lost. She was advised to continue the pilocarpin indefinitely in the left eye. I have not seen her professionally for eighteen months, but I am told the left eye still has good vision. I do not know whether she is using a miotic.

CASE 3.—Miss T., aged fifty-six years, was seen April 7, 1921. Her physician reported that she had had chronic glaucoma in the left eye for sometime and that lately he had thought the right eye was involved. A miotic had been used systematically in the left eye and occasionally in the right.

Previous physical history and examination were unimportant. She had never been seriously ill. She herself dated the left eye trouble back about five years, and attached little importance to the right eye.

Examination showed: Right eye, no bulbar injection; cornea hazy; deep anterior chamber; iris apparently normal; pupil about 4 mm., regular in shape, retarded light reaction; tension, + 2 to fingers (to tonometer, 90). Vision, 20/30; field as in Fig. 2, showing fairly good color perception, but contraction for form in the upper temporal quadrant. There was definite glaucomatous bending of the vessels, fundus otherwise negative.

Left eye, no injection; cornea steamy; anterior chamber less deep than right; pupil slightly smaller, 3 mm. in diameter. This may have been due to the greater use of a miotic in this eye, but at the first examination she had been without the drops for twenty-four hours. The lens and vitreous were hazy, and the view of the fundus unsatisfactory. However, glaucomatous bending could be made out. Vision, 4/200, probably eccentric fixation. Field showed, as in Fig. 2, a preserved portion in the lower temporal quadrant only.

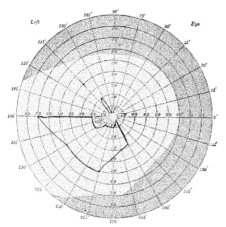

Fig. 3.—Miss T.   April 8, 1921.

Eserin, one grain to the ounce, was used in both eyes every two hours. The following day, April 8th, there was a slight field improvement in the left eye, as indicated by faint central perception for form (Fig. 3). Pilocarpin, four grains to the ounce, was substituted for eserin.

Tension under the miotic is illustrated by the following:

	TENSION	
	Right	Left
April 7: No miotic for twenty-four hours; pupil large 90		100
April 8: Eserin..... 26		33
April 9: Miotic omitted for twenty-four hours..........60		70
Reduced after use of eserin twenty-four hours to .30		35
April 11: After using pilocarpin forty-eight hours 36		50
April 12: After continuing pilocarpin twenty-four hours . 33		45

These tension readings seem to indicate that the miotic controlled the tension of the right eye to within little above normal limits, but that, in the left, the control was less.

I felt uncertain as to how her eyes would stand operative interference. On April 16th this was tested by an attempted iridectomy on the left, or poorer, eye. A spade knife was introduced about 2 mm. behind the limbus. I could readily tell when the point had passed the sclera and elevated the blade a little to avoid puncturing the lens. To my surprise the point of the knife appeared in the anterior chamber, covered with iris tissue. It is possible that the point made a peripheral opening in the capsule, but I doubt it. The knife was withdrawn a little, releasing the iris, and the section made wider by again pushing it forward. When I attempted to catch a piece of the iris the forceps cut through without grasping anything. Then I stopped. If I cut the capsule at all, I believe it was with the iris forceps. There was absolutely no bleeding. At the extreme periphery a small opening could be seen in the iris. It looked as though the iris had been torn from its ciliary attachment. The patient developed a low grade iritis which subsided under homatropin. The lens became totally opaque. Tension, which was 38 a week after the operation, was the same on May 2d, when she went home. The right eye, in which pilocarpin had been steadily used, had vision of 20/20−; tension, 28.

The most instructive article on atrophy of the iris which has come under my notice is in the Proceedings of this Society for 1915. It is from the pen of Dr. de Schweinitz, and is founded on three cases of atrophy, the form differing from those reported here. One was seen by Dr. de Schweinitz, the others were studied by Dr. Wm. Zentmayer and Dr. Casey Wood. Regarding the forms of this disease, de Schweinitz says: "The lightest degree of this phenomenon is seen in the diffuse atrophy which underlies the so-called heterochromia; more pronounced phases may be the sequel of various types of inflammation, as this occurs in recurring iritis and infective iridocyclitis. A common type of iris atrophy arises in consequence of increase of intra-ocular tension, and depends upon compression of the blood-vessels of the root of the iris, and perhaps upon compression of the ciliary nerves." Mention should also be made of Dr. Ellett's paper on "Heterochromia Iridis and Allied Conditions," in our own Proceedings of 1917, and of an experience similar to my own, personally narrated to me by Dr. Holloway. The three cases I am reporting evidently belong to those designated by Dr. de Schweinitz as a "consequence of increase of intra-ocular tension."

It will not be amiss to glance at some of the features of these reported cases and their relation to hypertension. de Schweinitz's patient was twenty-three years of age; Zentmayer's, twenty-seven; and Wood's, forty-four; all below the age when we would naturally look for primary glaucoma. To these may be added a patient of Dr. Stieren's mentioned in the discussion of de Schweinitz's paper. She was twenty-three years old. After two or more years of progressive atrophy, in the form of fenestræ without symptoms more striking than transient injection and photophobia, the patient developed hypertension. In an attempt to relieve this Stieren tried an iridectomy. He encountered the same condition I did. He said: ". . the iris was so friable that all efforts to draw it through the corneal section resulted only in tearing it to shreds." Later he successfully trephined the eye.

Casey Wood's patient had pain, inflammatory symptoms, plus tension, and finally came to enucleation. The iris was found to present, "subacute and chronic fibrinoplastic iridocyclitis; secondary glaucoma." Wood, whose original article I have not been able to review, quotes Harms to the effect that if the atrophic cases had been examined earlier, there would have been no glaucomatous signs; that the latter was an end result of whatever caused the iris changes. If this reasoning is correct, the glaucoma was secondary, a hypothesis apparently confirmed by the time of its appearance and advanced by de Schweinitz.

From a careful study of his case de Schweinitz thought the cause of the iris atrophy was probably tubercular, with a possible influence from intestinal auto-intoxication and some indefinite nerve disturbance. Zentmayer advances only vascular changes as a cause, and Wood, as quoted, presents nothing in the way of etiology. He regarded the hypertension as "an effort of the eye to rid itself of the irritating products of the primary affection." I hardly know what this means. Both de Schweinitz and Fuchs speak of hypertension in glaucoma as a cause of iridic atrophy, adding that pressure on the iris vessels and ciliary nerves is an active factor.

The essential difference between hypertension with and without iris atrophy probably lies in the fact that in atrophic cases a fibrinoplastic exudate compresses the vessels and causes atrophy, on the one hand and on the other, pushes the iris roots against the sclera, and brings about hypertension. It is not atrophy which produces hypertension, but inflammatory exudate which causes both. Cases which do not present iris atrophy as a complication have some other than a plastic inflammatory origin. With the diagnosis made, either before or during operation, we know that we have a degenerated eye to deal with; that a correct iridectomy is impossible; that any operative traumatism will probably be badly tolerated. The tendency to the formation of fibrinoplastic tissue obliges us to select a method of treatment which will inflict the least possible traumatism. In this connection we must consider the use of miotics. They were employed in the three cases reported, and with definite results. In neither were they given up until the tension went up in spite of their use. I was guided by the tonometer. Even with these elevations of tension vision, while it varied, was not falling off. Probably the ultimate result would have been the same with non-operative treatment, but I do not think it would have come as rapidly. The experiences have about convinced me that this form of hypertension is one in which

miotics will give us the longest lease of sight; that if, after
the corneal section for iridectomy, we find an atrophic iris,
we should stop at once, allow the section to heal, and then
rely on medical treatment.

Ophthalmology has had two instructive experiences in in-
terpreting mechanical devices for diagnosis. I allude to the
phorometer and ophthalmometer. They are useful instruments; but it is very important to know when to disobey
them. Possibly the same is true of the tonometer. Without
it, we would miss diagnoses of great importance, and fail in
many instances to discover early hypertension; but hypertension is a many-sided symptom, and from its discovery to
ultimate outcome demands agile thinking. Conditions back
of it, physiologic acuity existing in spite of it, anatomic conditions revealed by examination before and at operation, are
all as important as the hypertension itself.

DISCUSSION OF PAPERS OF DRS. DODD AND WOODS.

Dr. Arnold Knapp, New York: The reduced tension after
trephining to which Dr. Dodd has referred is due, I think, to
a fistula,—not a subconjunctival but a conjunctival fistula,—
because in these cases if you instill fluorescein and examine
the bleb with magnifying lens, you see distinct trickling of
green-stained fluid. In other words, there is a constant leakage of aqueous into the conjunctival sac, and I think that
explains why these eyes are so dangerous. I have recently
observed a case of spontaneous rupture of a cystoid scar in a
patient operated on for glaucoma. The symptom the patient
complained of was that the eye was leaking constantly, and
observing a red eye and the anterior chamber entirely empty
under pressure, the eye was bandaged for two weeks. Emptying of the anterior chamber occurred, and when I saw the
patient the tension was 7½ and the fistula was distinctly to
be seen. I thought the case was dangerous to leave in this
condition, and proceeded to excise the cystoid scar and cover
the defect by a conjunctival flap.

Dr. W. H. Wilder, Chicago, Ill.: While we may frequently encounter the dangers, whatever dangers they may be, of hypotony after trephine operations and other operations of this character, I think that such dangers are very much less than those of not getting a reduction of the tension.

After any of the various operations of sclerectomy, it seems to me the good results obtained are because of the establishment of an artificial system of drainage of the fluids of the eye, and unless we bring that about we are not accomplishing the desired result.

In order to secure adequate drainage, it is desirable to get as large and thick a conjunctival flap as possible, for a small flap near the limbus may result in a circumscribed bleb, and the escaping fluid will not drain readily into the surrounding submucous tissue. Elliot, in his later writings, emphasizes this point. I do not hesitate in the operation of trephining and also in the operation of iridotasis, of which I have now done quite a number, to make quite a larger flap, going back so that I may even open the capsule of Tenon, and it is essential that the ends of the incision by which the flap is made shall not approach too close to the limbus.

It is wise to keep close to the sclera in dissecting down the flap, but this should be done only over an area large enough to give access to the part of the limbus to be opened. A larger field is necessary when one is doing trephining than when doing iridotasis. I think this is an extremely important part of the technic, because unless we have a flap which is free for a considerable distance from the limbus, there will not be as free drainage or evacuation into the submucous tissue.

I have observed also that when the flap is too small, or even when made in this larger, more liberal way, that there will sometimes be a bleb over the trephine opening which is distinctly circumscribed, and in such cases the tension may increase, seeming to indicate that the aqueous is not escaping readily into the surrounding submucous tissue.

In a few instances of this kind I have, with strict antiseptic precautions, made a small opening into the conjunctiva, about 8 or 10 mm. from the edge of the bleb, and introduced a small, narrow spatula, one such as we use in cyclodialysis, pushing it beneath the conjunctiva close to the sclera and breaking down the adhesions that form the

5

edge of the bleb and so allowing the fluid to drain into the submucosa.

One little practical point I would like to bring forward that is suggested by the interesting case of Dr. Dodd's, which I had the opportunity of seeing and which illustrates that the human eye will stand a good deal of operating and still come out very well; that is, the original operator may have to repeat the operation or one of his confréres may have to repeat it, and I have found it a good practice, instead of putting the trephine opening in the vertical meridian, to put it to one side or the other so that there may still be an opportunity for the next operator whoever he is, to operate under the lid.

Dr. E. V. L. Brown, Chicago, Ill.: A judge with simple glaucoma, whom I think all the Chicago members, and many of you in other cities have seen, was operated by Holth, of Christiania, some ten years ago, and has maintained full fields, central vision, and normal tension in each eye ever since. At the suggestion of a colleague who contends that a high percentage of successful trephine blebs are fistulous, I tested out this patient with fluorescein only last week, and found a definite spontaneous leakage through a small break in the bleb of the right eye, and numerous porous thinnings in the other which emitted green-staining aqueous when enough pressure was made upon the bulb to make the bleb tense. Such eyes certainly are open to the danger of late infection.

Colonel Henry Smith, London, England: It seems to me in this question of trephining that we would need to revert a little to first principles. In the two schools of physiologists, one, the school which assumes that the performance of vital functions by physical or mechanical means, would hold that the result of trephining is by permanent drainage. The other would be the school which might be limited to myself—the school which believes that there is a vital factor in the performance of vital functions. We believe that this mechanical theory is entirely a mistaken view of how trephining acts. In the first place, if you have very high tension, you will have glaucoma; if you have very low tension, you will have atrophy of all the structures of the eye. Is there any means by which you can regulate the size which this trephine opening will remain? If it is too big, you will have a soft eye; if it is too small, you will have glaucoma. Are we to assume that the fibrous tissue of the sclerotic differs from the fibrous tissue of any other part of the body, that a small opening, say 4 mm. square, will remain permanently of the exact size that is required to maintain this tension of say 15 to 25 mm. of mercury? I think it is utterly irrational. Do a Cox incision for an inoperable stricture of the urethra and endeavor to establish a permanent fistula there. What is the result? There are 40 ounces of fluid to be driven through it with a strong pump behind it. That will close up and be the worry of the patient's life to have it periodically dilated. Do we expect a fistula will behave otherwise in the eye? Do a Talma-Morrison operation for dropsy of the peritoneum and you find that it will operate for a while, but it, too, will close up. This latter is essentially the same in principle as trephining for glaucoma. You pull out a strip of omentum and leave it subcutaneous to form a drain. The trephining has a place in surgery. I agree with Dr. Knapp that these cases that go bad are due merely to turning forward a conjunctival flap which is so delicate that it is liable to permanent fistulous communication with the conjunctival sac. As regards what is called the edema produced, I have been shown edema with probe. Apply the same probe to the other eye, and it will show the same edema in the other eye; apply to the back of your hand, and there you will have edema, too. You are likely to confuse this thing called edema. Let us take another instance. Open the lacrimal sac from the face and make a 6 mm. trephine opening into the nose from the facial opening through everything with a shoemaker's punch. You are astonished that this 6 mm. hole has become closed up at the end of three months. Do we expect that this little trephine opening in the sclerocornea will remain open? I have long held that the whole rationale of trephining—I call the LaGrange operation trephining; the whole of these so-called fistulous operations are trephining, they are of the same character—is wrong. I hold that it has a much sounder rationale than claiming a mechanical means for performing a physiologic function. If we assume that trephining established a drain for a limited time, which would be sufficient to

allow the physiologic equilibrium of the eye to become reëstablished, I think we would be claiming a much more rational
basis for the trephining.   I have frequently done an iridectomy on one eye and trephining on the other in patients who
I knew would come back to me in a year to have a cataract
removed, and to my surprise there was not much to choose
between the two procedures.   I was inclined to think that
the actual tension result was more favorable in the iridectomy, though I by no means turn down trephining, but in
doing trephining it is to my mind necessary to turn forward
the whole subconjunctival tissue so as to get a decent covering for the opening.   My own practice is to make a straight
horizontal incision in the conjuctiva, pull down the conjunctiva and subconjunctiva, and it will pull itself into position from the elasticity when we have finished.   The policy,
so far as I can see of it, of splitting the cornea is unnecessary,
and I personally think irrational.   If the conjunctiva is
pushed forward as far as a blunt spoon will push it, there is
ample space to get a trephine opening in well away from the
ciliary body.   The ciliary body is much further back in the
human subject than in some of the lower animals, and much
further back than the uninitiated would expect.

Dr. Dodd (closing): I was much interested in Dr.
Knapp's remarks in regard to fistula, and am sorry I did not
try the test which Dr. Brown suggested in my patient.   If
that is the explanation of the condition, we have an opening
which may become infected and dangerous.   As regards the
flaps, I make them much as Colonel Smith stated,—praetically a horizontal incision,—leaving it so that filtration may
occur under the conjunctiva at both sides of the opening.   I
found the closure of the trephine opening in this patient was
entirely due to the membrane which covered it, as the opening was in exactly the same condition that it was when I
made it eight years before, showing no growth into it from
the sides or from below.

THE ACTION OF ADRENALIN ON THE GLAUCO-MATOUS EYE.

ARNOLD KNAPP, M.D.,
New York.

On making the usual subconjunctival injection of novocain-adrenalin before operating for glaucoma, a dilatation of the pupil was frequently observed. As this dilatation must have been due to adrenalin, it suggested an investigation of the action of adrenalin in primary glaucoma to determine its effect on the pupil and on the intra-ocular pressure.

PUPIL.—In the normal eye the instillation of adrenalin has no effect on the pupil (Elliot, Schultz, Cords, Wessely).

Loewi found that adrenalin dilates the pupil in diabetes, in those suffering from Graves' disease, and in pancreatectomized animals; this constitutes the adrenalin pupillary reaction of Loewi and has diagnostic importance to show insufficiency of internal pancreatic secretion and hyperthyreosis.

According to Elliot, the irides of various animals do not all react in the same way to adrenalin. In dogs the injection of adrenalin caused a dilatation of the pupil. Wessely obtained a dilatation of the pupil in rabbits after instilling adrenalin in the conjunctiva. In dogs and cats this was never obtained, and it was possible only after subconjunctival injection.

Lewandoski found that the intravenous administration of suprarenal extract in a cat caused the same symptoms as an irritation of the cervical sympathetic; namely, mydriasis, retraction of the third eyelid, slight protrusion and slight enlargement of the palpebral fissure. The reaction in rabbits was much less. After section of the sympathetic and extirpation of the superior cervical ganglion, the same symptoms resulted, except that they were more pronounced.

Meltzer found that after extirpation of the superior cervical ganglion the pupil reacted more easily to adrenalin than it does in subganglion section of the sympathetic or in a normal animal. The instillation of adrenalin caused a maximal mydriasis, but the extirpation of the ganglion had to be done at least twenty-four hours before. In some animals, after three and one-half months, the action was still present, but less. Instead of extirpating the ganglion if all communications with the central nervous system are divided, adrenalin action is lost.

Auer says that the sympathetic, between the cervical ganglion and the eye, must carry two kinds of fibers, those coming from the central nervous system and those originating in the ganglion. This author believes that the postganglionic fibers carry inhibitory impulses to the pupil, which prevent the pupil from dilating. These are opposite to those conducted by the preganglionic fibers which dilate the pupil by stimulating the dilator muscle. Adrenalin contracts smooth muscle-fibers. If it dilates the pupil, the postganglionic fibers inhibiting the dilator pupillæ have been eliminated.

Langley drew attention to the similarity of adrenalin action to irritation of the sympathetic. If the pupil dilates to adrenalin, it shows increased sensitiveness to sympathetic stimuli or loss of inhibiting influences which come from the superior cervical ganglion or pancreas.

INTRA-OCULAR PRESSURE.—In glaucoma adrenalin was used at one time to influence intra-ocular pressure. Its action was not definitely determined, presumably as the tonometer was then not in general use. Some authors (Mac-Callan) warned against its use in glaucoma, as it was likely to increase the intra-ocular pressure.

Spengler believes that adrenalin causes an ischemia of the ciliary vessels, dilatation of the pupils, and slight reduction in intra-ocular pressure.

Rubert found that instillation of adrenalin or subcutaneous injections cause changes in the ocular pressure, at first a reduction, then a rise, and then a secondary reduction. In glaucomatous eyes an occasional increase is not to be denied, so that caution must be exercised.

Shahan and Post, in a study on "Heat in Glaucoma," found that cocain-adrenalin usually causes a drop in tension, followed by a rebound carrying the tension up to or above its previous level, while adrenalin alone causes a rise in tension, cocain a drop, but when combined, a more decided drop in tension resulted, which lasted for about one hour.

According to Leplat, adrenalin given subcutaneously raises the general arterial pressure. As for the eye, hypertonus was never observed, the ocular tension remained constant, and in two there was a reduction.

OBSERVATIONS.—I have examined a series of 65 cases of primary glaucoma, some of which had been operated upon, to observe the action of adrenalin on the pupil and on the intra-ocular tension. The adrenalin used was that of Parke, Davis, and Co., and it was fresh. After taking the tension with the Schiötz tonometer and measuring the size of the pupil, one drop of adrenalin was instilled every few minutes for five times. After one-half hour the measurements of the pupil and of the ocular tension were again taken. Cases with atrophic irides and posterior synechia were necessarily excluded.

I. After adrenalin instillation the pupil dilated regularly or eccentrically in 60 out of the 65 cases of glaucoma, varying from 1 to 5 mm. The degree of mydriasis was not so great if pilocarpin had previously been given.

II. In these 65 cases, after adrenalin instillation, the tension was unaffected in 40, decreased in 20, increased in 5.

The possibility of dilating the pupil for ophthalmoscopic examination with little prospect of increasing the tension is often of great advantage in glaucomatous eyes. The adrenalin mydriasis can usually be promptly corrected by miotics.

The reduction in tension which occurred in 20 of the 65 cases is particularly interesting.

Wessely believes that adrenalin causes a vasoconstriction which leads to reduced aqueous production and resulting hypotony. My observations lead me to believe that the hypotony results from the relief of mechanical causes, and that in some glaucomas there is a retention of aqueous in the posterior chamber, and by dilatation of the pupil by adrenalin this stasis is corrected. This was particularly noticeable in the case of S., where the pupils measured—right, $3\frac{1}{2}$ mm.,—tension, 22; left, $3\frac{1}{2}$ mm.,—tension, 34. The pupillary margin gripped the lens capsule like a crater, and the center of the iris was distinctly bulging. After adrenalin the pupils measured 6 mm. each, the tension was reduced to 16 and 22, and the iris contour was perfectly flat. Furthermore, in doing an iridectomy for glaucoma after the corneal incision and the escape of the aqueous with flattening of the anterior chamber, on excising the iris there is often an additional escape of a considerable amount of aqueous which seemed to have been retained in the posterior chamber. This confirms Curran's view, advanced in an article, "A New Operation for Glaucoma," that in glaucoma the passage of fluid through the pupil is impeded because the iris hugs the lens over too great a surface and dams back the aqueous. Curran attempts to drain from the posterior chamber into the anterior chamber by a peripheric iridotomy.

III. In 15 of these 65 cases subjected to adrenalin the glaucoma was only apparent in one eye. The other (normal) eye showed in 12 a dilatation of the pupil after adrenalin; in 3 there was no change; the intra-ocular pressure was unaffected in 12; in 3 the pressure was reduced. This suggests that a susceptibility to adrenalin may be present long before the usual clinical signs of glaucoma.

REFERENCES.

Elliot: Journal of Physiology, 1905, xxxii, 401.
Cords: Die Adrenalin-Mydriasis, Wiesbaden, Bergmann, 1911.
Schultz: Proc. Soc. Exp. Biology and Med., 1908, xl, 23.
Wessely: Zentralbl. f. Augenh., 1905, p. 130. Vers. Ophth. Gesellsch., Heidel-
　　berg, 1900,. 69.
Loewi: Wien. klin. Woch., 1907, p. 782. Also Arch. f. exp. Path. u. Pharm.,
　　1908, 59.
Lewandowski: Arch. f. Anat. u. Phys., 1899.
Meltzer and Auer: Amer. Jour. Phys., 1903, 1904; also Jour. Med. Research,
　　1903; also N. Y. Eye and Ear Inf. Rep., 1906.
Langley: Jour. Phys., 1901, 237.
Spengler: Zeit. f. Augenh., 1905, 33.
Rubert: Zeit. f. Augenh., 1909, 228.
Shahan and Post: Section Ophth., Amer. Med. Asso., 1920.
Leplat: Bull. d. le Soc. Belge d'Opht., 1921.
Curran: Arch. Ophth., 1920, p. 132.

DISCUSSION.

DR. J. W. CHARLES, St. Louis, Mo.: In the years 1916–17, having read that adrenalin only dilates the pupil when the sympathetic has been involved, I experimented with a series of cases as they came into the office, until a more serious work came up, and I only had about 60 to 70 normal eyes from which to report. I used the adrenalin pure, that is, 1/1000 P.D. I found no reaction whatever. Then I took all the cases of enlarged thyroid, from those in the very beginning stages upward, and I got 16 of those, some with exophthalmos, some having been operated upon, some the large colloid types, and I had no dilatation from any of these. The only dilatation I obtained in the series was in one woman who had a congenital ptosis on one side. In that case I did get dilatation on that side. As to the use of adrenalin in glaucoma, when we first had access to adrenalin some years ago, I had one case,—a man with an absolute glaucoma,—in which I tested it out. The reaction after vascular constriction gave him so much pain that I have never used it since.

DR. F. H. VERHOEFF, Boston, Mass.: When Dr. Knapp was in my clinic last week we had a case of sympathetic paralysis in a young boy. He had an injury to his back and neck, eight months previously, with definite paralysis of the right sympathetic nerve, large pupil, narrow palpebral orifice,

and some pallor of the iris.   Dr. Knapp suggested that we try
the adrenalin test.   We did this after he left, and found it
had no effect upon the pupil and no appreciable effect upon
the tension.   That may be due to the fact that this case had
gone eight months whereas, I suppose, the experiments on
animals are of much shorter duration.

DR. GEORGE S. DERBY, Boston, Mass.: Dr. Knapp states
that in patients with glaucoma in only one eye adrenalin
causes dilatation in the unaffected eye.   I had a case
which showed this: a man of sixty who had thrombosis of
the central vein in the left eye.   Last March he developed
glaucoma, with tension running up to 65 or 70.   The case
was seen in consultation by Dr. Knapp.   The eye was
operated upon, the tension recurred, and later came to
enucleation.   The tension in the right eye, which showed no
other sign of glaucoma, rose to 32 to 35, and it was impossible to keep it within normal limits by the use of myotics.
Following the enucleation of the glaucomatous eye the
tension in the so-called normal eye dropped to normal.
Nine days after enucleation the tension had dropped to 22
to 23 mm., and the adrenalin test was tried.   The eye was
not under a miotic at that time.   There was a very marked
dilatation of the pupil in that case.   I have tried the adrenalin test as described by Dr. Knapp in a number of other
cases, and in most of them the reaction has been marked.
There have been two failures in which there has been no
dilatation.   In one there was rather evident atrophy of the
iris; the other was a case of simple glaucoma and there was
no reaction.   It seems not impossible that this reaction may
take place, more especially in eyes that tend toward the
congestive type of glaucoma rather than the purely simple
type without any signs of congestion.

DR. MARK J. SCHOENBERG, New York: Dr. Knapp's observation on the action of adrenalin in the eye opens up the
doors to some further investigation as to the relation of
glaucoma to the general condition.   We all have the feeling
that glaucoma is due to the general condition.   It is not
only a local affair.   We know, for instance, that the sympathetic system is sensitized by the thyroid in some way, that
in disturbances of thyroid in hyperthyroidism the sympa-

thetic system is more irritable. On this is based the Goetsch reaction. Here we have a series of cases with ocular manifestations, glaucoma in which the instillation of adrenalin has a definite action upon the pupil, and we cannot interpret this action otherwise than the effect of the adrenalin upon the sympathetic nerve-endings and on the iris. If we would think a little further, then we would suggest that these cases of glaucoma which react to the instillation of adrenalin in the eye should be further investigated along the same lines. For instance, we should know whether this reaction is due to a state of sensitization of the sympathetic in the eye by the thyroid. If the thyroid is involved in cases of glaucoma, then studies of basal metabolism in cases of glaucoma are in line. Furthermore, the reaction of the skin or other parts of the body to local applications of adrenalin, or to subcutaneous intradermal injections of adrenalin should be studied to see whether other parts of the body react in the same way. Do we deal here in glaucoma with a state of disturbance or herperactivity of the thyroid? Any way, I believe Dr. Knapp's observation is one of the most important contributions to the study of glaucoma, we have had in a long while.

DR. E. V. L. BROWN, Chicago, Ill.: In connection with Dr. Knapp's statement that he made use of the pupil-dilating effect of adrenalin to study the fundus of glaucomatous eyes, and that he observed no ill effects, I would remark that I have used ordinary mydriatics cautiously in a considerable number of cases of simple glaucoma, for one purpose or another, and, too, have never observed any untoward effects.

DR. KNAPP (closing): My experience of dilating the pupil in glaucoma is necessarily limited. We have usually gotten along with using cocain. In this demonstration it was so easy to have a good look at the fundus that I thought it would be better to note it in the paper. I would like to say that my title was a preliminary one. The subject is an obscure one. It does open an interesting field and should be followed out by other members of the Society.

THE PHYSIOLOGIC MODE OF ACTION OF MYDRIATICS AND MIOTICS, EXPLAINING THEIR EFFECTS IN HYPERTENSION (GLAUCOMA).

CARL KOLLER, M.D.,
New York

We understand mydriatics to be those chemical agents which widen the pupil, and miotics those agents which contract the pupil. When we undertake to explain their mode of action we have, of course, to consider the anatomy of the iris, and the forces which normally determine the size of the pupil. This brings us at once face to face with controversies which are ages old, and, in spite of an enormous literature, have not as yet been fully determined and which, therefore, seem to stand where they stood decades ago. This may be seen when consulting the text-books as to the effects of mydriatics and miotics. In the following I shall limit myself to stating such facts as are obvious and accessible to the ordinary observer, facts which harmonize well with each other, so that the conclusions drawn appear well founded.

According to most text-books, mydriatics widen the pupil by paralyzing the sphincter and stimulating the radiating "dilator." To this stimulating action upon the dilator is ascribed the further increase of a pupil previously widened by paralysis of the oculomotor nerve. The existence of a dilator seemed necessary to account for a number of phenomena, and its reality was assumed even before the thin layer of radiating fibers on the posterior surface of the iris stroma ("Bruch's membrane") was anatomically found. Correspondingly, according to popular teaching, the miotics contract the pupil by stimulating the sphincter and paralyzing the dilator.

It is true that, for the quick reactions to light and accom-modative impulses the sphincter plays the most important part, but all the facts point to the conclusion that, for the habitual width of the pupil, the state of fullness of the iris vessels is the determining factor. For instance, everybody has observed that inflammatory congestion of the iris makes the pupil small, that is, the vessels are widened and filled; also, as is well known, narrow pupils are the rule in people whose cerebral arteries are pathologically distended (for instance, morphinists). But this aspect of the subject has been overshadowed by the prominence given to the effect of the different agencies upon nerves and muscle tissues.

To help our understanding of these vascular factors which affect the width of the pupil let us exclude from considera-tion for the moment all the physiologic and the pathologic factors, and look at phenomena which we know are produced by physical or mechanical forces alone. In death the pupils become wide, a fact especially apparent after an animal is bled to death. The blood has left the iris arteries, so that centripetal push in the vessels is no longer active, and the iris consequently follows the pull of the elastic fibers, which are arranged along the adventitia of the blood-vessels.

Further, if we take an animal, for instance, a white rabbit, previously exsanguinated, and inject methylene-blue into the aorta under pressure, we will notice that in the same instant that the ears become blue from the injection fluid, the pupils become as narrow as pinheads. What has taken place is that the pressure of the injection fluid has filled the iris arteries and erected, as it were, each sector of the iris, shoving it toward the center. Thus we see that the pupil can be widened by emptying vessels, and narrowed by filling them. This is in perfect accord with the fact that all states of cerebral congestion go with narrow pupils (sleep, mor-phinism, meningitic coma), whereas all states of cerebral anemia (syncope, epileptic seizure) go with wide pupils.

All the mydriatics known have a constricting effect on the iris vessels, though in a varying degree. In the case of atropin, paralysis of the sphincter is, no doubt, the predominating factor in widening the pupil; still the constricting action on the vessels is observed every day in its bleaching effect on an eye with "ciliary" or "pericorneal" injection. And it is not the ciliary arteries alone that are subject to this local effect of constriction. The shrunken mucous membrane of the nose, and the blanched pharynx of a person that has received an overdose of atropin by instillation, are proof of this. The flushed face and general hyperemia of the skin in atropin poisoning (which at the first glance do not seem to fit in with this) are produced by the systemic action of the poison on the central nervous system, whereas the vasoconstriction in question is purely local. Cocain has to a much higher degree the constricting effect on the iris vessels, and this can be beautifully demonstrated by injecting it subconjunctivally. If this is done at a place not far from the cornea, the iris will in about five minutes shrink in that very meridian in which the injection has been made, the pupil becoming eccentrically pear-shaped. A parallel to this enlarging effect on the pupil through vasoconstriction in the case of cocain is seen in the widening of the palpebral fissure. In explanation of this phenomenon a great deal has been said of smooth muscle-fibers in the lid (H. Mueller's fibers) and of smooth muscle-fibers behind the globe. The obvious fact is that the eyelids shrink by vasoconstriction. One can observe this equally well on a healthy eye as on an eye with paralytic ptosis, and on an eye whose upper lid is drooping, owing to inflammatory infiltration, as in trachoma.

Further, we know one agent which does not affect the sphincter at all, but widens the pupil, and that by vasoconstriction alone. This is adrenalin. Its effect cannot be demonstrated by instilling it, but only by bringing it in direct contact with the iris or by injecting it subconjunctivally.

The same asymmetry of the pupil mentioned in the case of cocain can be observed when adrenalin (1:10,000) is injected under the conjunctiva. One has to wait for the effect about fifteen minutes. After a further lapse of about a half-hour the pupil is less eccentric, almost round, but still wide, though it reacts well to light. After another half-hour it is of normal width again. This widening of the pupil by adrenalin is a strong proof of the vascular action in dilatation.

In a contrary way miotics, besides stimulating the sphincter, have a dilating effect on the iris vessels; one can directly observe this with a loop or corneal microscope. Proof of this we have in the action of dionin, which does not affect the sphincter, but contracts the pupil solely by congesting the iris. This miotic effect of dionin is little known, because difficult to observe. One can best demonstrate it on a pupil previously dilated with atropin. It does not last a long time, and one has to watch for it closely.

It is this vasoconstricting effect of the mydriatics and the vasodilating action of the miotics which account for many of the phenomena which we daily observe in our work. It is this vascular effect also which makes the pupil dilate bow-shaped between adhesions; so it is the vascular action which makes an iris with a coloboma move up toward the coloboma, no counterforce existing at that place, and exactly the same force which displaces the pupil of an eye inflamed after combined extraction upward, or rather pushes it up toward the incision.

The mode of action of mydriatics and miotics in hypertension is, of course, based upon their physiologic effects. But this comes about in a way different from that assumed in the Leber-Knies theory of glaucoma. This theory, so long dominant, and according to which the symptoms are still interpreted in the text-books, says that hypertension is due to retention of liquid in the eye owing to obliteration or clogging of Fontana's spaces.

If we but look at an eye with a mild attack of acute glaucoma, the state of the circulation in that eye is plainly discernible. The pupil is widened and usually irregularly oval; this bespeaks constriction of arteries, more so in some iris sectors than in others. The anterior ciliary veins, which carry blood from the ciliary body, and which leave the eyeball a little back of the corneoscleral junction, are widely distended and engorged, indicating that the intra-ocular veins, notably those of the ciliary processes of which they are collaterals, are in the same state of engorgement. This means that the circulation is sluggish. The cornea is edematous, the anterior chamber is shallow, both lens and iris being pressed forward on account of the increase of exuded fluid around the vitreous body. Of the presence of this fluid we get incontrovertible proof if we perform a posterior sclerotomy, and note that what escapes first is not vitreous, but a thin liquid, vitreous following after the thin liquid. I believe that Dr. Arnold Knapp first called attention to this fact. Taking all these signs together, the obvious interpretation is that in the acute glaucomatous attack the arteries of the iris and probably all ciliary arteries are constricted, carrying but little blood, whereas the veins are widened and engorged, which means that the whole circulation is stagnant. This stagnant circulation prevents the disposal of the increased amount of exuded liquid through the ordinary channels. According to the Leber-Knies theory, the lymph spaces of the iris angle are the only exit for the intra-ocular fluid. That this is one of the ways is certain, but it is equally certain that it is not the only way. In the healthy eye the anterior surface of the iris, a loose vascular structure, acts like a sponge, taking up the contents of the anterior chamber. That this is so can be seen after an operation or trauma, when blood in the anterior chamber is found absorbed after a few days, wherever it has been in contact with the iris; but a speck of coagulum left on the anterior lens capsule, removed from contact with the iris, may remain unabsorbed for weeks. It may not be amiss to mention here that this absorption from the iris surface is hastened by miotics and delayed by mydriatics, because the rapid circulation acts like a system of drainage ditches, in which the current takes up the moisture of the soil by side suction, due to the flow of the water.

If we keep in mind that in the acute glaucomatous attack the circulation is slowed up or stagnant, and that mydriatics slow up circulation whereas miotics speed it up, these adverse, respectively favorable effects become intelligible. Their effect is quite in keeping with what we know of the effect of other agencies on the glaucomatous attack. Sleep, administration of morphin, caffein, hot fomentations, in short, all means for increasing the flow of blood to the head, help to relieve glaucomatous hypertension; and it is known to every experienced ophthalmologist that exertion of the accommodation, for instance, reading, far from being harmful, exerts a favorable influence.

What, in the first instance, brings on the sudden prodromal or acute glaucomatous attack, we do not know; in all probability it is a certain toxicity, which in eyes of a definite architecture brings on an edema, comparable to the angioneurotic edema in other parts of the body.

In chronic "simple" glaucoma the condition is somewhat different, in that the accumulation of fluid within the eyeball is of purely vascular origin. But with regard to the action of mydriatics and miotics we see the very same effects in all kinds of hypertension, both primary and secondary ones, as, for instance, those caused by swelling of cortical matter after cataract extraction. Mydriatics slow up the circulation by producing anemia through constriction of the small arteries, whereas miotics, by dilating the small arteries, speed up circulation, and thus favor the absorption of abnormal quantities of transuded serum.

6

DISCUSSION.

DR. ALEXANDER DUANE, New York: Dr. Koller seems inclined to attribute pupillo-dilatation solely either to paresis of the sphincter or to vasoconstriction, being due in the latter case to stimulation of the vasomotor fibers of the sympathetic. But surely active pupillo-dilatation can be produced by stimulation of another set of sympathetic fibers passing through the long ciliary nerves. These and the sympathetic root of the ciliary ganglion are alike derived from the cervical sympathetic, but the course of the two is different. The cervical sympathetic sends one branch to the carotid plexus, and from this is derived the sympathetic root of the ciliary ganglion. It sends another branch, which is derived primarily from the ciliospinal center in the cord, to the Gasserian ganglion, and thence through the first branch of the fifth to the long ciliary nerves, and ultimately to the dilatator pupillæ. Cocain and adrenalin, according to good observers, act to stimulate the terminals of this branch and so cause a direct contraction of the dilatator. That these drugs may also act on the vasomotor nerve terminals is, of course, not excluded.

It must also be remembered that, apart from paralysis of the sphincter, pupillo-dilatation is in part effected by inhibitory impulses of peripheral origin conveyed to the pupillo-constrictor center in the third nerve nucleus; further, that pupillo-contraction may be produced by inhibition or paralysis of the pupillo-dilatator centers in the cord, or of their terminal connections, which are motor, not vasomotor.

The point I wish to bring out is that the continual variations in the diameter of the pupil are the result of a number of stimuli varying in origin and nature, and the mechanism of their production both in the case of pupillo-dilatation and of pupillo-constriction is doubtless partly muscular, partly vascular. It must often be difficult to tell which of the various agencies is most effective in causing pupillo-dilatation in glaucoma or similar conditions.

DR. F. H. VERHOEFF, Boston, Mass.: I have been for a long time convinced that the effect of atropin and miotics on intra-ocular pressure was not dependent upon their effect on the pupil, but my idea of their action on the intra-ocular vessels is exactly opposite to that of Dr. Koller's. Atropin in the general circulation produces vasodilatation, as evidenced by flushing of the face; miotics produce vasoconstriction. We should have to assume, if we take Dr. Koller's view, that their actions on the intra-ocular vessels would be exactly opposite to these when instilled into the conjunctival sac. I have assumed that when you instil atropin you produce dilatation of the small arteries in the eye and raise the intra-ocular pressure by increasing the pressure in the capillaries. On the other hand, if you use eserin or pilocarpin, you produce vasoconstriction and thus reduce the intra-ocular pressure. Of course, the effect of the general blood-pressure upon the intra-ocular pressure is a different matter. When you constrict all the small arteries in the body, you increase the blood-pressure, but at the same time you decrease, relatively, the capillary pressure.

Dr. Mark J. Schoenberg, New York: Dr. Koller's interesting paper is full of suggestions, but seems to me that some of his assertions lack the proof of proper evidences. For instance, he maintains that the habitual size of the pupil depends upon the amount of blood contained in the iris blood-vessels, and as a proof he offers the interesting fact that in cadavers even the pupils become smaller if a fluid is injected under pressure in the aorta. This experiment does not appeal to me as being a reasonable proof, since it does not exclude the possibility of the pupils contracting under the influence of the stimulation of the pupillary centers. Dr. Koller speaks of the dilatation of the pupils after death as due to the absence of blood in the iris blood-vessels, and of the contraction of the pupils in congestion of the brain as due to a filling up of the iris blood-vessels. But these phenomena could be interpreted in a different way. After death the impulses from the nuclei to the various sphincters cease and consequently general relaxation results: the anus, the muscles of the face, the muscular tonus of the entire body are relaxed. Is this general relaxation to be attributed to the exsanguination of the sphincter muscles, or is it rather due to a cessation of nervous impulse to these sphincters? The contraction of the pupils in congestion of the brain is not necessarily due to a congestion of the eyes, and the filling up of the blood-vessels of the iris. It is rather due to a state of irritation or excitation, either of the nerve in its course, or of the nucleus of the motor nerve. Dr. Koller's conception of the question of vaso-constriction by mydriatics and vasodilatation by miotics needs a great deal of corroboration before it could be accepted. So far the pharmacologic data do not agree with his views. For instance, if you perfuse the intestinal loop of a cat with a solution containing very small amounts of eserin, a very marked vasoconstriction will result. The opposite thing happens if we use atropin. If we perfuse lung tissue, which, as it is well known, does not contain vasomotors, with a very weak solution of eserin, we see the blood-vessels contract. It seems to me that Dr. Koller lays most stress upon the supposed vasodilating action of eserin on the iris, and does not mention the well-established fact that eserin has a direct action on the nerve-endings in the iris sphincter. Enucleate an eye of an animal, let it stand until you consider that there is no more blood in the blood-vessels of the iris, and put this eye into a very weak solution of eserin—the pupil will promptly contract. This action does not look as if the eserin has acted on the blood-vessels, but it seems to me to show that the eserin has acted upon the nerve-endings. We could go on to a number of other points mentioned in Dr. Koller's paper. For instance, the question of dionin. Is the contraction of the pupil after an application of dionin due to the hyperemia of the iris or to the pain? A foreign body of the cornea, or any superficial painful lesion of the cornea, will contract the pupil. Further work is necessary before it can be definitely stated what does contract the pupil after an application of dionin. Does dionin contract a pupil if the cornea is made completely anesthetic by using holocain previous to the application of dionin?

DR. C. F. CLARK, Columbus, Ohio: I would like to see this physiologic discussion diverted for a moment to the practical phases of the use of mydriatics in iritis and cyclitis. I think many of you have had experience similar to my own. Sometimes you will have a case of uveitis or cyclitis in which you find glaucoma as a marked symptom. My experience was, in my earlier years of practice, to avoid as far as possible the use of a mydriatic in such cases. I found later, however, that I was often forced to abandon eserin or pilocarpin and come to the use of atropin. Just when should we do this? By what means can we determine early in a case just when we should start in on the use of cycloplegics? I think our delay in the use of cycloplegics in the practical treatment of diseases of the ciliary body, iris, and uveal tract, because of a little increased tension, often deters us from using it at the proper time.

DR. KOLLER (closing): I only wish to reply to Dr. Duane's remarks. I did not say that the dilatation of the pupil is solely due to vasoconstriction, another reading of the paper will see that I was careful not to say so.

AFTER-CATARACT.

HENRY SMITH, C.I.E., LT. COL. I.M.S.
London, England.

The subject I propose to bring forward for discussion is the treatment of after-cataract. For the mildest form of after-cataract, needling is generally recognized to be efficient. There are many needling methods advanced, with very little to choose between them. In skilful hands any one of them seems as good as another. It is the more severe forms of after-cataract with which I propose to deal to-day. We are all familiar with the fact that needling is not satisfactory in the case of dense after-cataract. In these cases the iris is considerably tied down to the after-cataract. When an opening is made in them with needles, they have a very great tendency to resent our interference by flaring up with a violent inflammatory reaction. In any case they generally require to be needled several times before a permanent opening is secured. After each needling the opening we make tends to close up again. The inflammatory reaction which is very liable to follow in severe cases often results in the destruction of the eye. Needling in any case (mild or severe) is not the very innocent proceeding which many would have us believe.

In the last decade of the last century and in the early years of the present century needling was regarded as serious an operation as extraction of cataract. The same methods and the same precautions were taken then as are taken now. The trouble, in my opinion, is not due to direct sepsis, there are more evils in the world than sepsis. The more the iris is tied to the after-cataract by inflammatory adhesion, the greater is the inflammatory reaction following needling. The most severe form of after-cataract, according to my observation, follows the extraction of immature cataract by the capsulotomy method and also the needling of the jelly-like type of cataract which we often find in children and growing people. This stringy, jelly-like material does not seem to be absorbed after needling. I have come across cases in children and adults operated on by the above two methods with very dense after-cataracts, with the pupillary margin tied down all round to the after-cataract. These cases had had a long course of after-treatment, and when leaving, had been told that nothing further could be done and that the prospect of vision was hopeless.

Many of them had been operated on by highly skilled operators. These experienced operators had properly come to the conclusion that any needling interference would cause such an inflammatory flare-up as would in a few days utterly destroy the eye. These patients or their people were usually intelligent, and often came from very long distances. The unintelligent would have accepted the verdict that there was nothing more to be done; they were prepared to take risks, as they had no other prospect but to remain blind. In these cases there is always a posterior chamber. I do not interfere with them till all inflammatory reaction has settled down. I put them under the influence of a grain of blue pill four times a day, and continue for a few days after operation, in order to anticipate any further reaction induced by my interference.

I atropinize them heavily before operation. I make a liberal-sized iridectomy incision in the sclerocornea, so as to open up the posterior chamber. I do an iridectomy if one has not been done previously. If one has been done already, my wound is over one of the pillars of the coloboma, so that I can get a piece out of the iris there and thus open up the posterior chamber. I now insert a curved small dissector into the posterior chamber, and separate the iris from the after-cataract all round. This is not a difficult matter, as such adhesions are much less strong than the uninitiated would expect. This interference is associated with free bleeding from the iris which must be squeezed out repeatedly until it has ceased. It will now be observed that the atropin previously instilled has dilated the pupil; at this stage insert a good iris forceps to below the equator, allow the points to dilate widely, and press them into the after-cataract and fetch the whole after-cataract out with the forceps. If any pain follows within the next few days, I apply half a dozen leeches to the temples. There is no proceeding in surgery with which I am more satisfied than this one, and none more surprising to the patient. The results are eminently satisfactory; the pupil is again mobile, and the vision good. There was no one more astonished than myself in my first cases to see that this intervention was associated with little or no inflammatory reaction. In my opinion, in the relatively milder types of after-cataract the same proceeding should be adopted. The attachments of the iris to the after-cataract, if not released, as in the needling methods, are the cause of the inflammatory flare-up which is often so destructive.

DISCUSSION.

DR. W. E. LAMBERT, New York: While agreeing in a general way with what Colonel Smith has said, we all recognize the fact that the treatment of any secondary cataract is not such a simple proceeding as is generally considered. In my experience the use of the Ziegler knife in the simple membranous secondary cataracts has been very satisfactory, and it is a knife with which you can readily cut. In the types of dense after-cataracts, I agree that they are not suited for this method. We have been in the habit of using the de Wecker scissors, and the method Colonel Smith describes, of removing these dense after-cataracts, has been our practice for a number of years. Dr. Hunter, formerly one of our surgeons, devised a very unique little instrument called a duck-bill forceps, which I have found very useful in detaching cataracts from the iris. They seem most practical in getting a firm grip on these dense cataracts and extracting them in toto.

DR. BURTON CHANCE, Philadelphia: When Colonel Smith visited the Wills Hospital I asked him when he needled, early or late? I believe that he told me he did not disturb after-cataract for a long time. It has been the habit and custom at the Wills Hospital commonly to needle after the extraction of cataract before the patient is discharged. We use, frequently, a knife-needle which cuts but does not tear; and we do not hesitate to puncture deeply, making V-shaped cuts, in the manner described by Dr. Ziegler, always without reaction; indeed, at the end of three or four days the patient can be discharged. As to the use of that knife in congenital cataracts, some of us do not hesitate to go straight through both anterior and posterior surfaces of the lens, which very promptly causes a dissolution of the lens, and, in comparison to old methods, in an incredibly short time there is a perfectly clear pupil. In the dense adhesions of the iris to the capsule a similar bold thrust and cut through the membranes gives rise to a perfectly clear line of wound, which causes a separation, and is followed without recurrence of inflammatory reaction other than that which naturally occurs after puncture of the membranes. There is complete quieting of the eye and never, in my own experience and observation, septic infection afterward.

DR. T. B. HOLLOWAY, Philadelphia: I merely want to say that what Dr. Chance said about the Wills Hospital does not apply to my own clinic.

DR. G. E. DE SCHWEINITZ, Philadelphia: Ziegler's modification of the Hays' knife needle is an instrument which does not tear, but which cuts, as Colonel Smith desires a knife shall cut. With it even in dense, so-called after-cataract, not only where the iris is plastered to thickened material behind it, but also where the iris is not so plastered, it is quite possible to make very satisfactory openings. I quite agree, of course, that there are a few types of dense after-cataract in which this knife is not as useful an instrument as it is in those of lesser density. I served for many years in the Philadelphia General Hospital, where the ocular flotsam and jetsam of Philadelphia floats, and where you find in large numbers what the late Dr. Herman Knapp called "the end-results of uncured cases." There I naturally tried a great many operative procedures, among them the method to which Dr. Lambert referred. I only speak of this because Colonel Smith refers to the fact that, although the procedure appears to have a rough technic, and a good deal of manipulative effort is required, the results are extremely good. That is true in many cases, but, because anything Colonel Smith says comes with such weight of authority, I think it is not improper for me to refer to the fact that the extraction of thickened after-cataract is sometimes followed by disaster, to wit: detachment of the retina. This I have seen twice, and in consultation with colleagues in my own city. Therefore, as a note of warning, I am stating that it is not an operation which is devoid of danger. So far as my own experience is concerned, while it is not to be compared with Colonel Smith's, a large number of cases have come under my observation, and I have never seen a detachment of the retina after the Ziegler operation, nor secondary glaucoma, as in the old-fashioned needling.

DR. EDWARD JACKSON, Denver, Col.: I think that the attention drawn to some facts referred to in Colonel Smith's remarks is by no means unneeded. Certainly often a needling has not been a cutting operation. The late Herman Knapp emphasized that. But I believe that we can cut

with the rather long-bladed needle like the Hayes or Ziegler
needle. We can all try this experiment with the Graefe
knife; make puncture and counterpuncture, and if you try
to cut, without forward or back movement, you will encounter great resistance. It is scarcely a cutting operation.
But, if at the same time the knife is pressed against its edge,
it is pushed forward or back, it becomes a very perfect
cutting instrument. The instant the point of the knife-
needle touches the membrane,—and it should touch it at
the particular location best suited for it,—the needle is
pressed against the membrane and at the same time is
pushed forward, and then drawn back. You thus get a
clean cut with it, even on pretty tough membranes.

A good deal can be accomplished by carefully studying the
points of attachment of the membrane to the iris and the
adhesions, and trying to utilize these points—I am speaking
now of the knife-needle cutting operation—as points of
fixation for the membrane we want to cut, by cutting away
from them. That sometimes requires departure from the
technic Dr. Ziegler laid down in the way of placing our incisions differently.

There is one other point in reference to operation for
after-cataract, that is, the point of entrance into the anterior
chamber. If that is through vascular tissue, I believe the
danger of exogenous infection is slight. Of course, if operation is done on an infected patient, you may have an endogenous infection. I have never had serious inflammation of
the eye from any such operation. I have seen an eye lost
when the entrance was through a clear cornea. The eye did
well for a week, and the surgeon in charge, who was going
away, left it under my supervision. I noticed there was a
little point of infection in the corneal wound, and in a week
or so the eye was lost from that infection. In cases where a
good deal of violence has to be exerted on the eye, puncture
through the limbus with some bleeding into the limbus is a
safe procedure.

DR. JOHN W. BURKE, Washington, D. C.: Colonel Smith
said that he hoped that discussion of this subject would
draw blood, and it will draw blood from me. A case which I
had about a year ago, upon whom a simple extraction had

been done, I performed the operation described by Dr. Lambert. Vision was 20/20, but he had a transverse fibrous band in the pupillary area that made vision extremely poor when the pupil was contracted, as in sunlight or reading. He, being a doctor, realized the risks, but wished to have the capsule removed. The incision was made with a keratome above the band, then the band was grasped with duck-bill forceps, and gently removed. I did not cut any vascular tissue, the manipulation was very gentle, but on examining him after leaving the hospital I found the vitreous was solidly filled with blood. While I have not seen him for nearly a year I understand he has no vision, and I cannot consider the operation as unattended by risks, as Colonel Smith would lead us to believe.

DR. W. H. WILDER, Chicago, Ill.: It seems to me the desirable thing in this operative procedure is to accomplish the result with as little traumatism to the eye as possible, and the Ziegler knife has, in my experience, proved itself a more useful instrument in the simpler class of cases than the Knapp knife-needle. It does not always accomplish the desired result where the after-cataract is of long duration and has become thickened, is more or less parchment-like, and lacks elasticity. It seems to me we must use some other means in such cases.

I am rather surprised that the use of two needles has not been mentioned in the course of the discussion. By the use of two needles we have a method of dividing the capsule which causes less traumatism and dragging on the after-cataract than the operation with a single instrument If one introduces two Knapp needles from opposite sides of the cornea, making the one in the right hand penetrate the membrane a little to the left of the center, while the one in the left hand penetrates a little to the right of the center, by keeping their edges together he can make them act like a pair of small scissors when the handles are made to approach each other. By this means he can make a rent in the center of the membrane that will be further enlarged by spreading the blades with the least possible dragging on the membrane and the ciliary processes, for each little instrument pulls against the other.

However, I think it was the intention of Colonel Smith to direct our attention to a class of cases that are even worse than these, viz., the dense membranous after-cataracts to which the iris is probably adherent. To drag such membranes out of the eye in toto might cause serious hemorrhage or be followed by most severe reaction.

An opening made in such membranes with one or two knife-needles is likely to close up. In a number of such serious cases I have found the following operation useful: A narrow, rather long-bladed keratome is introduced into the anterior chamber at the limbus over the coloboma, and the point of the blade is made to penetrate the membranous cataract at a point corresponding to the lower edge of the pupil and near the edge of the iris. By a slight lateral motion this cut in the membrane can be enlarged from side to side. The knife is then withdrawn. An attempt may then be made to separate the attachments of the iris to the membrane on either side of the coloboma. If this can be done, the next step is made more easily. A small blunt Tyrrell hook is then introduced and made to seize the upper lip of the cut in the membrane. If the instrument is twisted on its axis one-half turn or more, it will secure a firmer hold. By this means the membrane is slowly drawn out of the corneal wound and a considerable piece of it is cut off with iris scissors. Such a procedure would probably cause less traumatism to the eye than attempting to remove the membrane in its entirety.

DR. G. ORAM RING, Philadelphia: The late Dr. Samuel D. Risley repeatedly told me that he regarded many of the operations required upon the posterior capsule, or upon the association of the capsule with the remains of lens substance, as among the most dangerous of our entire ophthalmic operative procedures. Those of us who have been fortunate enough to escape the disasters that sometimes follow in the wake of such operations are, probably, not inclined to view them with anything approaching the same degree of seriousness. The Ziegler modification of the Hays knife, if sharp and used as a pure cutting instrument, will certainly serve us in most of the cases, and for the tougher membranes I am, personally, fond of the de Wecker scissors. Supposing, despite our care, infection is apparent, to what procedure can we resort? Dr. H. F. Hansell, a few weeks ago, called my attention to one of his cases upon which an apparently uncomplicated incision was made upon the capsule under the usual antiseptic precautions. The following day the eye showed a moderate pericorneal flush, and the second day manifested definite evidence of a pronounced infection with pus in the anterior chamber. Dr. Hansell ordered 5000 units of diphtheria antitoxin, and subconjunctival injection of mercury cyanid, 1:10,000. The following day the pus had absolved, and the patient made an uninterrupted recovery, with corrected V. = 10/40.

DR. DORLAND SMITH, Bridgeport, Conn.: I want to add my mite of experience to the discussion of Colonel Smith's paper. While working with Colonel Smith in India in 1912 and in 1914 I saw some beautiful results by this method, even in desperate cases. Dr. Wilder has called our attention to the fact that this is perhaps the only method in some very dense cases. It does seem that there are cases which we can handle satisfactorily in no other way. I also want to confirm Dr. de Schweinitz's observation that the method is not without danger, and to report that I have just lost an eye by this method—an eye, to be sure, which had been through an iridocyclitis and was not in good shape. Nevertheless, the eye was lost from intra-ocular hemorrhage.

DR. EDGAR S. THOMSON, New York: It seems to me that the cases in which you have a dense membrane, are those which have had iritis, most probably due to some metabolic disturbance. In other words, the very case in which it would be desirable to pull out this membrane is the one which at times will least tolerate interference. The late Dr. Agnew, at the Manhattan Eye and Ear Hospital, advocated the hook operation, entangled the membrane, and withdrew it completely. We practised that operation for a long time. The reaction does not always occur, and the end results are so attractive when you get them that you are tempted to use the operation constantly. Every now and then, however, we get severe reactions due to traction on the ciliary body, and I have seen several cases of detachment of the retina and iridocyclitis from this operation. My choice is for the Ziegler knife needle or the de Wecker operation. It seems that the larger incision of the de Wecker operation is not a serious disadvantage.

DR. W. R. PARKER, Detroit, Mich.: I fully agree with the speakers who find that in the Ziegler knife we have a cutting instrument, and who hold that most of the cases of secondary cataracts can be opened satisfactorily by the proper use of this instrument. There is one type of case, however, mentioned by Colonel Smith, that I wish to speak of particularly. That is where you have a dense secondary cataract, with more or less firm attachments of the iris. One of the things I had to learn by experience in cataract work was the lack of dread of these posterior attachments. As a matter of fact, a posterior adhesion of the iris is not a very serious complication in the extraction of the lens. In the same way it is not necessarily a serious complication in cases of extraction of lens remnants. After a corneal incision is made, if you go in with iris replacer and sweep around the iris border, it is often surprising how easily these attachments may be broken.

DR. H. W. WOODRUFF, Joliet, Ill.: I expected to hear something said about a method suggested by Elschnig for the removal of pupillary membranes. He devised this operation for the removal of dense connective tissue, including the iris, when the pupil was more or less closed following traumation of the lens. It is also applicable to some of the worst forms of after-cataract. An incision is made with the cataract knife the same as if one were to make the regular cataract operation. Instead of completing the incision, the knife is withdrawn, leaving a bridge of sclera above, the two incisions being 3 or 4 mm. in length. Through these two openings a triangular piece of the membrane can be cut with the de Wecker scissors and then removed with the capsule forceps.

COLONEL HENRY SMITH (closing): The issue has been raised as to how early after cataract operations it is advisable to needle the after-cataract. My own experience is that to needle the after-cataract when the patient is normally leaving hospital, ten or twelve days after operation, is a very risky proceeding, no matter how mild the cataract may be. I have seen cases of the mildest type needled, and the man lose his eye. Almost inexplicable is the rapidity and violence of the flare-up. My advice would be six weeks at the earliest, and if a violent iridocyclitis has set in, such as the cases we have been talking about, wait until the last appearance of inflammation has subsided. Cases have been referred to me of detachment of the retina and hemorrhage after the proceeding I have advised. Well, in this variety there are cases and cases. There are cases which have had a violent iridocyclitis, an iris the luster of wash-leather, and no vision in the fundus, and if we operate on this class, we may expect anything. If there is no vision in the fundus it does not matter to the patient whether he has a detachment of the retina or not. Patients who have good recognition of light through the iris in after-cataract, such as you expect have a good fundus behind, then I think you will find that in these cases hemorrhages are not at all likely to occur. In regard to the drawing on the blackboard, the procedure looks a much bigger job than doing the original cataract. The incision I make would be sufficient to get in the forceps comfortably. In this case I would make the incision and take a piece out of the iris. The lower part of this after-cataract is not complicated with the original wound. The upper part of it is certain, in a large proportion of cases, to be tied down to the wound. Ziegler is quite right when he cuts across the membrane. It detaches as easily as the normal lens capsule can be expected to detach. You naturally use your common sense and cut off close to the wound, and you will find that there is no unusual violence in carrying out that procedure. When you detach the iris from the after-cataract, it will bleed and bleed very freely. If you squeeze it out carefully I do not think you will see any blood in the anterior chamber in a few days or a week afterward. If you go in and pull out the after-cataract before the bleeding has ceased, you may have some blood in it for some days afterward. I think we are more in harmony as to the dealing with that question than we would appear to be. It seems to me merely a question of the class of cases we are talking about. If we have a good fundus, we need not fear hemorrhage with detachment; if we have an eye which has had a violent iridocyclitis, we may have anything. The case with a healthy looking iris would look a risky case to most men, but it is not so. If the luster of the iris is healthy, there is astonishingly little risk in the proceeding I have advised. If the luster is unhealthy, it is not a proper case for any operation.

INTRACAPSULAR CATARACT EXTRACTION BY TRACTION ALONE.

ALLEN GREENWOOD, M.D.,
Boston, Mass.

A successful and uncomplicated intracapsular cataract extraction has long been the desire and dream of many ophthalmic surgeons. Since Colonel Smith's and his followers' contributions to the subject of intracapsular extraction there has been an increasing effort to perfect such an operation, even by men who have not had the advantage of the training under Colonel Smith. Some of Colonel Smith's students have, themselves, made alterations in his successful method. The principal complication which is likely to occur in attempting the exact procedure of Colonel Smith, and the one which has deterred most ophthalmic surgeons from adopting the method, has been the more than usual danger of a loss of vitreous. There are few ophthalmic surgeons who can view a gush of vitreous from an eye with an open wound with equanimity, and those who claim that moderate loss of vitreous is of very little moment are decidedly in the minority.

Let us consider for a moment the main cause of vitreous prolapse in any cataract operation. Barring out the prolapses due to the intractableness of the patient and those due to unnecessary dragging on the eye by dull knives and unskillfully used fixation forceps, we have left the most potent cause, namely, pressure on the eye exerted by the operator to cause the expulsion of the lens. The greater this pressure, the more the likelihood of a vitreous prolapse. When to the pressure that is ordinarily necessary to cause the expulsion of the lens in cases where the capsule has been previously cut, or the central portion removed, there is added the much greater amount of pressure necessary to break the zonule, then the danger of prolapse is markedly increased. The necessity of the excessive pressure used by Colonel Smith and his followers has prevented the general adoption of his method by any but the very few who have had the rare opportunity of acquiring the marvelous dexterity necessary for this procedure, which must be obtained if one is to perform this intracapsular method with any degree of safety. All those who express the lens in its capsule recommend that a spoon or hook be close at hand to aid in the removal of the lens if vitreous appears before the lens is out, thus acknowledging their unusual expectation of vitreous prolapse.

Shortly before the war the writer, who had tried intracapsular extraction by the pressure method and abandoned it, was favorably impressed with the method of rupturing the zonule with smooth-bladed capsule forceps, and then expressing the lens by the method employed by Knapp. In a few cases this method was tried with fair results, and some experimental work was done on animals' eyes. The war intervened to prevent any further experiences along this line.

Some time after returning to civilian practice the writer obtained a pair of the smooth capsule forceps devised by Dr. Verhoeff, with the intention of attempting to extract the lens, with little or no pressure accompanying its withdrawal, in its capsule by means of the forceps, hoping thus to reduce the danger of prolapse. An added reason for trying this lay in the fact that for some years, in doing extracapsular extractions, it had been the custom of the writer to take out the center of the anterior capsule with toothed capsular forceps. Therefore it was decided to attempt extraction by grasping the capsule near its center, or slightly above, so that if the capsule was torn it would be the central portion that came away. Experience seems to show that when the capsule is thus grasped the zonule can be broken all around more readily than when the capsule is grasped at the lower edge of the lens, and is less likely to tear. The results obtained have been most gratifying, and the first 25 cases form the basis of this preliminary presentation of the subject of intracapsular cataract extraction by traction alone.

The writer has not attempted any withdrawal of the lens in its capsule by traction alone by any other method than the use of the Verhoeff forceps, though the method of Hulen and Barraquer, of holding the lens by suction, seems very attractive when viewed in the light of Barraquer's results. In considering the method of extraction by traction alone as a measure of preventing loss of vitreous, one cannot help being impressed by Barraquer's figures. The ability to operate on 1000 eyes with a loss of vitreous in only 7 can probably be approached by only few operators. Even among those successful ophthalmic surgeons who always use the extracapsular method, such a minimum loss of vitreous is probably unattainable.

The writer has come to believe, from his own limited experience, that extraction of the lens in its capsule, without pressure, will in the future show less vitreous loss than in the common extracapsular method, where some pressure must be used to extrude the lens from its capsule and the eye.

Compared with Barraquer's 1000 cases and the hundreds of thousands of the Indian operators, and the hundreds of many of those who have published lists of cataract extractions, the few here presented are almost as nothing, but one cannot operate on 25 patients by one method without obtaining at least some fixed ideas as to the value of the method employed. The writer wishes to submit at this time his first 25 cases of extraction with the Verhoeff forceps, largely in order to induce, if possible, some of his hearers to give the method, as he employs it, a trial, so that a larger number of cases may in time allow us to come to a decision as to its practicability.

First let me, as briefly and concisely as possible, outline the method employed. The patient to be operated on is, of course, prepared in the usual manner, with careful attention to the patient's general condition and his or her tractability. It is my custom to use 10 per cent. argyrol for several days prior to the extraction and, at the time of the operation, to instil a drop of one-half per cent. atropin with the first drop of 4 per cent. cocain (my cocain solution contains 1:5000 solution of adrenalin). The cocain solution is used twice, at intervals of five minutes, and this is followed by two instillations of 1 per cent. holocain, at intervals of five minutes. The eye is then flushed out with a few drops of 5 per cent. solution of protargol, and the skin surfaces around the eye and those of the lids painted with 2 per cent. iodine. The speculum is then inserted, and careful attention is paid to the position of the speculum, and especially as to whether the assistant can properly hold up the lids away from the eye by its use. This, in my opinion, is one of the most important points in the prevention of blepharospasm and losses of vitreous, and must be found more so if the patient is at all intractable. I always train my assistant to take hold of the speculum in such a manner as to lift the lids away from the eyeball after I have completed my iridectomy, and maintain them so until I am ready to remove the speculum. In some cases it may be necessary to lift as soon as the section is made. The incision is made at the sclerocorneal margin with a keen Graefe knife with two or three movements, and slightly less than one-half of the circumference is included in the incision, which is deeply made, so that practically the entire wound is covered by a conjunctival flap. In the majority of cases it is customary at this stage to pass a suture through the conjunctival flap and then through the conjunctiva, just above the spot where it has been cut. The center of this suture is then drawn into a loop with a strabismus hook and laid to one side. This step in the operation only takes a moment, and is not attended with discomfort or annoyance to the patient. A medium-sized full iridectomy is then performed, and we are ready for the extraction of the lens in its capsule. It is at this stage of the operation that it is especially essential for the assistant to obtain his hold on the speculum and lift the lids away from the globe to be so retained until the operation is finished. The Verhoeff capsule forceps are then inserted into the anterior chamber and the capsule grasped about at its middle, or if anything, a trifle above the center. A gentle motion is then made from side to side, the extent of this movement being about one mm. each side from the center, and then the capsule forceps drawn straight upward. As the forceps begin to emerge from the eye they are pulled slightly forward and tilted forward. In the majority of cases the lens whose capsule has been thus grasped may be withdrawn from the eye without the necessity of the slightest pressure being made. The suture is then tied, if one has been introduced, and the pillars of the iris replaced. One always encounters a little more difficulty in replacing the iris where the vitreous body has come forward than in ordinary extracapsule extractions. The eye is then closed, the lids covered with sterile vaselin, with a considerable quantity placed in the hollow next to the nose. This free use of vaselin takes up any slight unevenness that may exist in the dressing. An ordinary double compress absorbent cotton eye dressing faced with linen cloth is then applied, a knit bandage fastened smoothly over this, and a Ring mask outside of all.

The writer is confident that this method of withdrawal

of the lens can be accomplished in the majority of cataract cases without endangering the integrity of the hyaloid membrane.

A very brief résumé of the results will be given without attempting to give a detailed account of each case. In 25 eyes the attempt to extract in the capsule was made, and in 3 the blades of the forceps slipped on the capsule and could not be made to grasp it. These three were then finished by using the capsulotome and extracting the lens extracapsularly in the usual way. Of the remaining 22 attempts, the capsule was torn in 1 and 21 were extracted in the capsule. In the first few of these 25 cases slight pressure was made to assist the extraction, and in 2 of these there was moderate loss of vitreous. After these two mishaps no pressure was made in any of the others, the traction on the capsule being solely relied upon. It should be stated that in the case where the capsule tore, the tearing occurred across the lower edge of the lens, and the entire capsule came away, leaving the lens to be pressed out. As might be expected, this loose lens was expelled with a minimum of pressure. The visual results so far have been 20/30 or better in all but three. Of these latter two were known to have had previous retinal and choroidal lesions, and one has retraction of the iris and vitreous opacities. The vision equals reading coarse print in one and 20/200 in the other, the poor vision of counting figures at six feet occurring in the patient having the largest vitreous loss. In the three cases where the forceps failed to grasp the capsule it should be noted that this occurred in fully matured cataracts of the sclerosed amber type, where the capsular sac was so thoroughly filled with lens that it put the capsule on a tension, making it extremely difficult to grasp it. Experience has shown that cases where intracapsular extraction by traction alone is best performed consist of the immatures, the posterior polars, and the Morgagnian cataracts. It is probable that there is less advantage to be obtained in attempting this operation where the lens is entirely opaque and there is little likelihood of retention of cortical material.

The principal advantages of extraction in capsule it is not necessary for me to enumerate, they being too well known. There is, however, in the traction alone method, the greatly added advantage that there is a lessened danger of hyaloid rupture and the presence of free vitreous in the anterior chamber. In none of the 21 successful cases was there the slightest evidence of iritis, and the healing was unusually rapid, the average stay in the hospital being eight days.

In view of my experience let me urge those of you who are accustomed to use toothed capsule forceps for removing the center of the anterior capsule to try the smooth-bladed ones, especially on your immature cataracts, and see if you cannot lift the lens out without pressure. If the capsule then tears, you are just where you usually are after using the toothed ones and can proceed accordingly. The above, of course, presupposes that you follow the method of grasping the capsule at its middle or just slightly above.

DISCUSSION.

COLONEL HENRY SMITH, London, England: I congratulate Dr. Greenwood on his success, although the figures are small. On his next 25 cases he may find a number with big soft cataracts in which you lift the capsule in practically every one. I saw de Wecker at work. With the vacuum method you will undoubtedly get a softer grip of the capsule than any forceps will do, and it is possible that you will get out a larger percentage of the lens with it. I agree with Dr. Greenwood that if you can lift them out this way, always providing you have good patients, you should have less escape of vitreous. The Indian method requires probably a little more technical training. This is the great stumbling-block to every operator by this method—the question of control of the eyelids. If the patient is unruly, you will have escape of vitreous and you will have escape of vitreous with de Wecker's method. He must have had a series of good patients to get so little escape of vitreous. I have never come across such patients. I would suggest to those not so familiar with the control of the eyelids that the drawing back of the brow is just as important as lifting forward the lids. A student or a nurse, can be trained in a short time. He may not become perfect. He presses back the brow with two fingers, and enters a single hook fairly close under the eyelid. If you lift the lid forward with the hook you will be able to see the whole fornix. If your assistant is able to show you the whole fornix right around, and to maintain it at that, you will find that you will prevent the escape of vitreous. It is not so much in the manipulation, as in securing control of the patient. An incision of 180° is safe and adequate, although a little less will do. In old cataracts, the pressure at the right place dislodges the lens at once without any force. Your aim is to press the cornea at right angles to the surface of the lens, and maintain it at that. Only sufficient pressure is to be used to rupture the few fibers below. The pressure is grossly exaggerated in the minds of most people. With the big soft cataract, no forceps or suction apparatus will lift out that cataract without lifting a piece out of the front of it. I should think you would average big soft cataracts in about 20 per cent. of the cases. When you have finished with the forceps and with other mechanical measures, I think you will be tempted to go the whole hog and adopt the Indian method to finish the remainder of it.

DR. C. F. CLARK, Columbus, Ohio: Will Dr. Greenwood, in his closing remarks, state how many were mature and how many were immature cataracts?

DR. T. B. HOLLOWAY, Philadelphia: I desire to ask Dr. Greenwood whether the statistics quoted include the first 100 cases or more that were operated by Barraquer. It has been necessary for me to review the literature of the lens, and I do not recall having seen such statistics. I make this inquiry because to the average operator in this country, 100 to 200 cataracts cover a considerable period of time and cannot be ignored.

DR. GREENWOOD (closing): Barraquer distinctly says,

in his report of 1000 cases, that he did not include his first cases until he perfected his instrument. His results on 1000 cases were after he had experimented on a good many cases. I wish to apologize to Colonel Smith and the Society for coming here with just a few cases, but my object was to induce those of you who do not wish to adopt the Indian operation at once, to try first with the smooth forceps on some of these cases. Even if you do tear the center of the capsule it is of no great moment. After it is seen how easily the lens comes out in the capsule and the freedom from iritis, you may pass over from this intracapsular method to that of Colonel Smith.

THE INSERTIONS OF THE OCULAR MUSCLES AS SEEN IN TEXT-BOOKS AND IN THE DISSECTING ROOM.

LUCIEN HOWE, M.D.,
Buffalo, N. Y.

The object of this paper is to call attention to individual variations in the insertions of the extra-ocular muscles.

After the medical student has finished the usual currieulum, and attention is turned to the clinical aspects of medicine, if he is attracted to ophthalmology, naturally he begins with the usual text-books. There he finds the classic descriptions of the insertions of the different muscles. These recall to his mind a part of what he once saw, although the remembrance of dissections had already grown dim.

The fact is that the descriptions of the insertions of the ocular muscles in the ordinary text-books are too short and too imperfect to give the details necessary for accurate thought or satisfactory work. When using the scalpel and scissors, the insertion of each ocular muscle can properly be divided into two parts, the primary and secondary.

The primary insertion is that part of the muscle which is distinctly a firm and well-recognized tendon. The secondary insertion, or rather insertions, consists of those fibres of connective tissues which pass from the muscle and its coverings to the globe or to adjacent tissues. Naturally we begin by studying the primary insertion of the different muscles, and we will find that although the descriptions given in the text-books do correspond fairly well with the average insertion of a given muscle, on the other hand, what we shall also see is that there are nearly always very decided variations from that average, both in the position of the insertion and in the line or arc which the insertion makes on the globe. Several years ago, when making a series of dissections of the ocular muscles, I measured the position, direction, and length of the primary insertions on a considerable number of eyes. It was not possible to find in the anatomies any method of making those measurements. While it was easy enough to use the edge of the cornea (when that was well marked) as one base line and measure backward to the edges of the tendon of each rectus, on the other hand, it was not so easy to determine what we call the equator of the eye.

Even after measuring to the position where that should be, one could not mark the equator well with ink or with any kind of pencil. The most practical way was to slip on to the globe a narrow rubber band just long enough to hold itself tightly in one position. That simple device made it possible to verify measurements from the cornea backward with other measurements from this rubber band forward. Also the band around the equator gave a base line from which to measure the position backward to the edges and exact positions of the divided tendons of the superior and the inferior oblique muscles. One great advantage of thus representing the equator of the globe (a great circle) by a rubber band and the junction of the cornea with the sclerotic (a small circle) is that, by projecting them on a plain surface like a sheet of paper, we can plot the exact position of the insertion of each muscle in any eye. Thus in the accompanying diagram, if the line A represents the junction of the cornea and sclerotic and the line B represents the equator of the eye, then the vertical line I would represent the internal line of a horizontal section. E would be its external line, Vs would be the upper line of a vertical section, and Vi would be the inferior line of the same section. With these lines of latitude and longitude, as it were, we can locate the position of any point on the globe.

Now such measurements have been made accurately upon some 20 odd globes, and 12 of these have been selected for demonstration here. Extreme variations from the average in

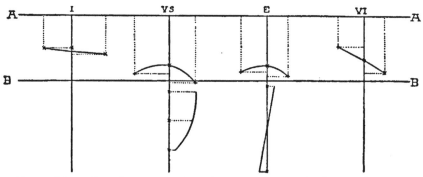

Lines of insertion of one eye plotted to a scale. A A, line of the cornea. B B, line of the equator. I, line where a horizontal plane cuts the inner portion of the globe. E, line where a horizontal plane cuts the external portion of the globe. VS, line where a vertical plane cuts the superior portion of the globe. VI, line where a vertical plane cuts the inferior portion of the globe. From the Muscles of the Eye—Howe, Vol. I, p. 33.

position or length were purposely excluded. Therefore, the groups here shown represent fairly well the principal insertions as distinguished from those which we find as the ideal insertions described in the text-books.

As for the secondary insertions of the ocular muscles, these more or less detached fibers of connective tissue can be easily seen if, after inflating the globe, we suspend it by holding up one of the muscles. We then see bands of glistening tissue stretching from the muscle to the globe. These are the ocular secondary insertions. Or, bending the muscle down on the globe, we see similar fibers of connective tissue stretching off toward adjacent tissue. These are the orbital secondary insertions. Or, still again, if we turn the muscle to one side or the other in the line of its insertion we see similar fibers stretching out to either side. They are the lateral secondary insertions.

These fibers were recognized and described in the more complete anatomies long ago, especially by Hans Virchow. Together, they were called the *adminiculum tendonis*.

It is probable that comparatively few ophthalmologists have ever carefully examined these secondary insertions, but it is certain that practically every one has recognized their existence. For, in making a tenotomy, after the tendon has been divided, the operator, often with a feeling of pride in his skill, and expecting that the former deviating eye will assume its normal position, wipes away the blood, removes the speculum, and directs the patient, perhaps, to sit up and open both eyes wide. But to the disappointment of the surgeon and every onlooker, the eye remains just where it was before the operation. It is possible to see distinctly the edge of the divided tendon, and perhaps the white sclera, but still the position of the eye is not improved. Then, with a suspicion that some fibers may still remain undivided, the surgeon applies more cocain, replaces the speculum, sweeps the hook a trifle deeper through the wound, here and there a little resistance gives way, and at once the globe swings into the desired position. The patient is gratified, and the surgeon remembers, as he did not before, that the ocular muscles have not only a primary, but a number of secondary, insertions.

THE ACTION OF THE OBLIQUES AND THE BEARING OF HEAD-TILTING IN THE DIAGNOSIS OF PARALYSIS.

ALEXANDER DUANE, M.D.,
New York.

The actions of the individual ocular muscles have been defined so clearly by a number of writers that it seems superfluous to restate them. Yet there seems reason for doing so, since some views, contrary to accepted teachings, still maintain currency and have led to what we cannot but regard as erroneous methods of diagnosis and treatment. For example, there is a wide-spread belief that the main function of the obliques is to rotate the eye on its anteroposterior axis. Some, indeed, aver that this is their only function, and others, who admit that these muscles do act to produce vertical and lateral rotation, nevertheless consider their predominant action to be torsion, just as they consider the predominant action of the superior and inferior recti to be elevation and depression.

On the other hand, the accepted and what, I hold, is the correct view, is that the main function of the obliques is elevation and depression and that their effect in producing torsion and lateral rotation is quite subsidiary and is shared equally with the superior and inferior recti. In other words, the superior rectus and inferior oblique are primarily elevators, the inferior rectus and superior oblique are primarily depressors, and in the case of each elevator, as in the case of each depressor, the torsion and lateral action of the rectus equals that of the oblique.

The accompanying diagram (Fig. 1), devised by the author many years ago, elucidates this view in all its ramifications.

In this figure the outer dotted line represents the field of fixation of the right eye projected on a tangent plane. C represents the fixation-point of the eye when in the primary position; D and E, its situation when the eye is abducted 20° and 30° respectively, B and A its position when the eye is adducted 25° and 50°. If the eye is directed toward E and

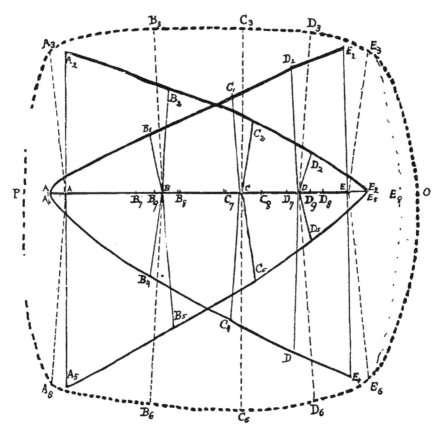

Fig. 1.—Field of fixation of the right eye.

is acted on by the superior rectus alone, it is carried straight up a considerable distance (to E_1). If it is directed toward C (*i. e.*, straight ahead), it is carried up to a less extent and is also carried moderately in (to C_1). So also at B it is carried up to B_1 and at A it is not carried up at all, but is simply adducted (to A_1).

Similarly E_2, C_2, B_2, A_2, represent the excursions that would be effected by the inferior oblique acting alone, and E_3, C_3, B_3, and A_3, the results produced when the two muscles act together. So also A_4, B_4, C_4, D_4, E_4, indicate the downward excursions effected by the inferior rectus, A_5, B_5, C_5, D_5, and E_5 those effected by the superior oblique, and A_6, B_6, C_6, D_6, and E_6, the effects produced by the two muscles acting together, under varying conditions of adduction and abduction.

The diagram also shows the torsion (tilting) action of the respective muscles. That is, at C, the superior rectus tilts the vertical meridian inward, the inferior oblique tilts it outward, and both acting together not only carry the eye straight upward (to C_3), but keep the vertical meridian strictly vertical, *i. e.*, gives it the direction C C_3. In looking up and out (to E_3) the vertical meridian is not affected at all by the superior rectus, which simply draws the eye up, and as it is now acted on strongly by the inferior oblique, it is tilted outward (taking a direction E E_3). Similarly when the eye is directed far up and in (to A_3), the vertical meridian is acted on solely by the superior rectus, which in-tilts it, so that it takes the direction AA_3. So also when the eye is directed down and in, the vertical meridian is out-tilted by the preponderating action of the inferior rectus (vertical meridian takes direction A A_6); and when the eye is directed down and out, the vertical meridian is in-tilted by the preponderating action of the superior oblique, taking the direction EE_6.

Such, then, is the accepted theory. How does this correspond to the facts? In other words, are the actions of the two obliques and of the superior and inferior recti, respectively, in producing torsion and vertical movement, such as are indicated in the diagram?

So far as torsion is concerned, this question is readily answered. The torsion effects indicated in the diagram are precisely those proved to exist by physiologic experiments with after-images. Indeed, they form the basis of what is

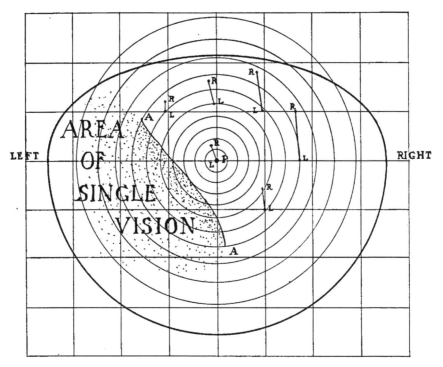

Fig. 2.—Complete traumatic paralysis of right superior rectus; diplopia taken on tangent curtain.

Miss K. S., aged twenty-six. Three tenotomies right superior rectus; last one two years ago. Left hyperphoria in primary position 10△; extorsion in right eye 5°; in left 0°. In looking to right, right eye drops, and if right eye fixes, left flies up. In looking straight up, right eye goes up fairly, and in looking up and left quite well, but in looking up and right lags more and more down. Movements of left eye normal in all directions of the gaze. Diplopia plotted on tangent curtain at 30 inches. R = image of right eye. L = image of left (fixing) eye. The circles indicate 5° intervals.

Note that the diplopia is carried far down into the right lower field, indicating a secondary contracture of the right inferior rectus. Note also that the characteristic feature is that the vertical diplopia increases to the right, so that when the eyes are carried 35° horizontally to the right it is as great as when they are carried 22° up and only 25° to the right. A, A. limits of field of single vision, indicating that diplopia extends 20° to the left of and 25° below the point of fixation P. B, B, limits of field of fixation.

known as Listing's law. In fact, this law is explainable and only explainable on the supposition that the superior and inferior recti have as much effect in tilting the eye as do the obliques.

For demonstration of the fact that the elevating or depressing action of the obliques is in the main equal to that of the superior and inferior recti we must resort to facts derived

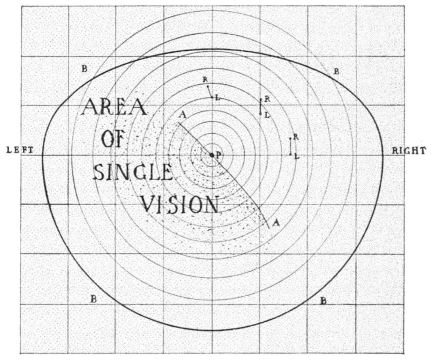

Fig. 3.—Same case six days after tenotomy of the left inferior oblique.

Note the large increase in the area of the field of single vision (A, A, now skirts the point of fixation P). Moreover, the diplopia is not only much less in amount, but now no longer changes rapidly as the eyes move to the right (movements of the eyes more comitant). Left hyperphoria in primary position 5.5△.

from pathology, and particularly from paralysis of the individual ocular muscles. The most convincing facts are those deduced from tests made before and after tenotomy of an elevator or depressor.

In drawing such a comparison we must add that a considerable difference will be noted between tests made immediately after the tenotomy and those made much later. In the later tests, owing apparently to a gradually developing contracture or overaction in the antagonist, there is super-added to the picture of a pure paralysis that of a spasm of the antagonist which may carry the diplopia and deviation far

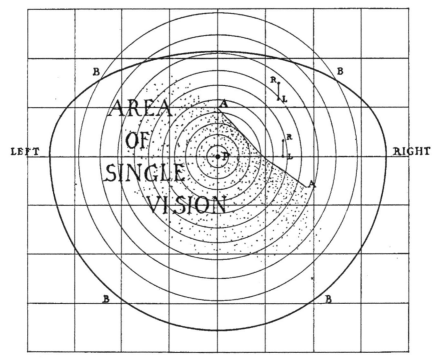

Fig. 4.—Same case four years after tenotomy of left inferior oblique.

Note that field of single vision has considerably increased (A, A, extends now 20° above and 25° to the right of the point of fixation P). Left hyper-phoria between 2° and 3°, as opposed to over twice this amount four years be-fore, and patient comfortable with a 1△ or 2△ prism. This decrease in the amount of range of diplopia due doubtless to secondary contracture of the left superior oblique occurring as a result of the tenotomy of the left inferior oblique.

into the field opposite to that which is characteristic of the paralysis *per se*. This is especially seen in complete paralysis of an elevator or depressor (see Figs. 2 and 4).

In paralysis of the right superior rectus the right eye lags below its fellow, and there is a corresponding vertical devia-

·8

tion and diplopia.   Diplopia and deviation increase *pari passu* as the eyes are carried up, and increase fast as the eyes

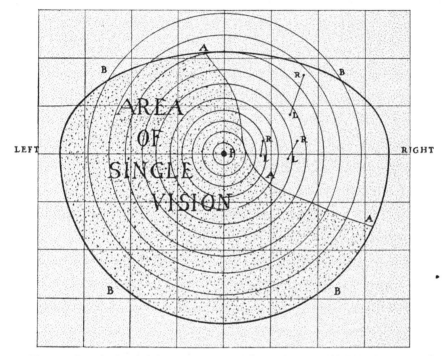

Fig. 5.—Paralysis of right superior rectus.   Relation of double images and limits of the field of single Vision.

Boy of twelve, in whom the condition, except as affected by operation, had remained unchanged during the whole period of observation (four years), and was evidently congenital.   Marked upshoot of the left eye when he looks up and to the right, and corresponding diplopia in the upper right-hand quadrant. L—R, L—R, double images; L, image of left or spasmodically deviating eye; R, image of right or fixing (paretic) eye; A, A, A, limits of the field of single vision, which presents the characteristic quadrantal defect up and to the right; B, B, B, B, limits of normal field of fixation.   Since the left eye is as much above the right as L is below R, we see that when the right eye is directed 45° up and to the right, the left one shoots above it by an amount equivalent probably to 10° or so of arc, and some distance above the normal limits of the field of fixation.   The upshoot of the left eye represents the excessive spasmodic deviation that regularly occurs in the sound eye when the paretic eye is used to fix with.

are carried up and to the right.   In the left upper portion of the field the deviation grows less and less as the eyes are carried toward the left and ultimately becomes nil.   In the lower field it is still present when the eyes are directed down and to the right, but to a greatly diminishing degree, unless marked contracture of the opposing inferior rectus has developed, in which case it may persist far down. With eyes directed down and to the lett, there is no diplopia. The lme bounding the field of single vision runs obliquely from above down and to the right. Theoretically there should be crossed diplopia, since the superior rectus is an adductor and its paralysis should produce divergence. As a matter of fact, the crossed diplopia may be slight or nil. For, as Mauthner pointed out, other conditions (divergence and convergence anomalies) may and often do neutralize the slight lateral diplopia produced. There should be and often is an extorsion (positive declination) of the affected right eye, amounting to from 3° to 4° to 10°.

The above facts are shown very clearly in Figs. 2 and 5.

From what happens when its muscular power is completely deficient we may infer what the superior rectus does when its power is unabated. It is evident, indeed, that it acts strongly to elevate the eye when the latter is in the primary position, and very much more strongly when the eye is abducted. But as the eye is adducted it evidently acts with constantly decreasing power, since the effect of its deficiency becomes less and less manifest. But the eye can be elevated just as fully in adduction as in abduction, indeed, a little more so. There must, then, be some other muscle reinforcing the superior rectus in this position of the gaze in order to effect the complete elevation that is actually obtained. That muscle can only be the inferior oblique, and as the action of this muscle· must be complementary to that of the superior rectus, we infer that it elevates the eye considerably in adduction, much less in the primary position, and little or not at all in abduction (cf. Fig. 1).

We may sum up the matter by saying that the field of action of the right superior rectus, so far as its elevating effect is concerned, is mainly confined to the right upper quadrant, and that of the right inferior oblique to the left upper quadrant of the field of fixation.

If we admit this, it follows that the right superior rectus and the left inferior oblique have a common field of action, namely, the right upper quadrant. In this common field, and elsewhere too, the inferior oblique, as Alfred Graefe long ago pointed out, moves the left eye in precisely the same way and nearly to the same amount that the superior rectus moves the right eye. Each acts to move the eye up, each rotates the eye slightly to the left, each tilts the vertical meridian to the left, and, what is of more importance, the elevating power of each increases as the eyes are carried to the right and decreases as they are carried to the left. So, also, the lateral and torsion actions of both muscles increase as the eyes are carried to the left and decrease as they are carried to the right. In other words, the muscles are complete associates. Similarly it appears that the inferior rectus of one eye and the superior oblique of the other are associates, as, of course, also are the internal rectus of one eye and the external rectus of the other; and each pair of associates has its own peculiar field of action.

This relation may be expressed schematically as follows:

	ASSOCIATES ACTING	
FIELD OF ACTION	Right eye	Left eye
Eyes up and right...............	Sup. rectus	Inf. oblique
	Ext. rectus	Int. rectus
Eyes down and right.	Inf. rectus	Sup. oblique
	Ext. rectus	Int. rectus
Eyes up and left................	Inf. oblique	Sup. rectus
	Int. rectus	Ext. rectus
Eyes down and left...	Sup. oblique	Inf. rectus
	Int. rectus	Ext. rectus

If this conception is correct it follows that—

1. In each of the four fields of action two pairs of associates (one vertical, the other lateral) predominantly act. If all four of these muscles are acting normally, the movements of the two eyes in this special field will be normal and comi-

tant. This will be so, even if the muscles acting in other fields are moderately incompetent, or even paretic. For example, in looking up and to the left, both eyes will move properly if the left superior rectus and left externus and the right inferior oblique and right internus are normal, even though there is a fairly marked paresis of the right superior rectus. That this is so appears from Fig. 5, which is typical of a great number of similar plots of diplopia, which have been made from our cases of paralysis and which confirm the truth of the statement just made. The statement, however, does not hold if a muscle acting in one of the adjoining quadrants is completely paralyzed or paralyzed for so long a time that contractures have developed in its opponent. See below (2).

2. Whenever a muscle is paralyzed, a diplopia and deviation develop which are always increasingly marked as the eyes enter the field of action of that muscle. In cases of incomplete and especially of recent paralysis the deviation is mainly confined to a single quadrant of the field of fixation (Fig. 5). But the field of action of any muscle occupies more than a quadrant of the field of fixation, so that regularly the deviation due to its paralysis extends into the adjoining quadrant also. Thus, as shown in Fig. 1, if the right superior rectus is paralyzed, the right eye, being elevated only by the inferior oblique, will rise to the extent indicated by the line A_2 B_2 C_2 D_2 E_2 and the deviation (difference between B_2 and B_3, C_2 and C_3, and D_2 and D_3), though much more marked in the upper right field, will be still present, though in diminishing degree, when the eyes are directed up and to the left. Furthermore, if the paralysis is old, so that a contracture of the opposing right inferior rectus develops, the diplopia and deviation may be carried well down into the lower right field. How both of these statements correspond to the reality is shown in Fig. 2, which again is typical of the findings in a great number of cases of complete paralyses.

This fact does not invalidate the statement that always the greatest deviation and greatest increase of deviation are found in the quadrant that we have named as the field of action for the affected muscle.

3. If, when the right superior rectus is paralyzed, it is made to fix, a strong secondary deviation is imparted to the left eye, causing it to rise unduly. Since this excessive impulse will be most marked in the field of action of the paralyzed muscle, *i. e.*, in looking up and to the right, it will affect the left eye most when the latter is also directed up and to the right. This is a fact very frequently verified in practice. In such a case, if the right eye fixes, the left will deviate up moderately when the eyes are looking straight up, and little or not at all in looking up and to the left. But as soon as the eyes are directed to the right, and moderately up, the left eye shoots sharply up and in.

4. If the statement we have made regarding the action of the inferior oblique is correct, this upshoot in looking up and to the right must be due to secondary spasm of this muscle. For, while the excessive secondary stimulus is doubtless conveyed equally to both elevators of the left eye, it produces little effect on the superior rectus, since in the direction of the gaze in which this muscle is most efficient (viz., up and to the left), the paretic right superior rectus is not much called into play, so that there is but little deficiency to make up for. On the other hand, in looking up and to the right it is evident that some muscle is acting intensely to elevate the eye. This cannot be the left superior rectus. It must be the left inferior oblique, which here is particularly able to act.

5. If this last statement is correct, then complete abolition of the action of the left inferior oblique should do away with the upshoot and largely compensate for the deviation. This, in fact, is the case. Some fifty tenotomies of the inferior oblique have now been done for paralysis of the

contralateral superior rectus. A typical effect of such a tenotomy is indicated in Fig. 3. Such a tenotomy not only produces the result stated, but shows conclusively what the action of the inferior oblique actually is. This may be stated as follows:

1. In the primary position it acts moderately to elevate the eye. The effect produced by tenotomy varies from 2△ or 3△ to 20△.

2. In adduction it acts as a strong elevator, its effect being measured by many degrees.

3. In abduction of the eye it elevates little and ultimately not at all.

4. Its lateral (abducting) action is very slight.

5. Its torsion (out-tilting) action varies greatly, in many cases seeming nil or negligible. In not more than one or two cases was it so great that a marked effect on torsion was produced by the tenotomy. In any event it is not decidedly greater than that possessed by the superior rectus.

A similar study of paralysis of the inferior rectus and superior oblique shows that the former is specifically the depressor when the eye is abducted, the latter when the eye is adducted; that the lateral action in each case is insignificant and often impossible to make out; and that the torsion may be slight or considerable, but is about as great for the rectus as for the oblique.

Thus we see that both physiologic tests and observations in cases of paralysis, confirm completely the accepted ideas of the function of the ocular muscles, as laid down by the great teachers from Graefe to the present day, and as they are shown in our diagram.

Head-Tilting as a Guide in Diagnosis. I should not perhaps have presented considerations that seem so obvious were it not for the fact that some authors, deservedly esteemed, still regard the torsion defects produced by paralysis of the obliques as the important guides in diagnosis, and in particular regard them as explaining the change in a vertical diplopia produced by tilting of the head toward one shoulder. That is, these authors say that if a vertical diplopia is present, and the images separate or come together according as the head is tilted toward one or the other shoulder, evidence is thereby afforded of a paralysis of one of the obliques. Now, it can readily be proved by applying the laws of projection and also by actual observation in cases of spontaneous diplopia that if we have a lateral or a combined lateral and vertical diplopia produced by deviation of the eyes (not by prisms), any tilting of the head to the right shoulder will depress the right-hand image, no matter whether this belongs to the right eye or the left and no matter to what muscular deficiency the diplopia is due. That is, if the diplopia is crossed such a manœuver will correct a right hyperphoria; if the diplopia is homonymous, it will correct a left hyperphoria. In cases of congenital and many cases of acquired paralysis such an attitude of the head is frequently adopted in order to bring the images on a level. If we examine such cases with the head in the ordinary position, we find a marked vertical deviation; if the patients tilt the head, as they are accustomed to do, this deviation disappears. A vertical diplopia of 30△ to 40△ can be corrected in this way; and in cases ot simple lateral deflection causing simple crossed or homonymous diplopia, a vertical diplopia of this amount can be produced in this way.

Therefore, the alteration in diplopia produced by tilting the head is no conclusive evidence of paralysis of an oblique. Nor is such conclusive evidence furnished by the tilting or the lateral separation of the double images, since the torsion action and the lateral action of the obliques are things that vary greatly and are often difficult to demonstrate. The real conclusive evidence is afforded by the development of a marked and increasing vertical deviation in adduction of the affected eye. In a paralysis of the inferior oblique the affected eye will lag down and there will be a vertical diplopia or a vertical screen deviation as the eye is directed up and in; in a paralysis of the superior oblique, the affected eye will lag up, and there will be a vertical diplopia or a vertical screen deviation increasing as the eye is directed down and in. From these criteria alone the presence and the amount of the paralysis can be sufficiently made out.

DISCUSSION OF PAPERS OF DRS. HOWE AND DUANE.

DR. ALEXANDER DUANE, New York: In considering the intracapsular attachments of the ocular muscles, one fact deserves attention. In specimens that I have dissected the inferior rectus is distinguished by the paucity of its accessory attachments except to its aperture of entrance into Tenon's capsule, and by the shortness of its intracapsular portion (5 mm., as distinguished from 10–12 mm. for the other muscles). This, I think, explains the disagreeable and uncertain results following tenotomy of this muscle. The latter, when divided, can readily retract to a point where it will no longer reattach to the sclera and may even retract beyond the capsule.

We cannot always affirm, from the character of the scleral insertions, the actions of the muscles. Fuchs, for example, from a number of dissections, found relations which would indicate that the external and internal recti would act as elevators or depressors or to produce torsion. Yet observation in cases of paralysis would indicate that this occurs in only extremely few cases, if at all.

Quite interesting are the extracapsular relations. The functional significance of these are not always evident. Thus the levator and the superior oblique are connected behind the eyeball by ascending bands of fascia, and near the trochlea the same muscles are so closely connected as sometimes to be almost fused. The only function that we can attribute to this connection is that of support, the levator in front and the levator and other muscles of the muscular cone behind being suspended in the orbit by these and similar bands.

Another connection, the purpose of which is not very clear, is that between the inferior rectus and inferior oblique, which are sometimes quite intimately fused together. As the muscles cross at right angles the connection does not effect any community of action; and this is also proved by the fact that tenotomy of the inferior. oblique produces no effect on the action of the inferior rectus.

Quite evident is the action of other fascial bands—the check ligaments and the palpebral bands. These serve to limit the free excursions of their respective muscles and also to retract the lids—the upper when the superior rectus is called into play, the lower when the inferior rectus acts. The presence of the palpebral ligaments also explains one difference between an ordinary paralysis of, say, the superior rectus and a paralysis due to a complete tenotomy. In the former case the flaccid muscle fails to exert even the usual traction on the palpebral band, hence the upper lid droops slightly. In the case of a complete tenotomy the muscle retracts and, pulling back the palpebral band with it, lifts the upper lid. In most of the cases of so-called exophthalmos after tenotomy the eyeball is not really prominent, but looks so because owing to retraction of the lid, the eye is wider open than the other.

These check ligaments and palpebral bands; their connections with the orbital fascia and with the canthal ligaments; the orbital septum; and bands running up from the eyeball and from the muscular cone to the levator and the superior oblique, form a series of supports, slight behind, very thick and strong in front, by which the eyeball and the muscles moving it are suspended in the orbit.

Dr. Howe (closing): I hope I have made clear the one point that what we find in the book is not at all what we find in life.

A CASE OF INTERMITTENT EXOPHTHALMOS.

W. GORDON M. BYERS, M.D.,
Montreal, Canada.

Apart from the rarity of the condition, the following case of intermittent exophthalmos seems worthy of recording, because of certain apparently novel clinical findings, and because of the additional light that these findings may throw upon the nature of the disorder.

Mrs. M., aged twenty-one years, consulted me on March 22, 1921, complaining of a sunken condition of the right eye, which bulged on stooping, and of a feeling that the eye would become "dislocated." Her dread of the globe falling out was carried on into the night, for the proptosis also followed lying on the right side, with pain, and the patient was frequently awakened to find the eye protruding as the result of having got into that position. A great deal of sleep had been lost in this way; and, to insure rest, she had tried various expedients with indifferent success—bandaging the eye; starting the night on the right side, and turning to the left just before passing into slumber; bolstering herself up with pillows in different positions, etc.

Mrs. M. complained greatly also of pain in the right temple, aching in character, "as if an abscess were present deep in behind the eye," and extending "like an earache" to the right ear, where it was felt sometimes to the inside of, at others to the outside of, the tragus; of pain over the whole top of the head, making her feel she would like to lift off the calvarium, and causing her often to unloosen her hair, "which she felt a burden;" of the right eye "feeling hot," as if it were reflecting heat onto the face; and of stiffness and tenderness on the right side of the face, in addition to the pain already described. Associated with all this discomfort was an almost constant headache. This was generally frontal

in situation, but it often extended to the whole head.   It
seemed to come from the eye, and made the patient feel
"utterly weary."

The changes in the right eye were first observed in 1915;
and since that time the variations have gradually become
more noticeable. The patient's father has thought that the
eye looked different from birth, and one can fancy that the
globe appears slightly sunken in a photograph taken at the
age of eight; but the evidence is not convincing. In any
case there was no consultation with an oculist until 1915. No
definite connection with trauma could be established.

In the family history the only thing of interest is that the
father has a congenital, raised nevus, about the size of a
large pea, just below the exit of the supra-orbital nerve on
the left side.

The patient is a healthy-looking woman, 5 feet 7 inches in
height, 155 pounds in weight. The right side of the face is
slightly, but definitely, smaller than the left; but apart from
this the general examination is entirely negative. There are
no venous enlargements of any sort in any part of the body,
and there is no orbital bruit.

The right eye (in the upright position) is sunken, showing
15 mm. with Hertel's exophthalmometer, as compared with
22 mm. for the left side; it lies somewhat loose in its socket;
and the palpebral space is slightly wider than on the left
side (22 for the right eye, as compared with 20 mm. for the
left eye). The fold of the upper lid is retracted.

Following stooping, pressure on the jugular, turning the
head to the left or to the right, on throwing the head well
back, and on holding the breath after forced expiration—
the right eye bulges in the way we have come to regard as
characteristic of intermittent exophthalmos. The degree of
proptosis varies with the degree of pressure exerted on the
jugular, and with the different positions in the order given.
Without pushing the effort to the limit, for safety's sake, an
exophthalmos of 25 mm. can easily be produced by pressure
on the internal jugular—a range for the globe of 10 mm.

The direction of the bulging and the rapidity with which it
occurs are nicely shown by the Maddox rod test: At rest
there are a left hyperphoria of 1° and an exophoria of 1°.
Following pressure on the jugular the right eye (as shown by

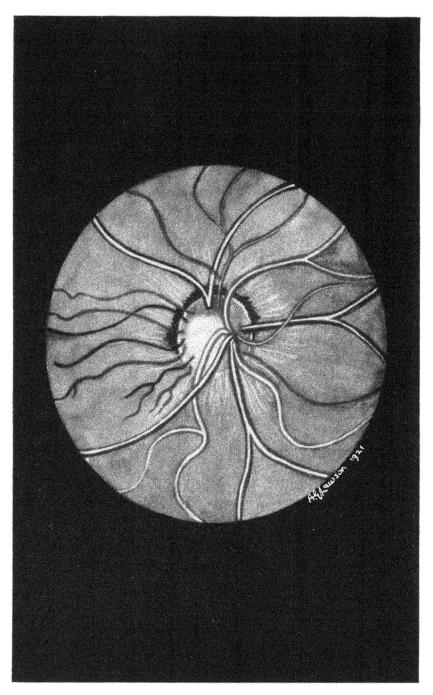

Fig. 1.—Drawing showing the distribution of the retinal vessels over, and in the vicinity of, the right optic disc.

the line of light) immediately begins to deviate upward and to the right, there being a change, with full proptosis, to 2° of right hypophoria, and 2°–3° of exophoria.

There is no limitation in the movements of the globe, and no diplopia in any part of the field (with colored glass and candle), either while the eye is at rest or during proptosis.

Returning to the routine examination of the globes, one notes an entire absence of congestion; the pupils are regular, active, and equal, and the media clear. Ophthalmoscopically, with entirely normal conditions on the left side, one sees the following changes on the right (Fig. 1): The fundus as a whole looks ruddier than normal—is, indeed, markedly congested. This applies especially to the disc, over and around which is a strikingly large number of venules and arterioles. The papilla shows a deep physiologic excavation and a broad band of pigmentation about its upper half. The arrangement of the larger vessels is highly irregular. A number of arteries and veins emerge from the periphery of the disc in the manner of cilioretinal vessels; and very generally the vessels bifurcate over the surface of the disc, instead of at the usual distance. Both veins and arteries, but especially the former, are fuller (larger) than normal; and the early ramifications give one the impression of a marked multiplication. There is, however, an actual increase in the number of vessels, in addition to the vascularization about the disc already mentioned. One has certainly an extramacular vein and artery of small size, and an extramedianal vein and artery of large size. A slight, but quite definite, edema of the circumpapillary nerve-fibers is discernible, as well as distention of the veins (but no pulsation) following pressure on the internal jugular.

The fields of vision are full, and central vision as follows: O.D., with + 2.25 sph. = 6/5; O.S., with + 2.00 sph. = 6/5. No increase in the hypermetropia during proptosis can be made out.

Tension: O.S., 11 mm. Hg; O.D., 8 mm. Hg. The intraocular pressure of the right eye rises 3 to 4 mm. Hg following pressure on the jugular with proptosis.

REMARKS.—The purpose of this paper is met by the statement that the following factors are now generally held to

unite in producing the clinical picture described in this report, and rather inadequately covered by the term intermittent exophthalmos:

1. A varicose condition of the orbital veins of, supposedly,
congenital origin.

2. Pressure on the internal jugular by the surrounding
parts, altered in their relationships by changes in the position of the body.

3. Inadequate collateral drainage, both forward and backward, in the event of blockage of the internal jugular.

The swollen and multiplied vessels in the right fundus of
my case imply a similar condition of the extra-ocular vessels,
i. e., a retro-ocular varix, and the irregular distribution of the
vessels certainly bespeaks a congenital origin. It is conceivable that the arterial overgrowth might be secondary to
heightened venous pressure following blockage; but this
hypothesis is ruled out by the low tension readings in this
case, taken while the proptosis was at its height.

In casting about for a cause of jugular constriction, it
occurred to me that a cervical rib, if present, might act in
this way; and x-ray photographs show, in fact, that a supernumerary rib is present on the side affected, and that it
moves to a certain extent in association with rotation of the
head. Dr. Cheney's notes are as follows:

"Plates were taken of the neck directly anteroposteriorly,
one with the head looking directly forward, and one with the
head looking sharply to the right. From the seventh cervical
vertebra the transverse processes are seen to extend slightly
farther than normal. On the right there is a cervical rib, a
little more than 1¾ inches in length, tapering away from its
vertebral attachment to a sharp point, which seems to rest
upon the upper part of the first rib. When the head is turned
toward the side, right, the space between this rib and the first
dorsal changes its shape and size, showing that, with the
movement of the head, this cervical rib moves."

The rib in this instance is not complete, but it is sufficiently large to account for a certain narrowing of the ring through which the vessels of the neck must pass, as well as for a heightening of the pressure upon the vessels which follow the positions that have been described. There is the possibility also that one may have here a strand of connective tissue passing from the tip of the rib to, or toward, the sternum. Cases of this nature have been described; but, of course, the band would not show on the plate. The chances of constriction, however, under these circumstances would be greatly enhanced; and this would still more apply to those cases in which the rib forms a complete osseous ring.

It is obvious that a supernumerary rib could not be regarded as the sole cause of intermittent exophthalmos; for cervical ribs are of not infrequent occurrence, and no connection has heretofore been established between the two conditions. Moreover, one can tie off both jugular veins without producing proptosis. There must, therefore, be additional factors at work; but if one grant the presence in these patients of an inadequate collateral drainage for the internal jugular, one has in the concomitant occurrence of this condition and of a supernumerary rib a probable cause for the present case, and by inference for a certain percentage of the cases of this type. It is not necessary in these circumstances to assume a congenital weakness of the veins; for venous dilatation would gradually take place as the result of pressure. On the other hand, an unusual arrangement of the vessels, such as one has in the present case, would act as a rare factor in favoring the development of an orbital varix.

The treatment of intermittent exophthalmos is in process of development. Tarsorrhaphy, as recommended by Hippel,[1] is merely palliative; and removal of the enlarged veins, as successfully reported by Löwenstein,[2] may be followed by such

---

[1] Archiv. f. Ophth., V. 95, p. 307.
[2] Klin. Monatsbl. f. Augenh., V. 49, p. 183.

disastrous consequences as to make one loath to carry out the procedure. The question of operation in this case is still under consideration.

In connection with this patient it is of interest to note that since undergoing an operation for a tubal pregnancy about a month after the foregoing report was written, Mrs. M. has been almost entirely free from the generalized headaches of which she complained; and that the proptosis, though still annoying, is not so easily produced or so pronounced as previously. We have here another instance of the influence of the pregnant state upon the vascular system as a whole.

DISCUSSION.

DR. WM. CAMPBELL POSEY, Philadelphia: Noting that Dr. Byers was presenting a paper on this subject, I looked up my notes on a case of the same which I reported before the A. M. A. in 1904, occurring in a young man. The affection, as is usual, was limited to one eye,—the left,—and had first appeared when the patient was but four years old, the eye protruding in stooping and recovering its normal position in the upright posture. Of late the patient had noticed that the eye could be made to protrude by merely holding his breath. No inflammatory symptoms. Finally, the degree of exophthalmos became so marked that there was danger of the eye being dislocated in front of the lids. The moment the strain was relaxed the eye went back into the orbit. No bruit. No change in fundus, except at time of proptosis the vessels became fuller and more cordlike, especially the veins. The condition has been variously known as "exophthalmos a volonte," "alternating enophthalmos, and exophthalmos" and "intermittent exophthalmos."

I was able to find but 39 other cases in the literature. All the monographs had been written by French and German observers. Dupont was the first to give a satisfactory description, in 1865, referring to four cases which had already appeared in the literature. At the time of my report but two cases had been reported by Americans—one by Sattler and another by Gruening. A paper by Hitschmann in 1900 was the best which had appeared up to the time of my report. The proptosis may reach 10 to 15 mm. Lacompte records a case where it actually proptosed between the lids. As in the case I reported, ptosis may appear when the exophthalmos is beginning to be marked and may attain a degree sufficient to cover the upper part of the cornea. The lids become distended and bluish. Any varicosities of the veins of the skin and conjunctiva become filled at the same time with the proptosis of the globe. Normal position, a slight enophthalmos at time of rest. Retinal hemorrhages have been noted by several observers.

A tumor may appear synchronously in the orbit, which may attain in size from a pea to a large bean, and may occupy any portion of the orbit. Some authors have grouped all three types of cases, *i. e.*, those with exophthalmos without a visible tumor, those with exophthalmos and an associated tumor of the orbit, and finally vascular tumors of the orbit without exophthalmos, under the one heading of intermittent exophthalmos; while others have arranged the cases according to the site of the various veins in the orbit. As the genesis of the three classes of cases is the same, and as the presence or absence of exophthalmos or orbital tumor is accidental in any given case, depending on the position of the dilated veins in the orbit, it is impossible to disassociate these groups in describing the disease, though for purposes of classification and description it may be well to do so.

DOUBLE LUXATION OF THE EYEBALLS IN A CASE OF EXOPHTHALMIC GOITER.

WALTER R. PARKER, B.S., M.D.,
Detroit, Michigan.

A. K., male, aged sixty years. German. Patient entered the Ophthalmic Clinic of the University of Michigan January 5, 1921. Family and previous personal histories were negative. The date of the onset of his present disease was indefinite. He had noticed a bulging of his eyes for several months, and had been very nervous at times. Seven weeks before the time of admission to the hospital he had observed a marked increase in the bulging of his eyes, followed by rapid failure of vision, with resulting blindness one week before admission.

9

Up to the time of the marked bulging of his eyes his occupation consisted in lifting bags of coal from a conveyor belt to trucks. The weight of each bag was from 80 to 100 pounds and he lifted about 300 each day.

Examination.—The patient was undernourished and obviously under weight. He had general weakness, tachycardia, tremor, and moist skin. Blood Wassermann, 1 +. X-ray examination, including the sinuses, was negative. Oral examination showed no foci of infection. The medical report was in effect that the patient had all the symptoms of hyperthyroidism. Basal metabolism—first test, 50 per cent. over normal; second test, 76 per cent. over normal.

V.R.E., light perception; L.E., nil. Both eyes were luxated, the lids being partially closed back of the equator of the globe. Ocular movements were present in all directions, though somewhat limited in degree. The lids were flaccid and could be easily separated from the globe. There was present a marked exposure chemosis in the portion of the globe not covered by the lids, and a slight mucopurulent discharge covered both eyes. The entire cornea in each eye was infiltrated and edematous, and a large central ulcer was present in both eyes. The cornea of the left eye had perforated. The exophthalmometer reading was: right eye, 24 mm.; left eye, 23 mm. Bacteriologic examination, staphylococcus albus.

Treatment consisted of rest in bed and high caloric diet. Enucleation of the left eye was advised, but permission was refused by the patient. The ulcers were treated with silver and argyrol. The discharge disappeared in about two weeks, in which time an attempt was made to reduce the proptosis by pressure. The cornea was smeared with vaselin, a rubber protective placed over the eye, and a bandage applied. In six weeks' time the proptosis had improved to such a degree that the lids could be closed over the eyeball. The patient's general condition so improved that after two and one-half months' stay in the hospital he had gained 25 pounds in weight and the proptosis had so diminished the lids could be closed.

Fig. 1 is a reproduction of a photograph of the patient on admission to the hospital, and Fig. 2 shows how he appeared two and one-half months later.

Luxation of the eyeball is of rare occurrence in exophthal-

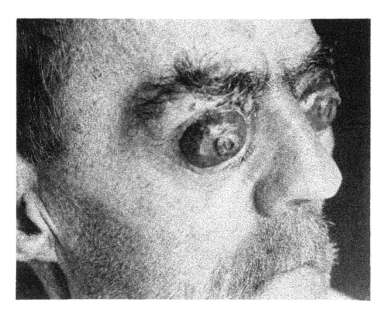

Fig 1.—Patient as he appeared on admission to the hospital.

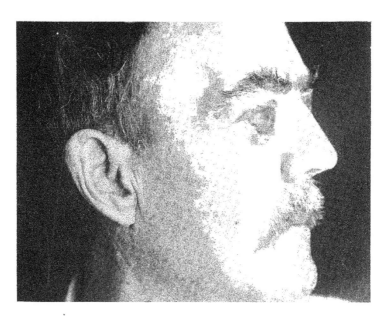

Fig. 2.—Patient as he appeared two and a half months after admission to the hospital.

mic goiter. While it is only an incident in the course of the disease, the treatment must be immediate and drastic or the effect on the vision may be most disastrous.

Our knowledge of the etiology of the cardinal symptoms of exophthalmic goiter is still too indefinite to permit of more than conjecture in regard to the causes of the disease. But, assuming that congestion of the blood-vessels plays a part in the exophthalmos, it may not be unreasonable to suggest that the lifting of 300 80- to 100-pound weights each day, as in the case reported, was one of the contributing factors in the causation of the extreme exophthalmos.

Treatment.—The general treatment of Graves' disease will not be considered at this time.

In regard to the local treatment that may be employed in these rare cases of extreme proptosis, I can merely offer suggestions resulting from the experience in the case reported and from information acquired from a somewhat incomplete review of the literature.

The treatment has included the use of the Buller shield, uniting the conjunctiva over the cornea; tarsorrhaphy alone, or in combination with canthoplasty or slitting the upper and lower lids, or with the removal of a considerable amount of fat from the orbit.

Mr. F. A. Juler* reported a case of purulent keratitis treated by tarsorrhaphy, resections of the cervical sympathetic and x-ray. One eye was lost, but vision of 6/12 was preserved in the other. When the patient, a woman aged thirty-six years, came under observation, there was extreme exophthalmos, hypopyon, and suppurative keratitis in one eye, while in the other the exophthalmos was not so marked and there were no inflammatory symptoms present. The right eye was removed after panophthalmitis developed. The cornea in the left eye became roughened, conjunctiva congested, and movement limited. The external canthus was

* Trans. Oph. Soc. U. K., 1913.

divided, and tarsorrhaphy performed after slitting the lids. The lids separated after the fourth day. One week later the cervical sympathetic was resected, the cornea covered with conjunctiva, and the lids were again united. After ten days the lids again separated. Mattress sutures were then introduced, but they also failed to hold, and the cornea became infected. Later canthotomy was performed and conjunctivoplasty repeated. The lids remained closed ten days, the cornea healed, and no further ulceration occurred. Final vision, 6/12.

Mr. Coulter, in discussing Mr. Juler's paper, reported the history of a case in which one eye was lost. As soon as the second eye showed signs of corneal involvement a tarsorrhaphy was performed and the lids were kept closed for months. Recovery with good vision. In the same discussion Mr. Paton referred to a case in which both eyes were lost in spite of the fact that a tarsorrhaphy was attempted three times. Each time the stitch pulled out. Von Poppen* reported a history in which the exophthalmos was extreme. He divided the outer canthus, but did not do a tarsorrhaphy. Both eyes were lost. Knapp succeeded in preserving the vision by suturing the lids, after making incisions after the manner of Harman. Sattler† referred to 40 cases of corneal involvement in exophthalmic goiter in which both eyes were lost; 9 cases had complete loss of vision in one eye and partial loss in the other; and 14 cases had complete opacity in one eye. While this list is in no way complete in regard to the number of cases reported, it is sufficient to indicate that the salvation of the cornea rests in some form of mechanical protection.

In order that the lids may be more firmly united, two suggestions have been made—one by Mr. Bishop Harman, namely, that in order to relieve the tension on the lids, a wide incision be made through the skin in the upper lid just below

* Deutsch. med. Woch., xxxvi.   † Graefe-Saemisch Handb.

the brow, in the lower lid just above the orbital margin. The raw surfaces present no difficulty, as the skin can be reunited if the expedient is temporary, or grafted, if permanent. Another mode of procedure is suggested by Foster Moore.* He successfully closed the lids in a case of extreme exophthalmos in Graves' disease by first removing a large amount of fat from the orbit through an incision made in the inferior fornix. While this procedure seems somewhat drastic, it appeals to the author as one that might well be employed in this group of serious cases.

DISCUSSION.

DR. H. M. LANGDON, Philadelphia: In 1906 there came to Dr. Morris Lewis' clinic at the Orthopedic Hospital and Infirmary for Nervous Diseases a woman, twenty-eight years of age, who seven years before had developed an exophthalmos which had increased to great proportions; seven months after the exophthalmos had first shown itself the other signs of hyperthyroidism developed. They were, however, rather moderate, tachycardia and slight tremor, but practically no loss of flesh; she was in good health, but the proptosis was about 22 or 23 mm., and was such that the globes had been spontaneously luxated between the lids twelve or thirteen times before she came to the clinic. While being examined by Dr. Lewis the globes came out between lids. There were normal central vision, fields, rotation, and convergence. The fissure was distinctly enlarged, von Graefe's sign was difficult to elicit. It was present about one in three times. She was placed in bed and ordinary rest treatment given. The general symptoms which were already slight, practically disappeared; the proptosis greatly lessened so that she could go about and do ordinary work as long as no luxation occurred. To me it was a mystery why the amelioration of the other symptoms was not accompanied by a lessening of the proptosis, which opens up the question of the reason for proptosis in these cases. It hardly appeals to one that an accumulation of orbital fat will explain all things; we do not have an accumulation of fat elsewhere in a hyperthyroid case, we have exactly the opposite. Why the selective action

* Lancet, 1920.

of the condition for fat of the orbit? It seems more likely to be of a vascular origin with probable formation of fibrous tissue in the orbit from the vascularity which would account for the exophthalmos persisting when all the general signs have disappeared.

DR. CARL FISHER, Los Angeles, Cal.: I think everyone must have given the subject of the possible causes of the exophthalmos in exophthalmic goiter a good deal of thought. The eyeball is held securely by the four recti muscles, and it takes a considerable force to push it so far forward that it is extruded between the lids. It has seemed to me that in these cases we must presuppose a weakening of the recti muscles—probably not as the sole factor, but as an important factor. I have seen sections of the recti muscles from eyes removed in cases of goiter. The condition found was a true parenchymatous degencration—not a simple atrophy. It is also true that the orbits in such cases are brimming with fat, whether secondarily or primarily I do not know. An exhaustive monograph by one of Landström's pupils has shown clearly that the Mueller-Landström unstriped muscle complex cannot produce more than a slight exophthalmos; from its insertions this is mechanically impossible, even if the unstriped muscles were strong enough to counterbalance the force of the recti.

DR. PARKER (closing): In looking over the records of published cases I find, with one or two exceptions, the eyes showing extreme proptosis were lost through suppurative processes, and after having experience of this one case I am struck forcibly by the comparatively simple procedure of dissecting out enough fat to let the eye go back before tarsorrhaphy is performed. Occasionally in health an eyeball can be luxated anteriorly by simply separating the lids. I had one such case under my observation, and another one which Dr. Cross has kindly sent me is shown in which the globe could be luxated and returned with ease. If a patient of this type, where the tissues are relaxed, were to develop an exophthalmos, it would seem not at all improbable that this condition might contribute to a more extreme exophthalmos than is seen in the average case.

LOSS OF VISION FROM SYMPATHETIC INFLAMMATION WITH RECOVERY FOLLOWING THE USE OF TUBERCULIN.

HARRY FRIEDENWALD, M.D.,
Baltimore, Md.

The diagnosis of sympathetic ophthalmia is ordinarily not very difficult. A penetrating injury of the eyeball, a rather characteristic inflammation of the eyeball, followed by an equally characteristic disease of the fellow eye, leaves little room for doubt as to the diagnosis of the affection of the second eye or its course. But all cases are not so clearly cut and we must agree with Schirmer[1] that an absolutely certain diagnosis of sympathetic ophthalmia is not possible, because conditions quite similar result from other causes. Schirmer points out that the correctness of the diagnosis is the more probable, the more it meets the following conditions: First, the first eye must present a uveitis of ectogenetic origin; second, the interval must be at least fourteen days; third, the second eye must show uveal disease involving all portions usually with profuse fibrinous exudate, with tendency to recurrences; though, much more rarely, it may also take the form of papilloretinitis; fourth, the general examination must show that there are no other causes of the affection.

Most prominent among the conditions with which sympathetic ophthalmia may be confounded is tuberculosis. There is marked similarity in the clinical course of the affections; and the histologic changes bear sufficient analogy to make the differential diagnosis very difficult.[2] Von Hippel has presented the pertinent question recently: Can the differen-

135

tial diagnosis between tuberculous and sympathetic uveitis be made with certainty upon the histologic findings alone, and without the knowledge of the clinical history, and his answer is that it cannot.

The case to be reported will show how difficult the diagnosis may become.

Miss K., of Penna., aged sixteen years, was brought to me for examination on December 3, 1918. Her physician informed me that she had had a definite Neisser infection of the vagina and that this had been followed by infection of the left eye. This eye became very severely inflamed on August 10th. She was taken to a local oculist who treated her for some time, when the inflammation disappeared, leaving a corneal scar, with iris adherent. The sight of the eye was greatly damaged. The right eye retained good vision until the last week of November, when it became so reduced that the patient was unable to read. She was obliged to leave school for this reason about December 1st.

The examination of the patient showed the following condition: Left eye: Slight congestion; a number of blood-vessels run over to the cornea; a small ectatic area at the inner margin, to which the previously prolapsed iris is adherent; several other scars, one in the inner and a small one in the outer part of the cornea; the remainder of the cornea was clearer but studded with deposits on membrane of Descemet. The iris showed marked congestion with bulging forward in the upper outer portion.

Right eye: There was more marked congestion than in the left eye. The cornea was studded with deposits on the membrane of Descemet. The surface of the iris was very irregular, showing bulging areas and depressions. V.L.E., movements of hand at 6 to 8 feet and fingers counted at 3 feet. V.R.E., 20/152, slightly improved with concave glasses. Tension R.E., normal, minus; tension L.E., normal, minus. Pupil of R.E., widely dilated, 6 to 6.5 mm.; pupil of L.E., 3 mm. and drawn over to nasal side. The patient was admitted into the Baltimore Eye, Ear and Throat Hospital and a general examination was made. It was found that she no longer had any vaginal discharge. A blood Wassermann proved negative. A von Pirquet was likewise negative. The urine contained neither albumin nor sugar.

The diagnosis made was sympathetic ophthalmia of the right eye, following a perforating ulcer of the left eye with prolapse of the iris, due to a gonococcic infection. The treatment was accordingly: atropin, 1 per cent., instilled into both eyes three times daily; salicylate of soda, together with bicarbonate of soda, each, 10 grains, three times daily. The patient was placed in a darkened room. On January 1st, vision in the right eye was recorded as 20/200. On January 2d and 3d, the same. On January 4th, 15/200. The sight slowly but definitely decreased from day to day. On January 13th the patient complained of the constant appearance of a flickering light before the right eye and was able to distinguish fingers at three feet with this eye, with the left at five feet. On January 23d I left the city, and my associate, Dr. Jesse W. Downey, assumed charge of the case. In spite of continued treatment, the vision became so poor that she soon had to be led about.* Having been practically blind for a number of weeks, on February 12th she was given 1/1000 mgm. of tuberculin (TR), although nothing had developed to suggest the diagnosis of tuberculosis. February 18th, 1/500 mgm.; similar amounts were given every third or fourth day until March 8th, when she left the hospital for her home. She was still unable to walk upon the street alone, but her sight had improved and after her return home, it kept improving steadily.

On my return to Baltimore I again saw the patient on August 10th. She had been coming to the city for tuberculin injection every week during April and May, every second week in June and July. The steady improvement of vision is shown in the following records:

April 9, 1919: V.R.E., 20/48; L.E., 20/121.
April 14th: R.E., 20/48; L.E., 20/96.
May 2d: R.E., 20/30; L.E., 20/121.
May 9th: R.E., 20/30; L.E., 20/96.
May 15th: R.E., 20/30; L.E., 20/152.
May 23d the ophthalmoscopic image had cleared suffi-

---

* The treatment mentioned was continued until March 8, 1919. She bore it without discomfort.

ciently to get a very definite view of the right disc, and the vision was—
    R.E., 20/19 partly; L.E., 20/121.
    June 20th: R.E., 20/24; L.E., 20/96.
    July 11th: R.E., 20/19; L.E., 20/96.
    September 9th: R.E., 20/19 partly; L.E., 20/192.
    October 15th: R.E., 20/24; L.E., 20/152.
    October 29th: R.E., 20/19; L.E., 20/152.

The tuberculin injections were continued with some irregularity about every week or two until the middle of January, 1920, when they were finally discontinued because there was no further improvement. The changes which occurred in the appearance of the eye were noted frequently. From these notes I shall take only the following excerpts: On January 29, 1920, the status was as follows: Right eye: There are still some deposits on the membrane of Descemet, though not as marked as in the past. The right pupil is about 6 mm. in diameter. (It is to be noted that no atropin had been used since the past July.) The right disc is fairly clear, not sharply outlined, but of very good color. The blood-vessels are somewhat tortuous. There is a stippling of pigment in the macula. In the periphery there are little white spots of choroiditis without pigment. They are seen throughout the periphery in all directions. The vitreous is fairly clear; there are dust-like opacities in the anterior portion of the vitreous.

The left eye shows the adherent leukoma near the inner margin of the cornea; the pupil is bound down firmly and is about 3 mm. in diameter. It is not possible to obtain the picture of the fundus. On May 7, 1920, the irregular arrangement of pigment in the macular region is seen much more clearly, as are likewise the peripheral patches of choroiditis, which are especially marked in the lower part of the fundus of the right eye. The left eye now gives a clear reflex, but no ophthalmoscopic details can be made out. The right cornea still presents a few large opacities in the center on the inner surface; the finer ones are slowly disappearing. The patient's vision is considerably improved with weak concave spheres. With −1.75 sph. V.R.E., 20/19; L.E., 20/192.

December 16, 1920, the right eye shows an absence of all inflammation, but there are about a dozen well-defined but small deposits on Descemet's membrane; the pupil is round and moderately dilated; the iris has become smoother. The left eye shows a fairly clear cornea, no deposits on Descemet's membrane; the entire pupillary area is covered with a thin layer of membrane; the pupil is not dilated and is somewhat irregular, with the iris completely bound down.

Under the circumstances of such remarkable recovery of vision following the treatment with tuberculin the question had again arisen as to the character of the inflammation. For this reason the patient was again referred to Dr. Harvey G. Beck, who made a complete clinical examination during December, 1919.

The report on the examination was that there were no definite clinical evidences of pulmonary or gland tuberculosis. (The pelvic organs showed chronic endometritis with salpingitis.) On January 24, 1920, an intracutaneous injection (1/10 of 1 c.c. of a 1:1000 dilution) of tuberculin (TR) was given. Twenty-four hours later there were redness and swelling at the seat of the injection, and this reaction increased during the following twenty-four hours. The body temperature did not rise during this period. It is interesting to note that the patient's temperature during January and February, 1919, when it was carefully recorded, morning and evening, showed occasional slight rises up to 99°. Dr. Louis Hamman, whose opinion was sought, regarded the patient, in view of the recent positive reaction to tuberculin, as "showing definitely some tuberculous infection, although it does not follow that the eye trouble is tuberculous. However, it makes the diagnosis of tuberculosis of the eye altogether reasonable, if the other clinical data points in the same direction." It would, however, be rash to accept the diagnosis of tuberculous uveitis upon this evidence and to discard that of sympathetic origin. A large number of cases of sympathetic inflammation are recorded as following gonorrheal conjunctivitis with perforating corneal ulcers.[3] The mode of onset, the interval between the affection of the first and the second eye, the low-grade uveitis, and the course leading to almost complete blindness, are quite in accord with the diagnosis of sympathetic inflammation. But I am the more reluctant to reject this diagnosis because we find a few other cases reported in recent literature in which tuberculin treatment likewise gave very remarkable results in sympathetic inflammation.

Bernheimer,[4] in 1912, published the history of a girl, aged nine years, with perforating injury and prolapse of iris of the left eye, followed five weeks later by unquestionable sympathetic inflammation of the right. Enucleation. Vision reduced to counting fingers at 1.5 m. Tuberculin injections were followed by gradual and permanent restoration of vision to 6/12. Bernheimer ascribes the curative value of tuberculin in cases of definite sympathetic inflammation, "with latent tuberculosis," not to a specific immunizing effect, but to the production of non-specific forces, and especially to increased phagocytosis, which tend to bring about the subsidence of the non-tuberculous ocular inflammation.*

In the same year Zirm[5] reported the history of a girl, aged sixteen years, who was operated upon for old traumatic cataract. Twenty-five days later sympathetic inflammation followed, which reduced vision to counting fingers at

---

* We are reminded that Berneaud has reported similar beneficial effect in sympathetic inflammation from |the parenteral injection of milk (Klin. M. f. Augenh., vol. lxi, p. 319).

1 m. Positive von Pirquet. Tuberculin treatment restored vision in two months to 5/20.

Stoewer,[6] in 1913, published two case histories: Male, aged twenty-one years, corneal injury with adherent iris, followed eight months later by sympathetic inflammation. After five weeks' treatment vision reduced to 1/60, when tuberculin treatment was begun, with restoration of vision to 4/50. Female, aged fifty-six years, sympathetic inflammation after operation for cataract, with recovery of vision of 4/12 following tuberculin treatment.

Berneaud,[7] in 1914, reported having had favorable results from tuberculin and salvarsan (but only then when injections were followed by rise of temperature).

Norman,[8] in 1915, cited the history of a girl aged four years; one eye lost by perforating ulcer of cornea; two months later the other eye developed sympathetic inflammation. First eye enucleated. In spite of vigorous treatment, including salicylates and mercury, the eye seemed doomed. Tuberculin treatment was begun, with gradual return of vision to 6/10, 8/10 doubtfully. No von Pirquet made, but enlarged cervical glands.

Kraupa,[9] in 1919, referred to a soldier whose left eye was severely injured. Exenteration on the eighteenth day. Sympathetic inflammation began two days later. Tuberculin treatment resulted in a complete cure.

The cases just cited, together with the experience of his own, leads the writer to conclude that the case he has reported may very properly be classified among the cases of sympathetic inflammation. He inclines to the view expressed by Bernheimer that the curative effect of the tuberculin treatment in some way depends upon the presence of latent tuberculosis, which has been demonstrated in most of the cases reported. These cases serve to emphasize again the marked similarity between tuberculous and sympathetic uveitis.

REFERENCES.

1. Schirmer: Graefe-Saemisch Handbuch, 2d Ed., vi, pt. 2, p. 130.
2. Arch. f. Ophth., xcii, p. 421.
3. Schirmer: Graefe-Saemisch Handbuch, 2d Ed., p. 61. Deutschmann: Ophthalmia migratoria, p. 89.
4. Bernheimer: Arch. f. Augenh., 1912, lxx, p. 5.
5. Zirm: Arch. f. Augenh., 1912, lxvi, p. 314.
6. Stoewer: Arch. f. Augenh., 1913, lxxiii, p. 155.
7. Berneaud: Münch. med. Woch., 1914, lxii, pt. 2, No. 29, p. 1650.
8. Norman: Ophthalmoscope, 1915, xiii, p. 179.
9. Kraupa: Zeits. f. Augenh., 1919, xlii, p. 112.

DISCUSSION.

DR. E. V. L. BROWN, Chicago, Ill.: Dr. Friedenwald's remarks bring to mind a case of my own in which the sympathetic nature of the trouble did not become evident for nine or ten months. The iris of the primary eye was then markedly tumified, and sections from the removed eye showed the changes characteristic of sympathetic disease. In this case both active syphilis and active tuberculosis, with positive lung findings and subcutaneous tuberculin reaction, were present; and, in addition, chronic gonococcal infection and abscesses in the tonsils and about the roots of teeth. A trephine for glaucoma secondary to iritis had been done the year before. When it came time to replace the conjunctival flap, the nurse had handed the operator a spatula taken out of a solution of carbolic and not well rinsed; when brought in contact with the conjunctiva, the flap turned white and shriveled to a size barely adequate to cover the trephine opening. Healing was uneventful. The fellow eye recovered 20/130 vision.

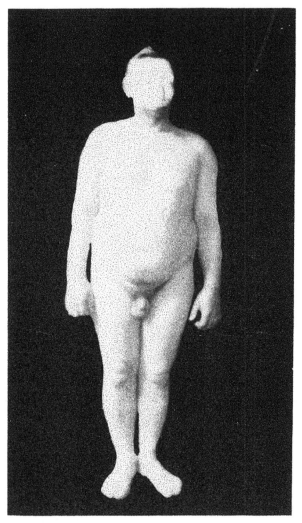

Illustrating short, heavy set, endocrine type.

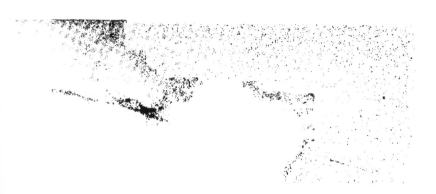

LOSS OF VISION IN ONE EYE RESTORED BY PITUITARY FEEDING IN A CASE OF COMPENSATORY PITUITARY HYPERTROPHY.

EDWARD STIEREN, M.D.,
Pittsburgh, Pa.

A preliminary report of this case was made to the Pittsburgh Ophthalmological Society December 6, 1920, and was published as a part of the Transactions in the American Journal of Ophthalmology, March, 1921.

At the time of the report the patient had been taking pituitary substance for about six weeks, the marked benefit in his general symptoms accompanied by an improvement in his field of vision being emphasized at that time.

Under continued exhibition of pituitary substance, central vision in the blind eye has been restored to normal, and interesting changes in the fields of both eyes have been noted.

The preliminary report is as follows: Male, aged forty years; printer. The right eye had gradually become blind in the past six months. In addition he complained of deep-seated pain in the right temporal and frontal regions, some loss of memory, and loss of sexual power.

When first seen, October 11, 1920, the pupils were normal in size and reaction; tension of each eye, 26 mm. (McLean). V.R.E., 1/40; L.E., 6/6—, with −1.00 sph. The corneæ, lenses, and media were clear. The temporal half of the right optic nerve was pale, and there was a narrow pigmented crescent at the temporal edge of the disc. The left nerve-head was normal. No nystagmus. Perimetric examination disclosed a complete temporal hemianopsia in the right eye; the field of the left was normal for form and colors.

Neurologic examination by Dr. W. H. Mayèr: Arm, abdominal, cremasteric, and patellar reflexes are present and normal. There is no Babinski. No evidence of any cranial nerve palsy nor any muscular twitching or tremor. His physical development is good, with a rather undue prominence of features, a definite thickness of his fingers, with a tendency toward the trident hand. He is short and heavy set, and has the straight lumbar spine so often noted in endocrine conditions. The thickness of the bone-shafts appears unusually heavy, both to palpation and x-ray examination, while the epiphyses are normal. There is a ring of fatty distribution in the abdomen above the umbilicus (Marie's sign). The gonads are well developed and show no abnormality. X-ray of the head shows a definite thinning of the floor of the sella; the anterior and posterior clinoid processes are indefinite and appear eroded.

Laboratory examination: Blood and spinal Wassermann negative; urine negative; blood count: hemoglobin, 95 per cent.; R.B.C., 5,000,000; W.B.C., 8,000; polynuclears, 49 per cent.; mononuclears, 26.5 per cent. The blood-sugar is within the normal point. The sugar tolerance test shows the patient to be able to ingest 500 gm. of glucose without functional glycosuria. Blood-pressure: systolic, 118 mm.; diastolic, 82.

From the above, a diagnosis of enlargement of the pituitary was made.

Following the observation of Timme that a hypertrophy of the pituitary occurs in a pluriglandular syndrome, and that the characteristic disturbances are due to an inability of the normal pituitary to combat antagonistic secretions elsewhere in the chromaffin and interrenal systems, it was decided to administer pituitary gland substance.

This was given as a test in the hope of relieving the overtaxed pituitary and ultimately permitting it to recede to nearer normal size. Whole pituitary gland, 8 grains every twenty-four hours, was begun October 21, and continued without interruption until December 6, 1920, a few days over a period of six weeks.

As a result there has been noted a gradual but undoubted improvement in several respects. The field of vision in the

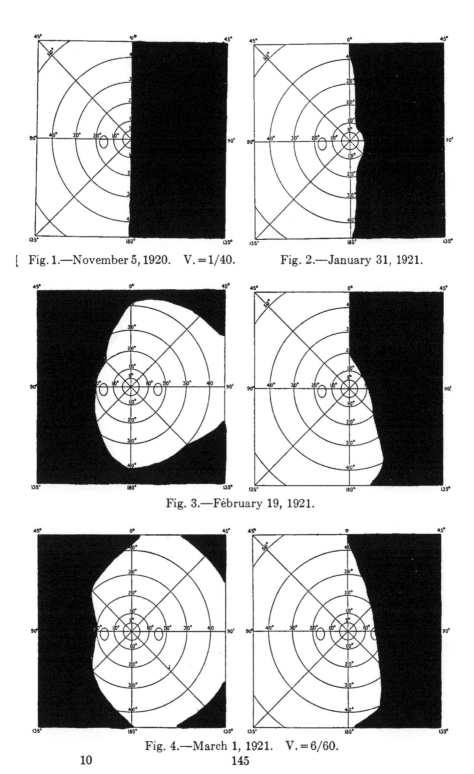

Fig. 1.—November 5, 1920.   V. = 1/40.   Fig. 2.—January 31, 1921.

Fig. 3.—Fébruary 19, 1921.

Fig. 4.—March 1, 1921.   V. = 6/60.

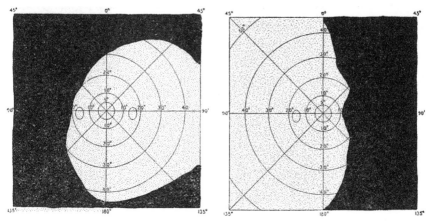

Fig. 5.—March 12, 1921.   V. = 6/40.

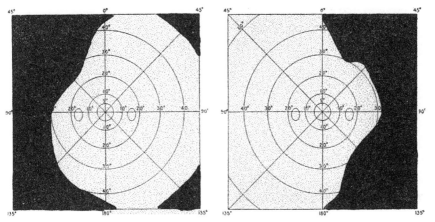

Fig. 6.—April 23, 1921.   V. = 6/8½.

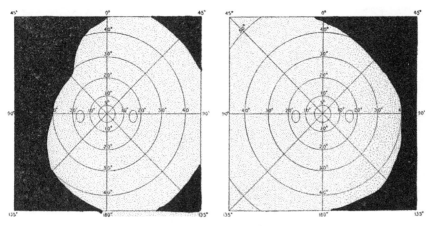

Fig. 7.—May 21, 1921.   V. = 6/6.

right eye has advanced almost 10 degrees from the fixation point on the nasal side—slightly less above and below. The headaches have been entirely relieved, and both the patient and his wife note an improvement in his mental and physical condition.

The therapy was continued in the same dosage, supplemented in January by bi-weekly hypodermic injections of 15 minims of pituitrin, until April 30th, when the pituitary substance was reduced to 6 grains per diem and bi-monthly injections of 10 minims of pituitrin.

Attention is directed to the fields taken at irregular intervals, which illustrate graphically the pronounced and steady improvement. Central vision improved in proportion to the field enlargements, as noted on the charts.

An interesting observation was the behavior of the visual field of the *left* eye. As stated in the preliminary report, the left field, October 11, 1920, was normal for form and colors. The field of this eye was not taken again until February 19, 1921, when the patient complained of a blurring of the vision or mist before the left eye, which he referred to the temporal side. Fields of both eyes were taken at this time, and it was noted that while there was a marked improvement in the right field, the left nasal field had become limited to within 20 degrees of the fixation-point.

This I believe is an original observation on the effect pituitary feeding may exert on the conformation of the gland in the sella. Central vision in the left eye has remained normal throughout the treatment.

A chronologic record of the vision of the right eye, corrected with −1.25 sph., follows:

October 11, 1920, V. = 1/40; November 5, 1920, V. = 1/40; January 31, 1921, V. = 1/40; February 19, 1921, V. = 1/40; March 1, 1921, V. = 6/60; March 12, 1921, V. = 6/40 +; April 23, 1921, V. = 6/8½; May 7, 1921, V. = 6/6½; May 21, 1921, V. = 6/6.

At the last ophthalmoscopic examination the pallor of the temporal half of the right disc had entirely disappeared and both discs had a normal, healthy appearance. The patient stated he felt better than he had in years. His headaches had entirely disappeared, he had no lapses of memory and could pursue a day's work without fatigue.

DISCUSSION.

DR. G. E. DE SCHWEINITZ, Philadelphia: A number of reports are on record of the relief of the symptoms of hypophyseal disorder as the result of such medication (Elsberg, Timme, and others in America, as well as physicians abroad), or at least improvement was coincident with the administration of glandular extracts. Two of the patients in my own practice whose histories have been recorded were unquestionably the subjects of dyspituitarism. Each of the patients selected received, in addition, in the one instance to thyroid extract, and in the other to thyroid and pituitary body extract, large doses of mercury by inunction; neither of them, if laboratory tests and clinical history can be trusted, was a syphilitic subject. In each the cure was perfect and has remained so for a number of years. What the influence of mercury was in these cases (assuming, as I think it is proper to assume, that the patients were not luetic) I do not know—an increase of the so-called antiphlogistic action of mercury by virtue of the action of the gland extracts, a synergic action in that the mercury and extracts aid each other in stimulating glandular secretion, with advantage, have been suggested. Timme believes that thyroid administration enhances the effects of specific treatment. All that I can say is—and on this I insist—that in any case of established or suspected disorder of the pituitary body the patient should be studied by the neurologist, the surgeon, the ophthalmologist, and the roentgenologist.

DR. HARRY FRIEDENWALD, Baltimore, Md.: How do you judge of the benefit of treatment?

DR. STIEREN (closing): I would like to corroborate Dr. de Schweinitz in all he has said in regard to his almost parallel cases. I think that all should be fed pituitary extract with the expectation of relieving many of them. The operative treatment is many times unnecessary, as the percentage of malignant growths is so small—less than 5 per cent. They are merely hypertrophies, as there are hypertrophies of the thyroid gland, due to overactivity, and the gland can be "rested" by feeding its extract.

In reply to Dr. Friedenwald, the only way you can judge of improvement is by the changes in the visual fields, as illustrated in the charts. In my opinion the left field in the case reported will improve as the right has done.

THE ESTIMATION OF COMPENSATION IN DISABILITY RESULTING FROM ACCIDENTAL LOSS OF VISUAL ACUITY.

E. TERRY SMITH, M.D.,

and (by invitation)

GEORGE E. TUCKER, M.D., AND ALEXANDER L. PRINCE, M.D.,
Hartford, Conn.

The present methods employed by Workmen's Compensation Insurance Commissions in estimating disability resulting from accidental loss of visual acuity are not uniform, and only infrequently are the age and occupation of the individual taken into consideration. The desirability of the general acceptance of a standard is evident, but unfortunately the various standards which have been suggested from time to time show such variation, and in some instances are so complicated by the introduction of more or less complex economic and mathematical principles, as to make the general adoption of these standards difficult.

A standard, in order to receive general acceptance, should retain a sufficient degree of simplicity, and yet should take into account certain factors which require consideration in accidental loss of visual acuity sustained in the course of occupation. The method presented here, we hope, will furnish a tentative basis for an acceptable standard. This method takes into consideration age and occupation, permits the determination of disability resulting from monocular and binocular loss of visual acuity, and yet retains sufficient simplicity to make its application practical.

Of the methods which have been proposed for the determination of a proper compensation rate in various ocular injuries, those of Würdemann and Magnus[1] and E. E. Holt[2] have received considerable attention. These methods, unfortunately, present a degree of complexity which makes their practical application somewhat burdensome.

H. S. Gradle, F. Brawley, and H. Woodruff [3,4] have proposed a method of estimating compensation for ocular injury in which four factors received consideration: (1) The vision of the injured eye; (2) the vision of the uninjured eye; (3) stereoscopic vision, and (4) cosmetic results. The first factor is computed in tenths, accepting as full vision the standard Snellen letter corresponding to 20/20. Should the vision of the injured eye be less than 5/100, the vision is counted as zero. The value as assigned to each degree of loss of vision is proportional to the Snellen chart fraction. These relations are shown in Fig. 1. The efficiency of the injured worker is computed by combining assigned values to the four factors mentioned above. In a sense, occupation is covered, inasmuch as workers are divided into two classes— Class A, including such workmen whose employment requires the ability to judge depth at arms' length or less, for example, a machinist, and Class B, including such workmen whose employment is of such character that the ability to judge depth at arms' length is not essential, for example, a trench digger. In our opinion occupations should be divided into more specific functional groups. Furthermore, as will be pointed out later, objection may be taken to the percentage of lost vision ratings assigned to the standard Snellen chart fractions.

A method similar to the above, and applicable to the New

York State Workingmen's Compensation Law, has been proposed by A. C. Snell.[5] In this method values are assigned to visual acuity, the visual fields, and binocular vision. The amount of vision remaining is then determined by dividing the sum of these values by a factor. No provisions are made for age and occupation, although, as the author points out, the more highly skilled worker automatically receives higher compensation for loss of vision by virtue of the fact that he receives higher wages.

The permanent disability rating schedule used by the State of California takes into consideration age and occupation in addition to the nature of the injury. In the case of eye injuries the Industrial Accident Commission of California has applied tentative standard ratings* for the Snellen chart fractions, as modified by other factors which impair vision. These other factors include blurring of vision, degree and character of any vision remaining, impairment of field vision, photophobia, dazzling, lacrimation, ocular fatigue, possibility of correction, cosmetic disfigurement, and whether the injured eye was the master eye or not.

The standard ratings are translated into percentages of total disability, instead of the usual percentages of vision as follows:

MONOCULAR LOSS OF VISION		BINOCULAR LOSS OF VISION		
ACUITY OF VISION	PERCENTAGE OF TOTAL DISABILITY	FIRST EYE	SECOND EYE	PERCENTAGE OF TOTAL DISABILITY
20/25	0	Nil	20/70	70%
20/30	5	Nil	Fingers	100%
20/40	10	20/30	20/30	10%
20/50	12	20/100	20/100	80%
20/70	14	20/200	20/200	100%
20/100	16			
20/200	18			
Light Perception	20			

* These ratings were transmitted to us, through the courtesy of Mr. W. J. French, Chairman, of the Industrial Accident Commission of the State of California.

When these ratings are translated into terms of percentage of lost vision, it becomes evident that the standard adopted by the California Industrial Commission is not in accord with the majority of visual acuity tables employed in other states (Curve A, Fig. 1).

In establishing a standard for making awards in ocular injuries it is believed that attention should be especially directed to loss of central visual acuity *per se.* In the last analysis the compensation commissioner is called upon to decide the remaining capacity of the injured eye as an organ the chief function of which is visual perception, and in order to simplify the problem such questions as to what should be allowed for contracted visual fields, loss of binocular vision, disfigurement, etc., may be considered of secondary importance. As Ginestons[6] points out, visual acuity is a primary element in the capacity to work, and no scale can be adopted that will measure ocular wounds and diseases in terms of incapacity. The lesions are too numerous, their disabling consequences too various. The experts should confine themselves to principles and let the interpretation vary with the particular case.

It is evident that, the percentage of total disability resulting from loss of visual acuity once established, it is a simple matter to add to the amount awarded certain percentages for various other defects which may be present. With this idea in mind, we have selected only central visual acuity, age, and occupation as the basis for the estimation of compensation in ocular injuries.

As Snellen chart fraction ratings have received general acceptance in the estimation of acuity of vision, these fractions have been adopted in the proposed standard.

On reviewing the estimates of various authors on the percentage loss of vision as derived by the Snellen chart method, there appears to be a considerable divergence of opinion not only as to the fraction which corresponds to so-called "industrial blindness," but also in the values assigned to individual fractions. As an illustration of the variations in the inter-

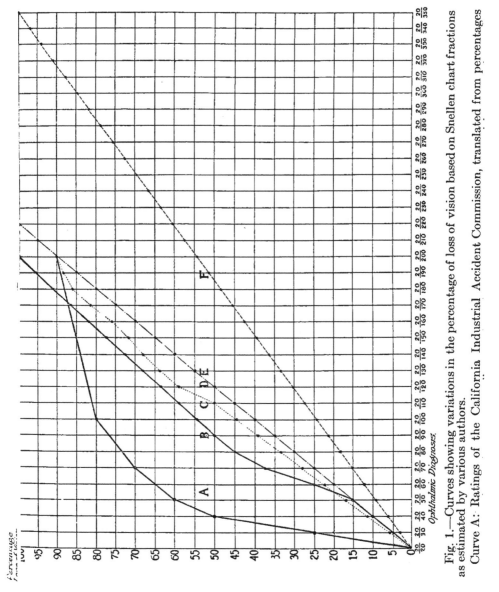

Fig. 1.—Curves showing variations in the percentage of loss of vision based on Snellen chart fractions as estimated by various authors.

Curve A: Ratings of the California Industrial Accident Commission, translated from percentages

pretation of Snellen chart fractions, the diagram (Fig. 1) is presented. In this diagram the ordinates represent percentage loss of vision, and the abscissa represents the ophthalmic diagnosis expressed in terms of Snellen chart fractions. These standards have been individually applied in certain states, and it does not seem logical that a given ocular injury should entitle the worker to considerably more or less compensation in one state than in another.

In considering the relation of visual acuity to percentage of disability, objection may be taken to standards in which it is assumed that this relation is linear. It does not appear reasonable that loss of occupational visual acuity should be directly proportional to the degree of vision indicated by Snellen chart fractions. In our opinion a progressive decrease of visual acuity affects occupational efficiency at a uniform rate until what may be termed the critical level of visual disability is reached, and it is at this level that the average worker is seriously affected in the pursuit of his ocenpation. Accordingly, in the preparation of our method, we have interpreted the Snellen chart ratings so that between 20/60 and 20/90, which we consider the critical level, there is a sudden rise in the percentage loss of vision ratings. These ratings when plotted yield an "S" shaped curve (Curve B, Fig. 1).

The selection of these Snellen chart ratings is based on the experience acquired by one of us (E. T. S.) over a period of several years. This experience covers a large number of cases, and dates back to the passage of the original Connectient Workmen's Compensation Law.

In rating accidental loss of visual acuity, the advisability of giving consideration to the age and occupation of the worker cannot be overemphasized. Some of the methods of estimating compensation for loss of vision do not consider age and occupation, and it is only in a very small number of states that attention has been paid to these two important economic factors. In the selection of a method for determining compensation ratings in relation to age, we have given consideration to the fact that while, after a certain age, the earning power of the average worker begins to fall, it is no less true that, with advancing years, the worker gradually loses the power to adapt himself to a new occupation. In the belief that the last factor is of greater importance than the first, we have selected the economic ratings established by Professor A. W. Whitney,[11] of the University of California, in the preparation of the proposed standard. This method of age rating has been adopted, and successfully applied, by the Industrial Accident Commission of the State of California.[12]

Ginestons,[6] in an article concerning work accidents, points out that in civil legislation occupational capacity plays the great rôle, and in the last analysis the estimation of compensation depends not on physiologic acuity of vision, but on professional or occupational acuity. The author consequently ranges occupations into three general classes: first, occupations necessitating ordinary visual acuity; second, occupations necessitating superior visual acuity; third, so-called visual professions, where perfection of the eye is essential to industrial efficiency.

This method of classifying occupations and other similar methods, proposed by various authors, specify the need of establishing functional occupational groups, but in the application of such methods, by compensation commissioners, experts are not always at hand to determine the specific visual requirements in a given occupation. It is therefore believed that each occupation should receive a distinct rating, based on the character of the injury sustained by the worker.

In our opinion the occupational classifications suggested by the Industrial Accident Commission of the State of California are at the present time the most adaptable to the needs of compensation commissioners. We have, therefore, selected this classification in the proposed standard. In this method occupations are divided into seven functional groups, a, b, c, d, e, f, and g; and each occupation is assigned to one group or another, according to its visual requirements. Group "a" represents occupations of lowest visual requirements, whereas "g" represents occupations of the other extreme. Objection may be taken to this classification as it lacks flexibility. For instance, laborers are assigned to the lowest visual requirement group (a), whereas it is conceivable that all laborers may not necessarily fall in this particular group.

A more definite occupational classification has been suggested by G. F. Michelbacher,[13] but unfortunately it is in the course of preparation and therefore cannot be utilized at the present time.

This author points out that instead of dealing with individual occupations, it is obvious that with a proper basis of grouping it will be possible to select a limited number of typical occupations, and by rating these, to cover the larger part of the entire industrial field. In other words, it should be possible to select a few representative occupations, to establish ratings for these and then to extend these ratings to the major share of occupations by analogy. A survey of the problem indicates that not more than 40 occupational groups are necessary. The method of establishing ratings for these groups of occupations may be done by sending trained investigators into the field to observe the work in the typical occupations, and thus to estimate the relative importance of visual and other functions.

Having selected Snellen chart, age, and occupational ratings, that in our opinion are free from serious objections, our efforts were directed toward combining this data in such a form as to make these standards applicable to the determination of monocular and binocular losses of visual acuity. To reduce the complexity of the method resort has been made to graphic presentation.

Our chart (Fig. 2) is divided into horizontal and vertical lines, the ordinates representing age (15 to 75), and the abscissa percentages of total disability. At the left-hand

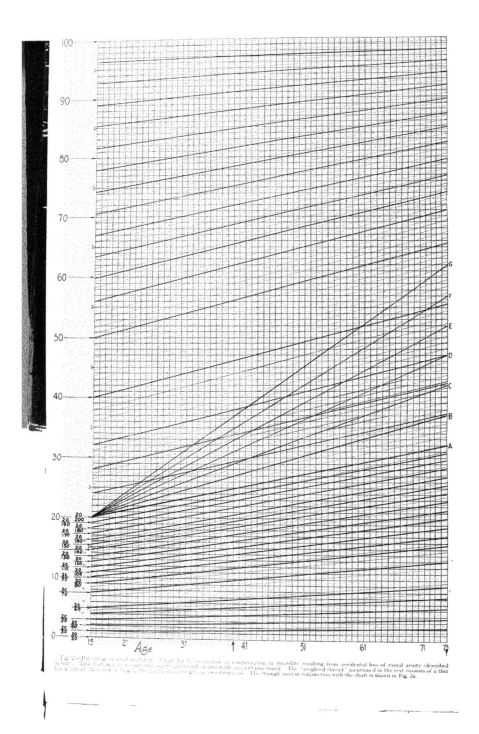

Fig. 2—Percentage of total disability. Chart for the estimation of compensation in disability resulting from accidental loss of visual acuity (described in text). This chart may be constructed conveniently upon a removable cardboard. The "weighted thread" mentioned in the text consists of a thin tough thread 12 inches in length, fitted with small weights at its extremities. The triangle used in conjunction with the chart is shown in Fig. 2a.

lower side of the table the Snellen chart fractions show the relation of these fractions to percentage loss of vision (small figures) and percentages of total disability. The diagonal lines, with the exception of those marked b, c, d, e, f, and g, represent the progressive increase in the percentage of total disability for any given loss of visual acuity, as the age of a worker increases from 15 to 75 years. These diagonals were plotted according to the computations of Whitney and Michelbacher.[14]

Briefly stated, the points used in plotting the diagonals were derived from two fundamental propositions (*a* and *b*) and an assumed standard (*c*), the latter established by the analysis of European, American compensation, and judicial experience, and data obtained through expert testimony.

These two propositions and the assumed standard may be expressed as follows: (*a*) a 100 per cent. disability is a 100 per cent. disability for all ages; (*b*) a zero per cent. disability is a zero per cent. disability for all ages; and (*c*) a 10 per cent. disability for a boy of age 15 is a 17.5 per cent. disability for a man of age 75.

The assumption that the adaptability of the worker varies according to this ratio was based upon a set of estimates collected on standard ratings for different age groups.

From such data it appears that, in the opinion of the experts giving the estimates, the rate corresponding to 10 per cent. disability at age 15 should be about 26 per cent. at age 75. The assumed standard, therefore, leans toward conservatism.

Using the above data as a basis for computation, Whitney and Michelbacher established the disability percentage relations between ages 39 and 75 by the following formula:

$$y = \frac{18\,x - 5\,x^2}{13}$$

where x = percentage disability at 39
and y = percentage disability at 75

(Age 39 was used as a basis because it was desired to have

the ratings under this age free from fractions of 1 per cent.)

Substituting for x the disability values .01 or .05 or .10, or any other value, the value of y, found by means of this formula, will give the rating for age 75.

By means of the diagonal lines plotted according to this formula it is therefore possible to establish the relative percentage disability for any given loss of visual acuity, at any age, at what may be termed a low grade occupation (Occupation A, California rating schedule classification, see Appendix, Table I).

For higher grade occupations a method of triangulation is used in which diagonals passing from the base to the apex of a triangle establish ratings for all ages and occupations.

The diagonals A, B, C, D, E, F, and G have been charted in Fig. 2 for the purpose of illustrating the influence of occupations on percentage of disability ratings in a case of total loss of industrial vision in one eye, with normal vision in the other.

APPLICATION OF THE PROPOSED STANDARD CHART FOR THE ESTIMATION OF THE PERCENTAGE OF TOTAL DISABILITY RESULTING FROM VARIOUS LOSSES OF VISUAL ACUITY.

I. Monocular loss of visual acuity.
   1. The following information is required:
      (*a*) Resultant vision after injury (corrected with glasses), and expressed in Snellen chart fractions.
      (*b*) Age and occupation of the injured individual.
   2. Insert pin on vertical line over age 15 at the point corresponding to the determined Snellen chart fraction. This pin will be at the left of the diagonal, representing the gradual rise of disability associated with increasing age in occupation A.
   In rating higher grade occupations:
   3. Insert another pin at right extremity of diagonal line where it meets the vertical line over age 75.
   4. Refer to table of occupations (Appendix, Table I)

and find the occupation and its corresponding index letter. Take sliding triangle (Fig. 2a) and place it so that its base coincides with vertical line over age 75, and so that line A at base of triangle is in apposition with the pin at the right-hand side and then

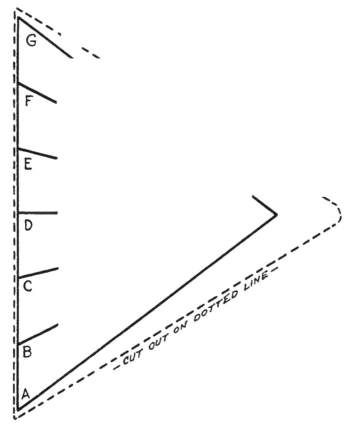

Fig. 2a.—"Occupational index letter" triangle used in conjunction with chart (Fig. 2). This triangle may be mounted on thin card-board.

insert another pin opposite the letter corresponding to the occupation.
5. Pass weighted thread so that it lies over the upper pin on the right-hand side and the single pin on the left-hand side. The thread will form a diagonal line which expresses the progressive increase of disability for that particular occupation between

ages 15 and 75. The point where any particular age line intersects this diagonal, carried horizontally to the left, will give the percentage of total disability assigned to that particular loss of visual acuity. (In the case of the lowest grade of occupations (occupational group A) it is not necessary to use pins, as the rating can be read off directly from the diagonal on the chart.)

EXAMPLE I: Laborer (Occupational Group A), age 25, monocular injury; resultant vision, 20/90.

(a) Insert pin opposite 20/90 on the vertical line above age 15. This pin will be at the left end of a diagonal line.

(b) Note point where vertical line above age 25 intersects this diagonal line.

(c) From this point follow horizontal line to left hand of chart and read off percentage of disability on scale. The percentage of disability is 11.2 per cent.

EXAMPLE II: Engraver (Occupational Group G), age 49, monocular injury; resultant vision, 20/60.

(a) Insert pin opposite 20/60, on the vertical line above age 15. This pin will be at the left end of a diagonal line.

(b) Insert another pin at extreme right of this diagonal.

(c) Place sliding triangle so that its base coincides with the vertical line over age 75, and so that point A on the sliding triangle is in apposition with the pin at the right-hand side of the diagonal, and then insert another pin opposite letter G (index letter of Occupational Group).

(d) Pass weighted thread so that it lies over the upper pin on the right-hand side and the single pin on the left-hand side. The thread will form a diagonal line which expresses the progressive increase of disability for that particular loss of visual acuity at any age for a worker in Occupational Group G.

(e) Note point where vertical line above age 49 intersects the "thread" diagonal.

(f) From this point follow horizontal line to left of chart and read off percentage of disability on scale.

The percentage of disability in this case is 24.5 per cent.

II. Binocular loss of visual acuity.

1. Obtain the following information:

(a) Resultant vision of each eye after injury (corrected with glasses).

(b) Age and occupation of injured individual.

2. Consider minor injury first unless loss of vision equal in both eyes. Insert pin on vertical line over age 15, at the point corresponding to the Snellen chart fraction found on examination of the eye having sustained the minor injury.

3. Read off the percentage of disability figure corresponding to the Snellen chart fraction ascertained for the eye having sustained the greater loss of vision.

4. Multiply this figure by 4, and add the product to the percentage of disability determined for the eye having sustained the minor loss of vision, then insert pin over the total thus obtained. This total represents the disability incurred for a particular binocular loss of visual acuity at age 15 in Occupation A. The diagonal extending from this pin represents the gradual rise of disability associated with increasing age in Occupation A.

5. Insert another pin at right extremity of this diagonal line where it meets the vertical line over age 75.*

6. Refer to table of occupations (Appendix, Table I) and find occupation of injured worker and its corresponding index letter. Take sliding triangle and place it so that its base coincides with vertical line over age 75, and so that line A at base of triangle is in apposition with the pin at the right-hand side, and then insert another pin opposite the letter corresponding to the occupation.†

* Table of occupation compiled from the schedule for rating permanent disabilities under the Workmen's Compensation, Insurance and Safety Act, effective January 1, 1914. Industrial Accident Commission, State of California. (Table not reproduced in Transactions.)

† In case the occupation index letter on the sliding triangle passes over the 100 per cent. horizontal line, insert the second pin at the junction of age 75 line and 100 per cent. disability line.

11

7. Pass weighted thread so that it lies over the upper pin on the right-hand side and the upper pin on the left-hand side. The thread will form a diagonal line which expresses the progressive increase of disability for that particular injury and occupation between the ages 15 and 75. The point where any particular age line bisects this diagonal, carried horizontally to the left, will give the percentage of total disability assigned to that particular loss of binocular visual acuity.

EXAMPLE I: Laborer (Occupational Group A), age 39, resultant V.R.E., 20/100; L.E., 20/100.

(a) Insert pin on vertical line over age 15 at the point corresponding to the Snellen chart fraction of one eye or the other, and note the corresponding percentage of disability. (Note: Keep in mind that in cases where the loss of vision is unequal, the eye having sustained the minor injury is considered first.)

(b) Since in this case the loss of visual acuity is equal in two eyes, add to this percentage of disability the same percentage multiplied by four (*i.e.*, $11 + (11 \times 4) = 55$).

(c) Insert pin on vertical line above age 15, opposite the total percentage of disability thus obtained (55). The diagonal extending from this pin represents the disability as influenced by age for that particular loss of binocular visual acuity in Occupation A.

(d) Note point where the vertical line over age 39 intersects this diagonal and carry this point horizontally to left side of chart and read off percentage of disability on scale. The percentage of disability in this case is 61 per cent.

EXAMPLE II: Chauffeur (Occupational Group C), age 30, resultant V.R.E., 20/40; L.E., 20/80.

(a) Insert pin on vertical line over age 15, at the point corresponding to the Snellen chart fraction 20/40, and read off percentage of disability on scale (2 per cent).

(b) Read off the percentage of disability figure (9 per cent.) corresponding to the Snellen chart fraction 20/80. Multiply this percentage by 4 and add to the product the percentage of disability determined for the eye having sustained the minor injury (*i. e.* (9 × 4) + 2 = 38 per cent.

(c) Insert pin at vertical line over age 15, opposite 38 per cent. This pin will be at the left extremity of a diagonal line.

(d) Insert another pin at the extreme right of this diagonal.

(e) Place sliding triangle so that its base coincides with the vertical line over age 75, and so that line A on the sliding triangle is in apposition with the pin at the right-hand side of the diagonal and then insert another pin opposite letter C (index letter of Group).

(f) Pass weighted thread so that it lies on the upper pin on the right-hand side and the pin on the left, opposite 38 per cent. The thread will form a diagonal line which expresses the progressive rise of disability for that particular loss of binocular visual acuity at any age for a worker in Occupational Group C.

(g) Note point where vertical line above age 30 intersects the thread diagonal and from this point follow horizontal line to left side of chart and read off percentage of disability on scale. The percentage in this case is 44.5 per cent.

EXAMPLE III: Carpenter (Occupational Group D), age 60, V.R.E., 20/200; L.E., 20/180.

(a) Compute percentage of total disability as in preceding example. The result will be 18.2 per cent. + (20 × 4) = 98.2 per cent.

(b) Place pin on vertical line over age 15 opposite 98.2 per cent. Note position of nearest diagonal line and insert another pin at corresponding point where this diagonal intersects vertical line over age 75. Place sliding triangle so that line A at base of the triangle is in apposition with the pin at the right-hand side.

(c) It will be noted that letter "D" (occupation index letter) lies above the 100 per cent. line, and since a disability cannot exceed 100 per cent. insert a pin at the junction of the vertical line over age 75 and the 100 per cent. disability line.

(d) Pass weighted thread from this pin to the pin on the left-hand side opposite 98.2 per cent. and note point where the vertical line over age 60 intersects the thread diagonal. This point is then carried horizontally to the left and the percentage of total disability read off. In this instance the rating is 99.5 per cent.

In the case of states where a definite number of weeks of compensation is awarded for total disability, it will be noted that this award when divided by 100 will give the number of weeks of compensation allowed for each 1 per cent. of disability. For example, in Connecticut total disability equals 520 weeks of compensation, consequently each per cent. of disability is awarded 5.2 weeks of compensation, and therefore 5.2 multiplied by the percentage of disability derived by means of the proposed standard will give the number of weeks of compensation to be awarded in each case.

It will be noted that in the application of the proposed standard the occupation of the worker does not influence the percentage of disability at age 15, but, as the individual becomes older, the occupation lines rise at a progressive rate so that, for example, a 23 per cent. loss at 15 becomes a 62 per cent. loss at 75, in the occupations requiring the highest visual capacity. At first sight this may seem unfair, but it is evident that at 15 a worker has seldom received sufficient training to be a skilled artisan. His earning power is correspondingly smaller, and his capacity to rehabilitate himself is much greater than in the case of a worker advanced in age.

In the computation of binocular losses of vision by means of our chart it should be noted that four times as much compensation is allowed for loss of vision in the eye sustaining the major injury. In other words, in binocular losses of visual acuity a much higher rate of compensation is allowed for the second eye. This is considered just, as binocular losses are far more incapacitating.

In the questionnaire submitted to the Milwaukee Oto-Ophthalmic Society by the Industrial Commission of Wisconsin[10] there appears a question of extreme importance, namely, what disability compensation should be given to a man whose vision has been impaired by accident but has been brought to normal by the use of a lens?

According to our experience in the State of Connecticut, award should be based on the resultant vision when corrected by a competent oculist by means of glasses. The Workmen's Compensation Law of the State of Connecticut, as revised June, 1919, expressly states that "reduction in one eye to one-tenth or less of the normal vision *with glasses*" is equivalent to total loss of vision. Accordingly, in the event where sight can be restored to normal by use of glasses the injured worker would not be entitled to compensation for loss of visual acuity, although in the presence of other defects of vision, such as loss of binocular vision, contraction of visual fields, aphakia, resulting from a cataract operation, etc., the worker would be entitled to a certain amount of compensation which would depend on the severity of the defect and his occupation.

The question arises as to whether there is what may be termed a major and a minor eye. Certain authors believe that the loss of the right eye for a right-handed person is more important than loss of the left. It is our belief that, except in a few occupations where one eye has been particularly trained, for example, in the case of the microscopist or the watch-maker, it cannot be said that there is a major or a minor eye, and even in these special occupations re-adaptation should take place rapidly.

Particularly in slight ocular injuries, there is always a

possibility of making excessive awards, owing to a pre-existing defect of vision. As pointed out by Harbridge,[15] employers would find it an advantage to keep accurate records of the condition of the eyes of all employees at the time that they are hired.

It is evident, however, that, until physical examination of employees is universally applied, the worker should receive the benefit of the doubt.

In conclusion, a review of the methods applied up to the present time for the estimation of compensation in ocular injuries serves to emphasize the need of establishing a national standard. Lack of conformity, particularly as it applies to injuries of the eye, has arisen, we believe, as a direct result of lack of central action. In many instances State Industrial Commissions have called the attention of the problem to committees of local oculists. The result has been a different standard in each case. It is our hope in presenting this paper before the American Ophthalmological Society to bring about the standardization of compensation awards in accidental loss of visual acuity.

That a man's vision should be worth infinitely more in one state than in another does not appear sound or just. Until the time comes when the problem can be attacked by experimental methods it behooves the different states to adopt a uniform standard, and it is believed that a standard, approved by the American Ophthalmological Society, would go far toward relieving the present situation.

We realize that the problem is beset with enormous difficulties, but its solution will not be hastened by divided effort. It is better to have an empirical standard, provided it is not unjust, than to have a number of opinions competing against each other. It is our belief that the existing diversity of opinion is dependent on the very fact that loss of visual acuity can be at present based only on economic and physiologic assumptions. In the last analysis, who can demonstrate that 20/70 means 30 per cent. or 45 per cent. or 50 per cent. loss of vision? Who can prove and convince others as to the economic value of the eye? Who can say what constitutes in each case absolute industrial blindness? The answer to these questions in the absence of experimental proof must be based on assumptions. These assumptions, of course, should be supported by as many facts as possible and should not deviate too widely from the path of logic.

REFERENCES.

1. H. V. Würdemann, with the collaboration of Dr. Magnus, Breslau: Ann. of Ophth., April, 1901.
2. E. E. Holt: Trans. Amer. Ophth. Soc., 1920, xviii, 298.
3. H. S. Gradle, F. Brawley, H. Woodruff: Report of the Committee of the Chicago Ophthalmological Society, read before the Society, December 18, 1916.
4. H. S. Gradle: Amer. Jour. Ophth., 1918, l, 487.
5. A. C. Snell: N. Y. State Jour. Med., July, 1919, xix, 277.
6. E. Ginestons: Annales d'Hygiene Publique et de Médécine Légale, 1915, xxiv, 75.
7. F. Allport, Jr.: Jour. Amer. Med. Asso., 1920, lxxiv, No. 3, 166.
8. N. A. Chapman: Wis. Med. Jour., June, 1918, xvii, 54.
9. W. N. Sharp: Amer. Jour. Ophth., June, 1920, iii.
10. S. J. Higgins: Report to the Wisconsin Industrial Commission, read before the Chicago Ophthalmological Society, May, 1919.
11. Manuscript, "Making of Permanent Disability Schedule," Industrial Accident Commission of California.
12. Schedule for Rating Permanent Disabilities under the Workmen's Compensation, Insurance and Safety Act, effective January 1, 1914.
13. G. F. Michelbacher: "A New Schedule for Rating Permanent Injuries," Unpublished MS.
14. G. F. Michelbacher: Proceedings of the Casualty Actuarial and Statistical Society of America, 1914-15, I, Nos. 1, 2, 3, 257.
15. Harbridge, D. F.: Ariz. Med. Jour., May, 1916, iv, 12.

DISCUSSION.

DR. GEORGE E. TUCKER, Hartford, Conn.: Workmen's compensation laws have been adopted by the several States on the theory that industry may rightfully be held chargeable for its damage to human machinery. Society has readily accepted this social relief legislation only after having become convinced that adding the cost of industrial injuries to the cost of production provides an economical and equable method for distributing this burden.

Insurance companies, fulfilling their rôle as distributors of benefits, are not so much concerned with the amount of awards allowed by administrative authorities if the premium rates are in accord with their interpretation of the benefit provisions.

The need for standardization of ratings of permanent disabilities is, perhaps, more apparent to those of us who are called upon to study large numbers of these cases, than to those who are only occasionally asked to guide a lay commissioner into a proper understanding of what a partial loss of function of an eye means in the way of loss of earning power. Ophthalmologists agree no more frequently than surgeons on the occupational value of the remaining function of injured parts.

As an illustration of the need for recognizing the importance of the factors of age and occupation in determining loss of earning power, the exaggerated case of the violinist, sixty-five years of age, who sustained third-degree burns of the tips of the fingers of the left hand while in the course of his employment, is in point. This individual became totally incapacitated from earning a livelihood as a violin player, whereas a day laborer of the same age, having sustained the same injury, would have suffered very little, if any, loss of earning power.

Our studies presented here to-day, we hope, may lead to further consideration of the standardizing of eye disability ratings.

DR. ERASTUS E. HOLT, Portland, Maine: The author asserts that "the present methods employed by workmen's compensation insurance commissions in estimating disabilities resulting from accidental loss of visual acuity are not uniform," and "the desirability of the general acceptance of a standard is evident," and he hopes his tables will furnish a basis for such a standard. As all the values given in his tables are based solely on the central acuity of vision without regard to the condition of the field of vision or the muscular functions of the eyes, how can he expect that such tables will furnish the basis for such a standard? He dwells upon the statement that central acuity of vision is the essential part of economic vision, ignoring the fact that the field of vision and the muscular functions are equally as important for economic purposes. If we find a loss of function only in the central acuity of vision, then we might use Dr. Smith's tables, but if we find a loss in the field of vision or in the muscular functions of the eyes we would be unable to determine that loss by Dr. Smith's method, because there are no tables constructed by which that loss can be measured. Hence the method presented for discussion is incomplete and empirical. Let us for a moment dwell upon the characteristics of a scientific method and the difference between it and an empirical method. For this purpose we might take any commodity, like wheat. If there were 100 bushels of wheat, and by the market price, or its competing ability among grains, this is worth $1.00 per bushel, the 100 bushels would answer to the factor of the multiplicand and the price would answer to the factor of the multiplier in the natural science formula, and the value of the wheat would be $100.00. If a fire destroyed a certain portion of the wheat and damaged the rest, namely, its sale, or competing ability in the grain market, we have a condition of the wheat similar to that of an employee who has lost the sight of an eye from a burn of the cornea from lime. The loss in the wheat by an empirical method, without going into any details, might be estimated as $32, or a 32 per cent. loss, or an estimation might be made that 85 bushels of wheat were not destroyed by fire and that it was worth 80 cents a bushel. Again, the number of bushels of wheat would represent the factor of the multiplicand, and the price it would sell for would represent the factor of the multiplier. When stated in the formula, we would have: $85 \times 80 = \$68$, the value of the wheat. Subtracting this from the cost of the wheat leaves $32, which is the same in amount as that estimated as a lump sum. Although in this last method the natural science formula was used to get at the loss, yet as a whole the method is an empirical one, because the remaining number of bushels of wheat, after fire had destroyed a portion of it, was not determined by any standard of measurement, neither was the price at which the damaged wheat would sell for in the market ascertained according to its actual market value. It was simply estimated or guessed at, and this method must necessarily lead to errors and inconsistencies, and if tested out in its entirety, leads to an absurdity. In the determination of the loss to the wheat by the scientific method, the first thing to be done is to find out how many bushels of wheat were not burned by actually measuring it by the accepted standard of measurement for grain, namely, the bushel. If, by this process, it was found that there were 82 bushels of wheat, this would again represent the factor of the multiplicand, and if it were actually determined that 82 cents was the best market price that could be obtained for the damaged wheat, this 82 would be the factor of the multiplier. $82 \times .82 = 67.24$, which, subtracted from the cost of the wheat, namely, $100, gives 32.76, equal to a loss in percentage of 32.76 per cent. It will be seen by these examples that whether you determine the value of anything by an empirical method or by the scientific method, its value must be based upon quantity and quality representing the factor of the multiplicand, and the price, or what it will sell for in the market, its competing ability, representing the factor of the multiplier, to obtain a product, representing its value, or its earning ability to the producer. This is true as regards the earning ability of a person. If, for instance, a floor-walker loses the sight of his left eye from a burn of the cornea from lime, leaving a conspicuous scar, he has lost .18 of the functional ability of his whole body, according to the standard of measurement set forth in "Physical Economics." If we subtract this .18 from the normal coefficient of F, the functional ability of the whole body, we have .82 for its remaining coefficient $(.82 F)$. As C, the competing ability of the floor-walker, depends upon the same identical functions of the body for its existence, it must also have for its "primary coefficient" .82 $(.82 C)$. As these two factors are the indispensable ones of E, the earning ability, we have the equation: $.82 F \times .82 C = E$, the statement of the earning ability of the floor-walker, after the loss of the sight in the left eye. Multiplying, we have .6724, representing the remaining earning ability of this employee, which, subtracted from 1, gives .3276, a percentage loss of 32.76. The percentage of loss to the earning ability of the floor-walker is obtained in a similar manner to the percentage of loss to the wheat, namely, by mathematics, the only way known to obtain the value of any physical force or any commodity.

There can be only 100 per cent. loss to the earning ability

of a person, and when this is graded by grading the 100 per cent. damage to the competing ability of that person, in the vocation followed, by mathematical laws which are as well understood as the multiplication table, the commission, or anyone else capable of understanding the compensation problem, can take up each individual case with the medical examiner and discuss every step of the determination, for each is made with mathematical precision and therefore may be readily understood by all concerned.

DR. SMITH (closing): The standardization of rates of compensation as applied to loss of visual acuity has interested me greatly since the enactment of the Workmen's Compensation Laws a number of years ago. The different methods suggested from time to time seemed so complicated and difficult to apply that I decided to work out a simple method. The difficulties multiplied so rapidly that I thought it well to associate with myself men who are continually engaged in the application of the different methods of determining compensation. I therefore asked Dr. George E. Tucker, the Director of Industrial Medical Division of the Ætna Life Insurance Co., and his associate, Dr. Prince, formerly Assistant Professor of Physiology in the Yale Medical School, to collaborate with me. The table we have presented is the result of our combined work.

The new features of our table are, first: A new standard expressing the relation of the Snellen chart fraction to per cent. loss of vision, taking into account the average occupational acuity of vision rather than physiologic acuity. Second: A method which can be applied to determine compensation in the presence of both monocular and binocular loss of visual acuity. Third: A simple graphic method which does away with the use of elaborate tables and mathematical formulæ, so complicated and irksome to most of us, that we shrink from using them.

When asked to estimate the damage to an eye, it has to be considered ordinarily as a visual organ, and we should first determine the loss of visual acuity sustained. After that is established, then we can add specific amounts for loss of binocular and stereoscopic vision, paralysis of eye muscles, etc. Dr. Holt's contributions to industrial medicine have

TABLE II

State	TOTAL LOSS OF VISION ONE EYE COMPENSATION				TOTAL LOSS OF VISION TWO EYES COMPENSATION			
	% of Wage	Limits per wk.	Duration weeks	Remarks	% of Wage	Limits per wk.	Duration	Remarks
Ala.	50%	$5-12	100		50%	$5-12	400 wks. then $5.00 per wk. or full wages until 550 wks. completed	Act effective, Jan. 1, 1920
Cal.	65%	Sliding Schedule			65% 40%		240 wks. thereafter Life	Act effective, July 22, 1919
Col.	50%	$5-10	Enucleation 139 Blindness 104		50%	$5-10	Life	Act effective, May 1, 1919
Conn.	50%	$5-18	104	Complete permanent loss of sight of one eye or reduction to 1/10 or less of normal vision with glasses	50%	$5-14	520 wks.	Total and permanent loss of vision in both eyes or the reduction to 1/10 or less of normal vision with glasses. Act effective, Aug. 1, 1919
Del.	50%	$4-10	113		50% $2-6	$4-10	270 wks. thereafter Life	Act effective, Jan. 1, 1918
Idaho	55%	$6-12	Enucleation 120 Blindness 100		55%	$6-12 $6	400 wks. thereafter Life	Act effective Jan. 1, 1918

TOTAL LOSS OF VISION ONE EYE

COMPENSATION

State	% of Wage	Limits per wk.	Duration weeks	Remarks
Ill.	50%	$7-12	100	
Ind.	55%	$5.50-13	150	Loss or 1/10 vision with glasses
Iowa	60%	$6-15	100	
2nd eye	60%	....	200	
Kan.	60%	$6-12	110	
Ky.	65%	$5-12	100	
La.	55%	$3-16	100	
Maine	60%	$6-15	100	Loss of eye or reduction of 1/10 V.
Md.	50%	$5-12	100	
Mich.	60%	$7-14	100	
Minn.	66⅔%	$6.50-15	100	
Mo.	66⅔%	$6-15	Enucleation 110 Sight 100	

TOTAL LOSS OF VISION TWO EYES

COMPENSATION

State	% of Wage	Limits per wk.	Duration	Remarks
Ill.	50%	$7-12 to $13.50	4 times annual earnings. Limit: $3,500 Thereafter 8% of total compensation	Act effective, July 1, 1919
Ind.	55%	$5.50 to $13.50	500 wks. Max. amt. $5,000	Act effective, May 15, 1919
Iowa	60%	$6-15	400 wks.	Act effective, July 4, 1919
Kan.	60%	$6-15	8 yrs	Act effective, May 26, 1917
Ky.	65%	$5-12	8 years Max. $5,000	Act effective, Aug. 1, 1916
La.	55%	$3-16	400 wks.	Act effective, July 31, 1918
Maine	60%	$6-15	500 wks. Max. $4,200	Act effective, July 3, 1919
Md.	50%	$5-12	Max. $5,000	Has partial loss of vision provision. Act effective, Nov. 1, 1916
Mich.	60%	$7-14	Max. amt. $6,000	Act effective, Aug. 14, 1919
Minn.	66⅔%	$6.50-15	410 wks. thereafter $6.50 per wk. to 550 wks. Max. $5,000	Act effective, July 1, 1919
Mo.	66⅔%	$6-15	240 wks. thereafter Life	Act effective, Nov., 1919
	40%	$6-15		

TOTAL LOSS OF VISION ONE EYE

COMPENSATION

State	% of Wage Limits per wk.	Duration weeks	Remarks
Neb.	66⅔%	$6-15	125	
N. J.	66⅔%	$6-12	100	
N. Y.	66⅔%	No limit	128	
Ohio	66⅔%	$6-20	No fixed schedule 5.2 wks. = 1% disability.	
Okla.	50%	$8-18	100	
Ore.		$25 a month — 40 mos. or $850 lump sum.		
Penn.	60%	$10-12	125	Complete permanent loss of sight of one eye or reduction to 1/10 or less of normal vision with glasses
Terr. Hawaii	50%	-$12	128	
Tenn.	50%	$5-11	100	Complete permanent loss of sight of one eye or reduction to 1/10 or less of normal vision with glasses

TOTAL LOSS OF VISION TWO EYES

COMPENSATION

State	% of Wage Limits per wk.	Duration	Remarks
Neb.	66⅔% 4%	$6-15 thereafter $4.50-12	300 wks. Life	Act effective July 18, 1919
N. J.	66⅔%	$6-12	400 wks.	Act effective, July 4, 1919
N. Y.	66⅔%	$5-15	Life	Act effective, May 13, 1918
Ohio	66⅔%	$6-20	For life	Act effective, July, 1920
Okla.	50%	$8-18	500 wks.	Act effective, June 29, 1919
Ore.		$30-50 per mo. for life		Act effective, July 1, 1913
Penn.	60%	$6-12	500 wks. Max. $5,000	Total and permanent loss of vision in both eyes or the reduction to 1/10 or less of normal vision with glasses. Act effective, Jan. 1, 1920
Terr. Hawaii	60%	$3-18	312 wks. Max. $5,000	Act effective, Oct., 1917
Tenn.	50%	$5-11 $5 per wk.	400 wks. thereafter 550 wks. Max. $5,000	Total and permanent loss of vision in both eyes or the reduction to 1/10 or less of normal vision with glasses. Act effective, July 1, 1919

State	TOTAL LOSS OF VISION ONE EYE COMPENSATION				TOTAL LOSS OF VISION TWO EYES COMPENSATION			
	% of Wage	Limits per wk.	Duration weeks	Remarks	% of Wage	Limits per wk.	Duration	Remarks
Texas	60%	$5-15	100		0%	$5-15	401 wks.	Act effective, Mar. 28, 1917
Utah	60%	$7-16	Enucleation 120 Sight 100		0%	$7-16	For 5 yrs. thereafter	Act effective, July 1, 1917
					5%		Life	
Vt.	50%	$3-12.50	100	Complete permanent loss of sight of one eye or reduction to 1/10 or less of normal vision with glasses	0%	$3-12.50	260 wks.	Total and permanent loss of vision in both eyes or the reduction to 1/10 or less of normal vision with glasses. Act effective, June 1, 1919
Va.	50%	$5-10	100		50%	$5-10 $4,000 max.		Act effective, Jan. 1, 1919
W. Va.	50%	$5-12	132		50%	$5-12	Life	Act effective, May 13, 1919
Wis.	65%	$6.50-15.60	140		65%	$6.50-15.60	Max. 15 yrs. Min. 9 yrs.	Act effective, Sept. 1, 1919

been very valuable, but the application of his laws are rather difficult for most of us, because they are quite complicated. He speaks of a 125 per cent. loss of vision as being beyond the realm of reason. The German at the present time allow 125 per cent. for total loss of vision, considering that the individual is not only totally disabled, but that economically, in the average case, he is a burden upon the community. It may not be mathematically sound, but praetically it is so.

AN UNUSUAL CASE OF CONJUNCTIVAL IRRITATION.

H. H. BRIGGS, M.D.,
Asheville, N. C.

Male, aged twenty-seven years, while walking in the woods, felt a mass of foreign matter strike the right eye, followed by the usual burning and itching sensation. The intense symptoms soon subsided, and the patient thought that the foreign body had been dislodged. The next morning, however, the lids were swollen, and the uncomfortable symptoms continued to the third day, when he consulted me. In the interim several unsuccessful attempts at removal had been made by various laymen.

Examination revealed the palpebral fissure narrowed, the lids swollen, and the inner canthus filled with a stringy mucus. The upper lid, elevated with difficulty on account of the swelling, showed a dark-red, velvety conjunctiva, much moie swollen than that of the lower lid or of the bulbus. The general appearance did not suggest a foreign body in the cornea, which appeared normal, or of the conjunctiva, and there was no evidence of any ciliary or other intra-ocular inflammation. No foreign body was found at first, but on account of the history, the search was resumed, when, by oblique illumination of the everted upper lid, a tiny cream-colored body was seen moving over the conjunctiva. Before it could be removed it passed around a fold of the conjunctiva and was temporarily lost, but again everting the lid and exposing the culdesac, six similar objects were located and removed. The conjunctiva was irrigated and 1 per cent. silver nitrate solution applied to its entire surface. The symptoms quickly subsided, and in three days the eye was normal.

Under the low power of the microscope the object proved to be a larva, composed of 12 segments. Its length, estimated as being about ¼ mm., was about twice its breadth. The two ends appeared so symmetric that it was with difficulty that the head could be distinguished from the caudal extremity. Definite identification was not made, but morphologically it answered to that of the gall-gnat, Cecidomyia Trifolii, of the family Cecidomiidæ.

Whether the insects entered the eye in the larval stage or as ova developing into larvæ in the interval prior to their removal, I do not know, nor shall we ever know whether the ocular symptoms were caused by mechanical irritation or by some chemical substance excreted.

The case is reported for the reason that it cites an unusual cause of conjunctival irritation. It is of little scientific value, and perhaps of no practical value, for a similar case may never present itself to any of us.

One can conceive of such a small larva entering the eye, passing into the lacrimal sac, and, if anaërobic, as seems probable, might there thrive and increase in size until it could neither pass into the nose nor back into the eye and furnish another possible cause for an acute dacryocystitis; or passing into the nose, find its way into the nasal accessory sinuses, including the Eustachian tube, middle ear, and mastoid cells. By way of analogy, we have the intestinal tract, liver, lungs, and blood-channels harboring worms and insects which enter the body in the oval and larval stages.

A MODIFIED ACCOMMODATION LINE AND PRINCE'S RULE.

ALEXANDER DUANE, M.D.,
New York.

Some years ago I presented a test for the accommodation—a black velvet disc on which was mounted a little white card with a fine black line on it. This served the purpose well, but as it was difficult to make and soon got soiled, it made a rather expensive test-object. Experiment showed that practically the same purpose was served by the same fine black line engraved on a simple white card. This is held in any ordinary clip, so that it can be carried back and forth along the accommodation rule. These cards can be made cheaply and thrown away as fast as soiled.

The accommodation rule is simply a Prince's rule, lighter and rather more closely graduated than the ordinary, and with a notch at the end. When the notch is placed so that the bridge of the nose fits into it, the prong on either side can readily be set so as just to touch the trial-frame on the patient's correcting glasses, which themselves should be placed 14 mm. in front of the cornea. When the rule is thus placed, the test-card can be run along either edge to measure the accommodation of the right and left eye separately, and along the top to measure the binocular accommodation, all three measurements being made rapidly without withdrawing or shifting the rule.

I may add that I have lately used the accommodation card and rule not simply as a test, but as an exercise when the accommodation and convergence are deficient. For this purpose I make the patient fix as sharply as he can on the line and bring it up as close as possible until it blurs, this, first, with the right eye, next with the left, and finally with both. I not infrequently give the patient one of these cards to exercise with at home making him practice in this way monocular and binocular accommodation, and with the latter the convergence also. The effect of this simple exercise is often very good.

The cards and accommodation rule are made by Gall and Lembke, 5 West 42d Street, New York.

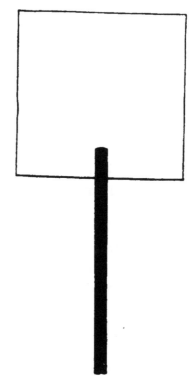

Accommodation
rule. × 0.3.

Accommodation line held in a simple clip.

ILLUMINATED EYE SPUD WITH MAGNIFIER.

Dr. George S. Crampton, Philadelphia, exhibited an illuminated spud designed to throw a convergent pencil of light upon the area under examination, which is viewed through a strong magnifying lens supported at the proper distance by means of a rod with ball-and-socket joint.

Another lens with central perforation into which a spud, knife-needle, or other instrument is fixed is made of a short section of barometer tubing about 5 mm. in length and 7.15 mm. in diameter with a central lumen of 1.5 mm. This thick lens not only forms an ample mounting for the spud, but in turn is firmly spun into a seat in the end of a metal tube in which there is a miniature lamp. The light from the lamp surrounds the instrument as it leaves the tube to converge upon the cornea, thus obviating all shadow. The electric current is supplied, either by a standard fountain-pen battery in the handle of the instrument or through flexible cords from a separate source, such as a dry battery in the pocket, or the house circuit through a rheostat. When the blade of the instrument is not in use, it is covered with a cap so that it can be carried in the pocket.

The tube with the perforated lens and

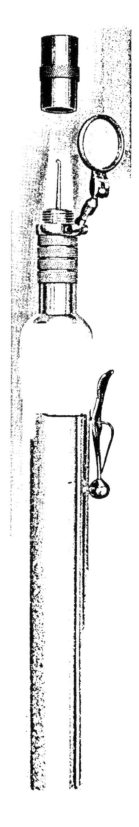

spud can be unscrewed and replaced by another carrying the illuminating and magnifying lenses, but no cutting instrument. This combination gives one an excellent means of examining the cornea under the high magnification of a one-inch lens.

Another attachment in which the light tube carries a tapered, bent rod of glass is used as a sclerascope, and still another tip carries special cilia forceps astride the pencil of light by means of which the palest cilia are plainly seen under magnification.

For use in the removal of wild hairs by galvanism a fine needle is mounted in the lens and attached to a source of current other than that supplying the lamp.

The casing is made of duralumin, an aluminum alloy having the tensile strength of mild steel, although almost as light as aluminum. The instrument is manufactured by the Lenox Instrument Company of Philadelphia.

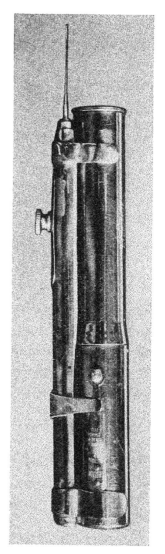

Foreign-body spud illuminator, with spud exposed.

FOREIGN-BODY SPUD ILLUMINATOR.

Dr. W. Holbrook Lowell, Boston, Mass., exhibited a "fountain-pen" light, with contact switch, to which is attached a smaller parallel barrel, equal in length, with a sliding member in this superimposed barrel. The spud is fastened in this sliding member. When pushed forward over the electric bulb with the light on, the spud point and cornea are well illuminated and the light is where you want it when you want it. The spud is protected when not in use by sliding it back into the barrel.

The writer is indebted to Mr. Sach, of F. H. Thomas and Company, Boston, for his interest and zeal in carrying out the writer's ideas.

DISCUSSION.

DR. WM. CAMPBELL POSEY, Philadelphia: Dr. Lowell is probably unaware that some years ago Dr. Snell, of Rochester, devised a similar apparatus to remove foreign bodies from the cornea, with an illumination of the spud by a small electric globe, and presented the same before this Society.

FORCEPS FOR TENDO-MUSCLE LENGTHENING.

Dr. W. Holbrook Lowell, Boston, Mass., exhibited a modification of his forceps for tendo-muscle lengthening. The space between the jaws of the instrument is 3 mm., which is regarded as ample. The instrument is made by Codman and Shurtleff, of Boston.

CORALLIFORM CATARACT AND ASTEROID HYALITIS.

Dr. F. H. Verhoeff demonstrated sections of a coralliform cataract removed by Dr. Zentmayer, and a microscopic specimen of the vitreous humor from a case of asteroid hyalitis.

TONOMETRIC CHART.

Dr. E. C. Ellett presented a chart for making a graphic record of tonometric readings. It resembles a temperature chart, with the normal indicated by a heavy black line for

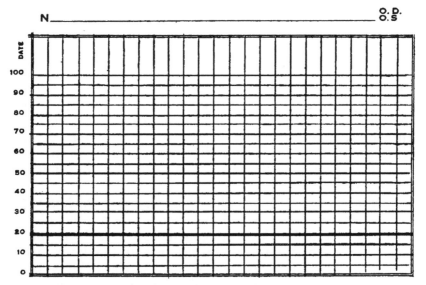

Tonometric chart. (Reduced ¼ in size.)
Use black ink for the Schiotz Tonometer. Normal (20) indicated by heavy black line.
Use red ink for the McLean Tonometer. Normal (40) indicated on chart by red line.

the Schiötz tonometer, and a red line for the McLean tonometer. The lighter lines correspond to intervals of 5°, the date of the observation being indicated in a space at the top of the chart.

A CASE OF MOOREN'S ULCER.

ARTHUR J. BEDELL, M.D.,
Albany, N. Y.

Mooren's ulcer is sufficiently uncommon to warrant the presentation of another case in the hope that in discussion points may be brought out which may offer some new line of treatment for one doomed to blindness unless the process is soon checked. It is because of this that the following case is reported to you:

On January 14, 1920, J. W., aged fifty-six years, a strong, healthy-appearing man, weighing 185 pounds, was so burned with acetic anhydrid that all lids, surrounding face, the entire conjunctiva, and superficial cornea were involved. There was marked congestion and swelling, with blisters on the lids, and a thick, white, adherent, membrane-like conjunctival and corneal burn.

Immediately after the accident his eyes were washed with boric acid solution. He was then taken home, and his physician, Dr. Frederic C. Conway, called, to whom I am much indebted for asking me to see the case within five hours after the injury. The man was sent at once to the Albany Hospital, where the eyes were put under atropin, castor oil, and ice compresses. Healing progressed well. There was very little pain, much oozing from the conjunctiva, and rapid exfoliation of the burned tissue. By February 13, 1920, the right vision was 20/40 and the left 20/30. Both corneas were practically clear, although the conjunctiva surrounded each with a thick roll resembling a moderately vascular pterygium. There was also a partial symblepharon of the right upper lid and inner portion of the globe. On February 28, 1920, he returned to work with vision in each eye 20/15, with correction, Jaeger 1. He was not seen until June 1, 1920, when +2.50 sph. was given for near work.

He had no annoyance until August 21, 1920, when he showed a slight epithelial roughness to the lower inner side

Right

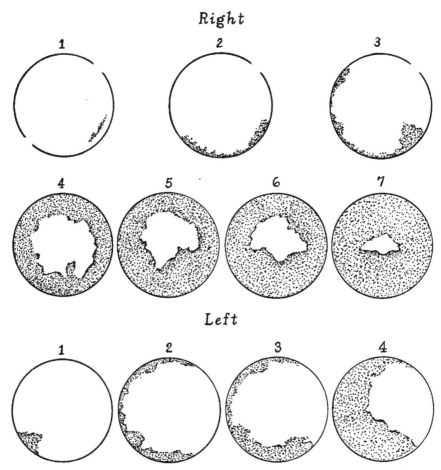

Left

The stippled areas represent corneal involvement, superficial epithelial infiltration in Fig. 1, but in the others destruction to the middle of the corneal stroma. The white shows uninvolved cornea.

Right Eye: Fig. 1, August 21, 1920; Fig. 2, October 16, 1920; Fig. 3, November 22, 1920; Fig. 4, December 4, 1920; Fig. 5, December 17, 1920; Fig. 6, January 22, 1921; Fig. 7, February 24, 1921.

Left Eye: Fig. 1, November 22, 1920; Fig. 2, December 17, 1920; Fig. 3, February 24, 1921; Fig. 4, May 25, 1921.

of the right cornea, about 1.5 mm. from the limbus. The cornea was then insensitive, but the eye was not painful. By October 16, 1920, there was a definite limbus ulcer, with moderate congestion of the scleral vessels near it. The margin of the ulcer was irregular in outline, the advancing edge undermined almost 0.5 mm., with a distinct gray infiltration of the overhanging part. The epithelial layer, Bowman's membrane, and about one-half of the true stroma were destroyed. Blood-vessels from the conjunctiva extended over the denuded area up to the progressive line. Cultures showed nothing characteristic, although the pneumococcus predominated. Optochin was used with seeming improvement for two days, when the ulcer progressed.

By November 22, 1920, there was a semicircle of corneal loss, as shown by the diagram, and the left eye for the first time presented evidence of corneal infiltration at the lower nasal side. December 17, 1920, the right eye showed a still greater loss of cornea and the left eye a crescent of encroaching ulceration. On January 22, 1921, the right eye was cocainized, the ulcer cureted, cauterized, and a conjunctival flap brought from above over the cornea. The ulceration was not checked, and by February 24, 1921, all that remained of the superficial cornea of the right eye was a densely gray ovoid area in the center. Dr. C. S. Merrill saw the patient several times, and we agreed that every time I cauterized the ulcer destruction seemed more rapid. On March 16, 1921, the patient saw two other members of this Society, both of whom agreed to the diagnosis of Mooren's ulcer, although one considered the condition stationary. Both expressed an opinion that the accident had nothing to do with the disease. Considering we know so little as to the cause of the condition, and as the case was one in our compensation courts, I believe their deduction unwarranted.

By May 4, 1921, the remaining part of the superficial cornea of the right eye had melted away, and now, May 25, 1921, the right cornea shows an irregular surface, with the conjunctival overgrowth extending almost to the center. The remaining portions of the cornea are vascular, with an irregular surface from the many depressions and elevations between the vessels. The conjunctiva of globe and lids is smooth, but somewhat vascular, with a slight mucopurulent secretion. Beneath the vascular cornea the iris can be distinctly seen, and a slightly irregular, 3 mm. pupil well outlined. Vision equals fingers at 18 inches.

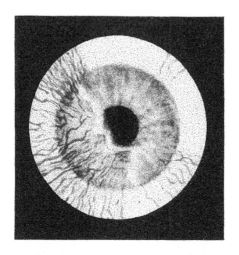

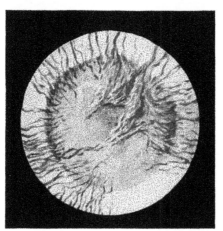

Upper figure, R. E., February 24, 1921, showing the extension of the conjunctival vessels over the elevated limbus to the margin of the remaining superficial layers of the cornea, which are already opaque.

Center figure, L. E., April 14, 1921, the vascularization extending over the cornea up to the advancing ulcer. Margin of the ulceration infiltrated and so undermined that the destruction of the layers of cornea is evident.

Lower figure, May 16, 1921. Complete vascularization of the right cornea, showing the two layers of blood-vessels, the deeper being more evident to the lower and outer side. The more superficial remains of the conjunctival flap to the upper inner side.

The left eye shows no injection of the eyeball to the upper outer quadrant, corresponding to the remaining clear portion of the cornea. The other parts of the bulbar conjunctiva are vascular, and the conjunctival vessels extend by branching over the denuded cornea up to the line of the advancing ulcer. This irregular margin is definitely undermined, with a slightly gray, 1 mm. infiltration beyond the actual edge. The anterior chamber is normal. Iris clearly detailed. Pupil 3 mm., reacting to light and accommodation.

The treatment of the condition has been zinc sulphate, formalin solution varying from 1:5000 to full strength, the galvanocautery, the thermophore, ethylhydrocuprein, mercurochrome, eserin, atropin, hot compresses, ice compresses, fixation abscess, the extraction of many infected teeth with apical abscesses, bandaging, conjunctival flap, and curetment of the cornea. This last procedure involved not only cureting the ulcer margin, but also the entire corneal surface. It hardly needs to be stated that each change of treatment was carefully considered.

The diagnosis of Mooren's ulcer was made because of the insensitive cornea, the undermining infiltration of the irregular, overhanging, lip-like ulceration, the vascularization of the cornea following the progressive ulcer, the lack of pus in the region of the ulcer margin, and the clinical course of the disease. There is, of course, no confusing this with the destruction of a serpiginous ulcer in which the advancing margin is always filled with pus-cells.

As in many other cases of this disease, insensitiveness of the cornea has been an early prominent symptom. While pain has been complained of often, my patient never spoke of pain even after the fixation abscess. The Wassermann and tuberculin reactions were negative. He has had no pus in nose or tonsils, and as far as can be determined he is, with the exception of the eye condition, perfectly well. Last year in his thesis, Feingold carefully and thoroughly discussed the pathologic changes occurring in this disease, so it is unnecessary for me to even refer to them in this paper.

To summarize: Eight months after a very severe conjunctival burn of both eyes ulceration of the cornea began, first in one eye and then in the other. Despite all treatment the ulceration progressed so that the first affected eye now shows a vascular cornea, with no change in the anterior chamber and vision reduced to fingers at one foot. The second eye is going just as the first. No therapeutic measure has been of avail, and without new trauma, change in his general health, method of life or surroundings, except the accident, this progressive condition has involved both eyes.

DISCUSSION.

DR. E. C. ELLETT, Memphis, Tenn.: I have notes of two similar cases:

CASE I.—A man, aged sixty-five years, was seen September 8, 1915, with an inflammation in the right eye of six weeks' duration. There was not much pain. There was a large, tongue-shaped ulcer at the outer edge of the cornea, with vessels passing to it from the conjunctiva. Pupil active; V. = 15/20. A month later the ulcer was somewhat larger, 6 x 8 mm. long, axis vertical. The corneal edges of the ulcer and the conjunctiva adjacent to the ulcer were undermined about 2 mm. The conjunctival undermining was only apparent at the limbus, where the ulcer touched it. Smears and cultures were negative. Various remedies, including the cautery, did not help matters until all the overhang was trimmed off on November 19th, and the cautery applied. This was repeated on a limited scale during the next month, as new points of undermining were found. On January 30, 1916, the entire ulcerated surface was covered with epithelium. The ultimate visual result was 20/30 mostly, with a high degree of astigmatism. The general physical examination revealed arteriosclerosis and high blood-pressure.

CASE II.—A man, aged fifty years, seen June 2, 1916, gave a history of an acute inflammation of the right eye on May 25th. On May 27th the lid was painted with nitrate of silver. V. = 20/100. An ulcerated groove was found parallel to the limbus, and about 2 mm. from it, extending one-quarter of its circumference. The whole center of the cornea was cloudy, and stained except for a rim about 2 mm. wide all around. Smears and cultures were negative. The epithelium ceased to stain except a crescent at the nasal edge, and this broke down and the epithelium then was found to stain again over most of the cornea. The epithelium became loosened around the edge of the staining area, and could be pushed back toward the limbus, but the central epithelium was not loose. Gradually a circular ulcer formed, isolating a central elevated area of nearly normal-looking cornea, but the circle of ulceration was never complete, but broken at the nasal side. The ulcer traveled toward the center, the elevated portion getting smaller, and when quite small, it was cut off, leaving a clean, horseshoe-shaped ulcer 1.5 mm. in diameter, with opening at 2 o'clock. Both edges of the ulcer, *i. e.*, the central and peripheral, were undermined. The process took about four months, the little island being cut away in October. The cornea was not healed until January, when the whole membrane was partly opaque, with iris visible up and out. The pupil was occluded, and the conjunction of the lids had a shark-skin look. In May the conjunctiva was normal. V. = l. p. The patient subsequently became insane, and died in an asylum in 1920.

DR. CHARLES W. KOLLOCK, Charleston, S. C.: I wish to place on record another case in a negro who consulted me several months ago. At that time there was an islet of clear corneal tissue, similar to that which Dr. Ellett has described. It was situated in the center of the cornea, and about 0.5 mm. above the surrounding tissue. There may have been a very gradual dwindling of the spot, but the change was almost imperceptible, so that when I last saw him I was uncertain whether any change had occurred.

Treatment at various times consisted in giving, internally, Fowler's solution of arsenic, iodid of potassium, and mercury. Externally, tincture of iodin, 20 per cent. solution of argyrol, and a solution of nitrate of silver were applied without any appreciable beneficial effect or otherwise. Unfortunately, no bacteriologic examination was made, and as the man stopped coming to me, I cannot report the final outcome.

DR. MARCUS FEINGOLD, New Orleans, La.: There is very little to be said about any suggestions as to the treatment of these cases. A good deal has been suggested, a great many things have been tried, but the hopes have been shattered almost every time, exactly as in the case under discussion. Still two reports in the recent literature hold out a possible ray of light in this discouraging field, and to mention these I rose in reply to Dr. Bedell's question. Koeppe* tells of two cures of Mooren's ulcer by tuberculin injections, and in the case of Eyer† the ulcer healed during an attack of facial erysipelas. A trial with tuberculin would be almost harmless, but, of course, we dare not produce erysipelas; it is a force which, once called into play, might cause unlooked-for damage. We might possibly accomplish a similar result by streptococcus vaccine. Parenteral milk therapy, as suggested by Eyer, who sees in the fever of the erysipelas of his case the curative factor, can certainly be tried with little risk. An interesting feature in the present case was, as I understand it, the utter absence of pain; as a rule, the suffering is intense. An explanation for this would be interesting.

DR. BEDELL (closing): In answer to Dr. Feingold's question in regard to pain, I mentioned that the patient had anesthesia of the cornea from the beginning, even in the first stage of infiltration. He never has had pain. He is a rather curious individual. For instance, at one time we used fixation abscess in his left flank, injecting 1 c.c. of sterile oil of turpentine, yet he made no complaint. As to tuberculosis, we ruled it out as far as we could by the subcutaneous injection of increasing doses of old tuberculin; having at no time local, general, or focal reaction. Wassermann reaction negative. When the long list of treatments are noted, the hopelessness of the condition will be appreciated.

* Zeitschrift f. Augenh., vol. xxxviii, 1917, p. 301.
† Klin. Monatsbl. f. Augenh., vol. lxiii, 1919, p. 28.

SARCOMA OF THE CORNEA. CASE REPORT.

GEORGE S. DERBY, M.D.,
Boston, Mass.

The patient whose case I desire to report is Mrs. A. M., aged seventy-nine years, coming from Stoneham, Mass., seen early in January, 1921. The right eye had watered for ten or fifteen years, and there had been a chronic conjunctival inflammation. About ten years ago one of the silver preparations was injected into the right lacrimal sac. Following this the right cheek became discolored, and there is now a very marked, grayish-brown discoloration, which shows that the silver had penetrated beyond the sac into the tissues of the face.

There is an entropion of the right upper lid, with contraction of the tarsus. The conjunctiva is scarred, much reddened, and shows some argyrosis. There is a question of one or two small granules. In the lower culdesac there are a number of small adhesions and scars, probably of old trachoma. There is a marked peribulbar injection. The cornea is opaque and vascularized throughout. Slightly to the inner-lower side of the center of the cornea is a grayish-red tumor, about 3 mm. in height and 6 mm. in its greatest cross diameter. Its margin is everywhere considerably removed from the corneal limbus. No details of the iris or of the fundus can be made out. The eye perceives shadows.

The left upper lid shows a little thickening, with some redness of the conjunctiva. Left cornea, iris, and media normal, as is the fundus. There are a few medullated nerve-fibers. Vision in the left eye with the correcting glass is 6/6—.

Enucleation of the right eye was advised, and was carried out on January 11th. The eye was then turned over to Dr. Verhoeff, who reported a melanotic sarcoma of the cornea.

"*Pathologic Report.*—The globe is normal in size and shape,

191

except that the cornea is slightly collapsed as a result of the formalin fixation.

"Arising from the cornea, a little to one side of the center, there is a tumor, almost hemispheric in shape, with slightly constricted base and smooth surface. It is light gray in color, 3 mm. in height, and 6 mm. in greatest cross diameter. The base is 4.5 mm. in greatest diameter, and its margin is everywhere more than 2 mm. from the corneal limbus. The interior of the eye appears normal.

"*Microscopic Examination.*—Horizontal celloidin sections were made through the eye and tumor, at various levels, some of them passing through the middle of the tumor, and others passing through the tumor where the latter is nearest to the limbus. Staining in hematoxylin and eosin.

"The tumor is found to be a slightly melanotic spindle-cell sarcoma. Near the periphery on each side almost all of the cells are spindle-shaped and arranged in fairly definite bundles. In the central portion an arrangement into bundles is only occasionally recognizable, and many of the cells here are irregular in shape, large in size, and often multinucleated. No cells resembling Langhans' giant cells, however, are seen. Cells in mitosis are abundant in this portion of the tumor. In general the tumor is very slightly pigmented, but in places many of the tumor cells contain pigment and those often display the branching processes of typical chromatophores. The pigment bleaches readily by the method of Alfieri, and is evidently autochthonous in origin.

"Blood-vessels are not abundant in the tumor. All of them have thin walls to which the tumor-cells are closely applied. The connective-tissue stroma of the tumor is inconspicuous.

"The tumor is partly covered with a thick layer of epithelium continuous with that of the cornea. Over the central portion the epithelium becomes thinned out and finally completely lost. Beneath the site of this erosion the tumor shows a marked chronic inflammatory reaction, being pervaded by granulation tissue, and infiltrated with chronic inflammatory cells and a considerable number of pus cells.

"Beneath the central portion of the tumor the anterior third of the corneal tissue has been replaced by tumor cells.

"Extending to the tumor from the limbus all around, be-

Section of eyeball.

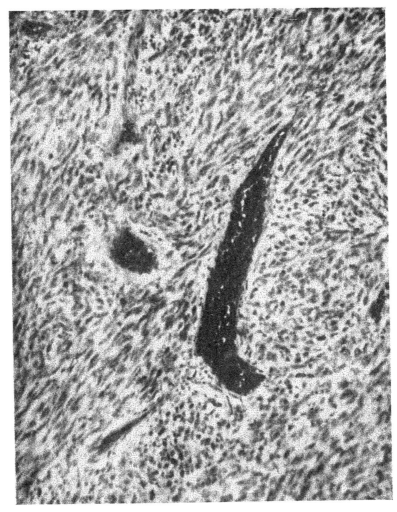

Microscopic section of tumor.

tween the epithelium and Bowman's membrane, is a vascularized pannus richly infiltrated with plasma cells and lymphocytes. In places this has destroyed Bowman's membrane. The epithelium over it is thickened and shows a keratin layer.

"In some sections the tumor cells have invaded the pannus for a short distance, but nowhere do they reach as near as 2 mm. from the limbus.

"The interior of the eye, except for ordinary senile changes, is normal. The iris is heavily pigmented, as is also the choroid, but the tissue of the corneal limbus does not contain an unusual amount of pigment.

"*Diagnosis.*—Melanotic spindle-cell sarcoma of the cornea."

According to Parsons, there is great doubt as to the true status of recorded cases of corneal tumors. All of the newgrowths are vascular to a greater or less degree, and derive their vessels from the limbus. The most doubtful of all are the malignant ones, especially the epitheliomata and the endothelial type of sarcomata. None of the cases cited by him is regarded as being above suspicion as to diagnosis. "The avascular fibrous stroma of the cornea, like tendons and aponeurosis, might be expected to enjoy relative immunity from malignant growths, while it is always impossible to exclude invasion from the periphery from which the blood supply must necessarily be derived. The resemblance of embryonic connective tissue in inflammatory granulations to sarcoma and the loss of the iron reaction in old hemorrhagic pigmentation form insuperable barriers to certitude of diagnosis in the present state of knowledge. Nevertheless, malignant proliferation of the fixed corneal corpuscles cannot be definitely eliminated. Should it occur, the disposition of the corneal lamellæ might be expected to give rise to a quasialveolar arrangement."

Sarcoma of the cornea is extremely rare. The following cases are cited by Parsons: Rumschewitsch, Blanquinque,

13

Chantiniere, Gonin, Rogman, and Fumagalli, six in all, cases in which the growth extended to or over the limbus being excluded. In addition, I find a case occurring in a child of eight months reported by Addario in 1912. This was a growth measuring on the surface 6 or 7 mm. by 2 or 3 mm. and 4 mm. thick. Microscopic study disclosed a melanotic sarcoma, which had begun in the center of the corneal parenchyma and had destroyed Bowman's membrane, but had shown little tendency to extend backward.

In 1913 Dean reported the history of a woman of sixty-three years. The brownish tumor, 5 mm. in vertical and transverse diameter and 2 mm. thick, occupied the central part of the upper half of the cornea, extending a little below the median line. In no place did it extend nearer than 1 mm. to the limbus, but the corneal tissue above was traversed by blood-vessels. Microscopically, it was a somewhat pigmented sarcoma, originating probably from the superficial layers of the substantia propria of the cornea.

In 1917 Meanor's case of sarcoma was demonstrated before the Pittsburgh Ophthalmological Society by Dr. E. J. Willets. This was a dark-red growth of the cornea in a man of sixty-eight years. When first seen, the growth is said to have been confined to the cornea, while at the time of demonstration there were several pigmented spots in the neighboring conjunctiva. A small piece was removed from the cornea and presented the appearance of a typical melanotic sarcoma under the microscope.

In the case reported by Black and Crisp before the Colorado Ophthalmological Society in 1914, the tumor involved the conjunctiva, and thus must be excluded from the true corneal growths. Thus, with the growth reported here, I have been able to find but ten cases, which shows the rarity of the condition.

In the case reported there is some question as to whether the conjunctival scarring, the diseased tear-sac, and the corneal vascularization represented an old trachoma. If it did, then there may be some doubt as to whether the tumor developed from the corneal stroma or from the remains of the pannus. In this connection Parsons cites a second case, reported by Rumschewitsch, in which a corneal growth occurred in a girl of fourteen who had advanced trachoma. Parsons does not regard this case as a true sarcoma, but as a pannus showing an unusual degree of hyperplasia. That the same criticism cannot apply to the case which I present to you is, I think, clear from the microscopic examination.

REFERENCES.

Parsons: Pathology of the Eye, vol. i, 259–261.
Addario: Ann. di Ottal., xli, 33, 1912.
Dean: Annals of Ophth., xxii, 764, 1913.
Willetts: Penn. Med. Journ., xxi, 421, 1917–18.
Black and Crisp: Annals of Ophth., xxiii, 394, 1914.

MELANOSARCOMA (MELANOMA) OF THE CHOROID OCCURRING IN BROTHERS.

ADOLPH O. PFINGST, M.D.,
Louisville, Ky.

Inasmuch as malignant growths of the eye occurring in more than one member of a family have, to my knowledge, never been recorded in medical literature, the report of two cases which recently came under my observation may be of interest.

CASE 1.—W. B. G., farmer, aged forty-four years, consulted me in February, 1919, with the history that he had noticed a dimness in vision of the left eye a year previously, and that the vision had decreased so that by June of that year he could just about differentiate between light and darkness. Diagnosis of retinal hemorrhage was made at the time by the late Dr. Wm. Cheatham. The patient had never had eye trouble of any kind and gave no history of an injury to either eye. His general health had always been perfect. Family history extending back two generations was negative as regards malignancy. His mother died at the age of thirty-six years of heart trouble following rheumatism, and his father was in good health at eighty years. He has, besides the brother included in this report, one sister, aged fifty, and a brother, aged thirty-seven years, both in good health.

Examination showed a robust, well-developed man of healthy complexion, with light brown eyes. The right eye was normal and had perfect function. The left showed an extensive detachment of the retina on the temporal side and upward. Tension was normal. The retina on the nasal side was responsive to light. This man absented himself for a year, when he returned with the history of severe pain in the left eye of two weeks' duration. He was found to be in an acute attack of glaucoma, with hazy cornea, shallow anterior chamber, increased tension, etc. The interior of the eye was not recognizable. Würdemann's transilluminator showed darkness on the temporal side. Based upon the increased tension and the knowledge of a previous detachment of the retina, the diagnosis of intra-ocular tumor was made, enucleation advised and allowed.

The removed eyeball was fixed in 5 per cent. formalin solution. Anteroposterior section extending through the optic nerve and the middle of the cornea revealed a globular mass about the size of a pea close to the entrance of the optic nerve on its temporal side. The tumor mass had a light, chocolate-brown color. The retina was entirely detached. The specimen was sent to Dr. Stuart Graves, of the University of Louisville, for microscopic report.

CASE 2.—Farmer, aged forty-seven years, while at my office on April 1, 1920, with his brother, whose eye had been removed a few days previously, made an inadvertent remark that he felt sure that he had in one of his eyes the same trouble as his brother. He based this belief upon the fact that he had noticed a hair-like body before the left eye for six or eight weeks, and that his vision was obscure on one side. As this history was given in a passing way, no attention was paid to it and no examination was made. A few weeks later, while on a visit in Washington, he consulted Dr. Wm. H.

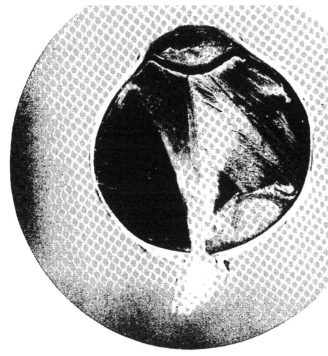

Fig. 1.—Anteroposterior section of case No. 1, showing small tumor near optic nerve.

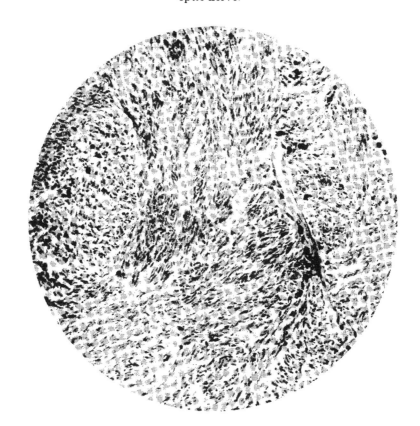

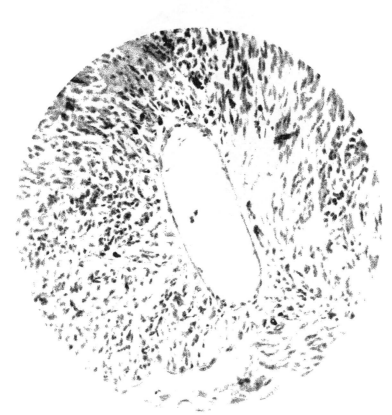

Fig. 3.—(× 230) Greater magnification of same tumor, showing same features
and delicacy of blood-vessels.

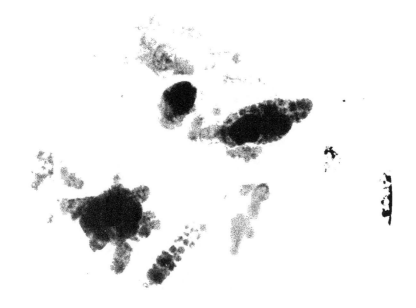

Wilmer, who made a diagnosis of intra-ocular tumor and advised enucleation. Personal history in this case was negative; no history of traumatism or of any inflammatory eye disease. Family history same as brother.

Examination, which was made at my office on April 20th, revealed by focal illumination a mass in the vitréous chamber on the temporal side, and close behind the lens, which seemed to be protruding from the ciliary body and which extended to the edge of the normal pupil. Würdemann's transilluminator showed the temporal half of the eye darkened. Tension was normal. There was no inflammatory reaction; the exterior of the eye was normal. Vision was reduced to perception of light on the nasal side of the retina. The right eye was normal. Vision, 20/15.

The left eye was enucleated on April 23d and placed in formalin solution. Anteroposterior section disclosed on the temporal side a black, globular mass, about one-half inch in diameter, of smooth contour, and covered with retina. It seemed to spring from the choroid anteriorly and to extend backward beyond the equator of the eye and far into the vitreous cavity. The specimen was submitted for microscopic report.

PATHOLOGIC REPORT BY STUART GRAVES, M.D., LOUISVILLE, KY.

CASE 1.—The specimen consists of one-half of eye, 26 mm. in diameter. It has been cut in the middle of the plane of optic nerve, dividing the latter; in cut surface, springing from the junction of the retina and nerve, extending laterally from the nerve 11 mm., and extending into vitreous 5 mm., is a chocolate gray, rather spongy tumor. The opposite half, when split at right angles, reveals apparently the same kind of tumor, but about three times as large.

Microscopic description: Sections show the tumor to be made up almost entirely of spindle-cells, supported by very scanty stroma and few blood-vessels, those present appearing more as blood-channels lined with endothelium and without normal vessel-wall. The tumor-cells lie in interlacing bundles and contain rather elongated, oval, pale nuclei. In the cytoplasm of some cells there is an abundance of brownish, finely granular pigment, but these pigmented cells are irregularly distributed and, when the section is viewed under low power, are comparatively scanty. Mitoses are very few.

Microscopic diagnosis: Melanoblastoma (melanosarcoma).

Case 2.—Gross description: The specimen consists of half of eye, 27 mm. in diameter. Springing from one wall and involving one-half of the vitreous chamber is a dense, homogeneous mass of dark brown, almost black, substance. This neoplasm extends from the region of the ciliary body, which seems to be involved in the tumor mass, backward about 22 mm. to a point about 12 mm. anterior to the optic nerve. The retina is separated and pushed to one side by this mass. A layer of vitreous humor, 4 mm. thick, is present between the dense mass and the separated retina. Specimen split at right angles to anteroposterior axis shows the dark mass to be rounded, about 12 mm. in one diameter and 20 mm. in the other.

Microscopic description: Sections of this tumor show a general structure similar to that of first case, but the pigmentation is so exceedingly abundant that even a thin section appears almost black and the cell structure is largely obscured; under the high power the outlines of cells can be seen, and these outlines frequently sharply circumscribe the pigment deposit.

It becomes manifest at once that these cases offer nothing of especial interest regarding the points of origin of the growths or their histologic structure, nor does the individual case present any unusual clinical features. However, the occurrence of identical growths in brothers at about the same time of life is so very unusual that a report of the cases for the sake of future reference seems warrantable. It would seem that as long as the etiology of malignant growths remains as obscure as it is to-day any data that might eventually be of value in determining this problem should be placed on record.

It is well known that after these many years of research

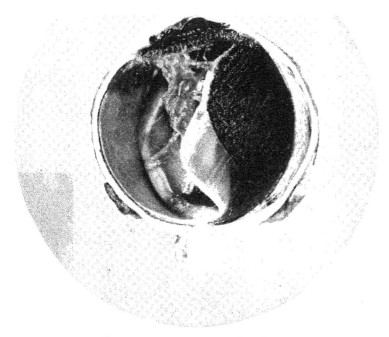

Fig. 5.—Anteroposterior section of case No. 2, showing large tumor far forward.

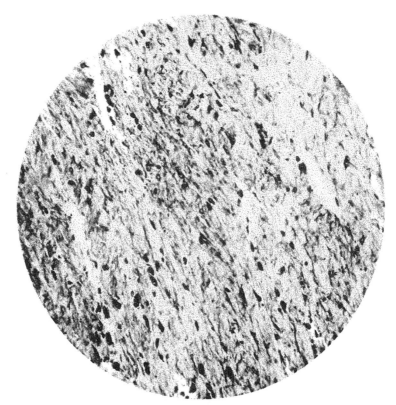

Fig. 6.—(× 120) Showing general structure of more abundantly pigmented
tumor.

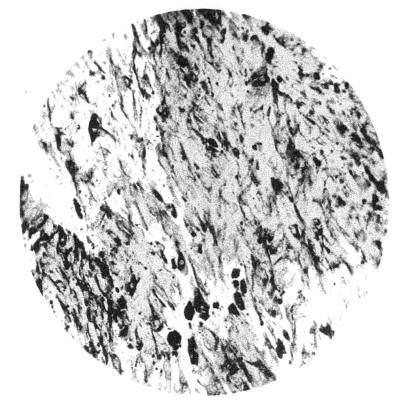

Fig. 7.—(× 230) Greater magnification of same tumor, showing more clearly
spindle type of tumor cells and relative scarcity of stroma.

nothing definite has been established regarding the causative agent of malignant growths or, in fact, of tumors in general. The much-quoted hypothesis promulgated by Cohnheim that tumors develop from superfluous masses of simple or complex tissue misplaced during embryonic development, although not universally accepted, still has many adherents who look upon the frequent origin of new-growths from congenital abnormalities, such as the development of melanomata, from pigmented moles and pigmented spots in the uveal tract of the eye as the chief support of this theory. Cohnheim also saw in the frequent development of malignant growths at the mucocutaneous junctions strong supporting evidence of his embryonic theory. While Cohnheim's hypothesis does not explain why the displaced embryonic cells may lie dormant for years and finally either atrophy or produce new-growths, the assumption is warranted that the primary cause of neoplastic growths may be assigned to some cell disturbance either of an embryonic nature or of a later development, and that the various conditions assigned by pathologists as probable causes are merely determining or exciting factors in the individual case. Whether the disarrangement of cells always takes place during embryonic development or whether Ribbert's modification of the embryonic idea that the isolation of the cells which eventually produce the growth probably occurs in adult life through the irregular growth of the tissue, it must be remembered that every group of misplaced cells does not form a tumor, the development probably depending upon favorable conditions of nutrition and the activity of some exogenous influence.

In recent years it has been suggested that the growth of these dormant misplaced cells is ordinarily prevented by the existence in the organism of some chemical or biologic influence of an unknown nature, but probably emanating in the ductless glands, and that a perversion of this internal secretion, either by an overproduction or an insufficient absorption, annuls the inhibitive influence over cell growth. It is suggested by the exponents of this theory that the misplaced cells, relieved of the retarding influence of the conjectural endogenous substance, become susceptible to exogenous influences, which then serve as the determining cause of tumor development. While the theory seems reasonable, it must be admitted that it is not based upon adequate facts.

Much time and thought have been given the endeavor to determine the relation between tumor development and certain external exciting influences. All efforts to transmit malignant growths by inoculating living tumor cells or the filtrate of the tumor in the human have been futile. We know too that there is at present no direct evidence of a bacterial cause of tumor development or of any other definite extrinsic influence, and yet we are all familiar with the many instances in which injurious influences of all sorts preceded the development of tumors, making the causative relation between them extremely suggestive. Nevertheless, we cannot conceive of such injuries causing tumor growth without assuming the existence of some abnormality in the tissue involved. The irritants which, by Virchow, were called formative irritants, and which are now looked upon merely in the light of contributory factors in tumor development, are not necessarily the result of one direct violence, but may be due to long-continued influence of mechanical, chemical, or bacterial irritation, associated with inflammatory infiltration. Common examples of this kind are seen in the pipesmoker's epithelioma of the lip, malignant uterine growths following long-continued acrid discharge, etc.

In considering the exogenous causes of tumor development, it is quite natural to look to parasites, either of animal or vegetable nature, as etiologic possibilities, though up to the present time growths have not been produced experimentally by inoculation nor have bacterial inclusions been demonstrated in cells of new-growths. McCallum[1] believes that bacteria, in order to cause cell growth, must be so included in the growing cells as to multiply with them and accompany them wherever they go, since otherwise it would seem impossible that they could maintain their stimulating effect upon the cells which have been transplanted to distant organs.

Some twenty years ago pathologists believed to have found within the protoplasm of tumor cells bodies which they considered as protozoa. As late as 1913 Rohdenburg[2] expressed the belief that the existence of blastomycetes in malignant tumors could be regarded as certain and irrefutable. However, later observers have proved that the variously described inclusion bodies were due to degenerative changes in the cell protoplasm, and that they bore no etiologic relation to the tumor. Where protozoa were really observed, it subsequently developed that the growths containing them were granulation tissue and not sarcoma.

The incidence of heredity in the development of neoplasms, especially as regards the development of malignant growths, has perhaps received more discussion than any other phase of the subject. Although evidence is accumulating in recent years, based upon experimental study with mice and other lower animals by Dr. Maud Slye and others, indicating that malignant growths can be transmitted by transplantation of tumor cells in animals, and that the several generations following the occurrence of the disease in an animal are prone to develop a like condition, we have as yet no corroborative evidence in the human in which all inoculation efforts have failed. The frequent appearance of similar growths, especially of a malignant type, in different generations of a family, would make it appear to the casual observer that there is quite a family predisposition to tumor formation, yet statistical proof to warrant this belief is wanting, and it is now pretty generally conceded that heredity does not play a notable part in tumor development. As it is practically impossible to obtain complete family histories through more than two or three generations, and as collected figures represent the minimum rather than the maximum of familial growths, there is difficulty in drawing accurate conclusions, hence statistical proof regarding heredity is necessarily unreliable. As evidence of the uncertainty of such statistics, Warthin[3] relates his observations that among 3600 cases of neoplasms of all kinds seen at the University of Michigan from 1895 to 1913, complete family records could be obtained but 13 times. In view of the statistical data indicating an infrequent hereditary tendency to the development of neoplasms, and based upon the great frequency of growths, especially those of a malignant type, it is a reasonable assumption that the cases of tumor producing potentiality in families rather followed the law of chance, and that their development in different members of a family was coincidental.

Melanotic sarcoma (melanoma, melanoblastoma) of the uveal tract represents the most frequent variety of tumors of the eyeball occurring in adults. According to Fuchs' statistics, it occurs in 0.07 per cent., and Wintersteiner in 0.05 per cent. of ophthalmic cases. Most cases are observed between the fortieth and sixtieth years. All reported cases of melanoma of the uveal tract have been primary growths: no instance of such metastatic growths of the eye have been recorded. As far as is known they are always malignant, and they frequently give rise to metastases by way of blood and lymph. They spring from any portion of the tract, but most frequently from the choroid, and are believed by Ribbert[4] and others to be the result of proliferation of the neoblastic cells and a differentiation of many of the cells into pigmented cells or melanoblasts. The cells are of a definite type, usually spindle shaped, and are characterized by the production of pigment within the cytoplasm in the form of granules, varying in color from a light brown to a black. The great majority of sarcomata of the uveal tract are pigmented, though the origin of leukosarcoma in the pigmented coat of the eye is not uncommon. Whereas malignant tumors have been known to occur in the eye even before the time of Hippocrates, little or nothing was known of their pathology until the early part of the twentieth century, when the advent of the microscope opened up a new era in the study of malignant growths. But even with this important adjunct added to our methods of research, the etiology of tumors of the eye is as obscure as it was years ago.

Applying the theories of the cause of tumors to melanoma of the choroid and ciliary body, it would seem that tumors develop in the eye under conditions similar to those which have been thought to influence the development of neoplasms elsewhere, and nothing is definitely known of their specific etiology. Borst,[5] like Cohnheim, believes that during embryonie growth a superfluous and imperfect tissue develops in the uveal coat. He believes that an overproduction of pigment takes place in the misplaced tissue, which predisposes to cell proliferation and to the formation of new-growths. Others[6] believe that some form of inflammation in the uveal tract results in the production of scar tissue, from which the neoplasm takes its origin. Fuchs,[7] who approved this theory, classes these inflammations with the traumatic causes in his count of 11 per cent. of cases among 259 sarcomata of the uveal tract in which he assigned trauma as the cause of uveal growths. If these cases were eliminated, a history of trauma could not be elicited in many instances of tumors of the interior of the eye. The large number of tumors of the uveal tract that have been reported and the infrequent instances in which trauma was assigned as the causative agent and the position of the uvea protected from all kinds of traumatic influences seems to controvert the theory of trauma acting as an exciting cause of the development of eye tumors.

The protected position of the middle coat of the eye would also lend little support to the parasitic theory of tumor development, even as a contributory cause.

As far as our present knowledge goes, there is little evidence of heredity influencing the development of ocular growths. Regarding the influence of heredity on the development of melanoblastoma of the eye, Wintersteiner[8] points out the fact that the entire ophthalmic literature contains but two cases that were suggestive of a hereditary influence in the development of eye tumors. One of these cases, reported by Silcock,[9] which has been frequently quoted, occurred in a girl of twenty years whose eye was removed on account of melanosarcoma of the choroid. Her mother at the same age had one of her eyes removed for the same reason, while her maternal aunt died of a malignant growth of the breast and the maternal grandfather of a melanoma of the choroid. Notwithstanding this pronounced case, Wintersteiner concludes that heredity is not an important factor in the etiology of neoplasms of the eye.

Whether the occurrence of two identical growths springing from the same structure in the eye and developing in brothers at about the same time of life will prove to be of future value in determining the etiology of eye tumors is problematic. For the present it would seem that heredity played no part in their development, and that their occurrence must be looked upon as one of those rare coincidences that are at times encountered in the practice of medicine.

REFERENCES.

1. Text-Book of Pathology, 1921.
2. New York Med. Jour., March, 1913.
3. Arch. Inter. Med., 1913, 546.
4. Ribbert: Ziegler's Beitrag zur Path.-Anat., 1893.
5. Die Lehre v. d. Geschwulsten, 1902.
6. Hauke: Arch. f. Ophth., 1899.
7. Sarcoma d. Uveal-Tractus, Wien, 1892.
8. Wintersteiner: Geschwulste d. Uveal-Tractus, Erg. d. allg. Path., Lubarsch u. Ostertag, 1040.
9. Brit. Med. Jour., 1892, 1079.

REPORT OF A CASE OF PRIMARY TUBULAR EPITHELIOMA OF THE LACRIMAL SAC.

WILLIAM CAMPBELL POSEY, M.D.,
Philadelphia.

About two years ago E. H., at that time aged seventy-four years, who had been under my care for some twenty years or more on account of myopia with increasing choroidal and retinal disturbance, came complaining of lacrimation in the right eye. Examination revealed what appeared to be a small mucocele of the sac, there being nothing unusual in the swelling to excite the suspicion of any complicating condition. Operation was refused, and refused at several subsequent visits, when he returned on account of progressive failure of vision. Upon each of these occasions a marked increase in the size of the swelling was noted, but the swelling was always confined to the region of the sac; the skin, which showed no sign of discoloration, was freely mobile over the sublying mass. There was no pain—nothing to excite the suspicion of any unusual condition. Finally, yielding to the solicitations of members of his family as well as to my own urging, the extirpation of the sac was consented to.

I must confess that notwithstanding the unusual size of the swelling (it now equaled a horse-chestnut in size) the suspicion of it being a neoplasm never occurred to me, for I had upon several occasions removed mucoceles of the sac of the same, if not greater, size, and, moreover, in my entire experience, I had never encountered a tumor of the sac; to be frank, I was but vaguely aware of the reported existence of such growths.

In the extirpation of the sac, by Meller's method, the

anterior surface of the upper portion of the sac ruptured, giving exit to a quantity of thick pus, but a quantity inferior to what might be expected from a sac of such apparently voluminous contents. Further dissection revealed a marked thickening in the walls of the sac, especially below, with a marked rugosity of the mucous membrane lining it, the thickening of the membrane being so pronounced that an unusual degree of polypoid overgrowth was thought of. So far as could be ascertained, the extirpation of the sac was complete and the operation was concluded by the customary sounding and curettage of the lacrimonasal duct. Healing was prompt and uncomplicated.

The closer scrutiny of the sac following its removal at once awoke the suspicion of malignancy, for its walls were now seen to be much thickened, and the mucous membrane lining it to be covered with granulations and polypoid overgrowths more or less characteristic of carcinoma. A pathologic study of the sac was accordingly made and was pronounced by Dr. Holmes, the pathologist of the Bryn Mawr Hospital, in which institution the operation was performed, to be a typical tubular epithelioma of the sac.

The subsequent course of the case has been uneventful. Fearing a recurrence of the growth, Dr. Pancoast* of the University Hospital applied radium tubes to the operated area upon three different occasions, and although two years have passed since the tumor was removed, there has been no recurrence.

In his exhaustive treatise on tumors of the eye Lagrange attests to the rarity of malignant tumors of the sac, citing but four instances of sarcoma of the sac, occurring curiously

* Mr. H. reported April 29, 1919, with a diagnosis of carcinoma of the lacrimal sac of the right eye. We gave him the following treatment: 40 mgm. radium, ½ mm. silver capsule, plus rubber tube, for one hour. We saw him again on May 10, 1919, and decided he must have more treatment. He came in on May 21, 1919, and received 50 mgm. radium, ½ mm. silver capsule, plus rubber tube, for one and one-quarter hours. This was the last time we saw him.

enough in the practice of four Italian ophthalmologists—De Vincentiis, Sgrosso, Moauro, and Silvestri. The report of two cases of epithelioma by Piccoli and Seggel were also cited.

A short synopsis of the notes of two cases of primary tumors of the sac reported by Rollet* is as follows:

Case 1.—Man, aged sixty-five years. Supposed lacrimal tumor of ordinary nature. Sac extirpated and sectioned on account of an abnormal hardness; the cavity was found to be filled with a cancerous mass—an atypical epithelioma.

Case 2.—Female, aged sixty-one years. Small mucocele of sac, which proved to be a sarcomatous polyp.

Both cases presented a concomitant dacryocystitis.

Rollet referred also to a case seen by Bistis, in which the tumor was the size of a small nut. Histologic examination showed a network of investment belonging to the sac proper and transformed into fibrous tissue. The tumor was divided by connective-tissue septa into small islands which contained epithelial cells. Small hemorrhagic areas were also present. A diagnosis was made of carcinoma developing from the epithelial investment of the sac.

We are indebted to Pasetti for the most comprehensive paper upon epithelioma of the sac† which has yet appeared, with a review of some of the cases just referred to, and the report of one additional. This case, occurring in a male aged seventy-three years, had many of the characteristics that I have reported, the tumor appearing as an enlargement of the sac the size of a small nut, with the overlying skin normal and readily movable over the mass, which was of hard consistency, without any sensation of fluctuation. Upon section after its extirpation the tumor appeared dense, without trace of the cavity of the sac, except in its central portion, where upon pressure there was noticed a slight purulent secretion. Pasetti goes into the minutiæ of the histologic

* Arch. d'opht., June, 1906.　　　　　† Ann. Di Ott., xlii, 42, 55.

examination of his own and other reported cases, and concludes as follows:

"From what we were able to learn from these few observations of epithelioma of the lacrimal sac, all have been made up of cylindric cells. All have exhibited marked malignancy. The commencement is insidious, without the appearance of subjective symptoms different from those caused by a harmless chronic dacryocystitis or from a simple stenosis of the lacrimal apparatus. Recurrence is frequent."

Pasetti asserts that the experience derived from these cases should be of great importance in daily practice, for although tumors of the sac are rare, the surgeon should always have the possibility of their occurrence in mind, and should advise extirpation in all suspected cases, rather than other forms of operative procedure. Despite apparent complete removal, recurrences are not uncommon.

An interesting case of epithelioma of the sac cured by Roentgen-rays was reported by Guibert and Gueriteau.* The growth had appeared primarily as a pimple at the root of the nose of a man fifty-six years of age, some fifteen years before consultation, but at the time of observation by the authors had broken down, the anterior wall of the sac having been entirely destroyed by the ulceration, so that "the sac became wide open in front," the resulting excavation being the size of a large kidney bean. Eight x-ray treatments were applied over a period of four months, and a complete cure attained. The radiographer in charge of the case notes that improvement was only attained after fairly intense radiodermatitis had been produced, and he states that although the general trend of opinion is very strong against the production of radiodermatitis, it is his own belief that improvement can only occur after fairly severe burns of this nature.

* Clin. Opht., March 10, 1905.

GLIOMA RETINÆ TREATED BY X-RAYS, WITH APPARENT DESTRUCTION OF THE TUMOR AND PRESERVATION OF NORMAL VISION.*

F. H. VERHOEFF, M.D.,
Boston, Mass.

The first attempt to treat a glioma retinæ† by radiation was made in 1914 by Axenfeld,[1] who employed x-rays and mesothorium. The result at first seemed successful, although a cataract developed which required operation, but recurrence of the growth took place within three years after the beginning of the treatment, and the eye was enucleated. Subsequently other unsuccessful attempts have been reported by Kusama[2] (3 cases), Janeway[3] (2 cases), Knapp[4] (1 case).

In each of Kusama's cases both eyes were in the second stage, and were treated by exposures to x-rays and radium. Shrinkage of all six tumors took place, accompanied by shrinkage of the eyeballs. Death from metastases occurred in each case—one in eleven months, another in eighteen months, and in the other case in twenty-seven months, after the beginning of the treatment. In two cases there were general metastases, while in the other the patient died with symptoms of intracranial involvement. Kusama believed that the phthisis bulbi was due to direct action of the radiation upon the eye, but to me it seems possible, if not probable, that it was secondary to degenerative changes in the tumor,

---

* From the Massachusetts Charitable Eye and Ear Infirmary.

† The term glioma retinæ is a misnomer, because these tumors never produce neuroglia, and are highly malignant, but it is so commonly employed that any other term would lead to confusion.

for it is well known that glioma retinæ may undergo extreme necrosis, and thus cause degenerative changes in the eye, and even marked phthisis bulbi. I have examined microscopically the eye from such a case, reported by Dr. T. O'Connor.[5] Kusama concluded that in his cases the treatment by radiation hastened the occurrence of general metastases. This conclusion also seems doubtful to me, because, disregarding the effects of the radiation, the chances of general metastases occurring were enhanced by the facts that the cases were bilateral and none of the eyes was enucleated.

Janeway treated six cases of glioma retinæ with radium. Two cases were later reported in detail,—one by Schoenberg and the other by Knapp,—while two others could not be followed. In the two remaining cases, which were in advanced stages, no improvement followed the treatment.

In Knapp's case a glioma was discovered in the second eye four and a half years after removal of the first. The tumor consisted of two main masses and was of considerable size. Treatment with radium was followed by temporary improvement, but after six months the tumor began to enlarge and the eye was ultimately enucleated. Neither of the eyes in this case was examined microscopically.

Duncan[6] treated with radium recurrences in the orbit after enucleation in three unilateral cases with apparent success, although eighteen months was the longest period of observation.

Up to the present only two cases have been reported in which an eye containing a glioma retinæ has been treated with radiation with apparent success. In Hilgartner's case (cited by Schoenberg[7]) the right eye was completely filled up with the growth, while the other contained only a small growth. After eighty-four exposures to x-rays the right eye shrunk and the growth in the left eye resorbed. In Schoenberg's[7] case, the second eye was treated with radium three times in twenty-six months, beginning three weeks after removal of the first eye. The tumor in the second eye consisted of a grayish-white mass occupying an area a little larger than the lower nasal quadrant of the eye-ground, and a smaller grayish mass, 4–6 P.D. in size, in the upper part of the fundus. As the result of the treatment the tumor underwent retrogressive changes, but it is not stated that it became reduced in size. At the end of three and a quarter years after beginning treatment the patient had vision of 20/100 and the glioma appeared as a "degenerated, necrosed mass." A posterior cortical cataract was observed at the end of two and a half years.

In the following case that I have to report the tumor was much smaller than any other yet treated by radiation, and the result at the present time, over three years after the treatment was begun, is remarkably successful.

CASE.—Harry G., aged seventeen months, was referred to me by Dr. John Kerrigan on November 22, 1917. One week previous the mother had observed a white reflex from the pupil. Two brothers, aged twelve and eight, and a sister aged six, had normal eyes, and the family history was otherwise negative. On examination the right eye showed a typical picture of glioma retinæ at the end of the first stage—shallow anterior chamber, dilated pupil, moderate increase in tension, and a vascularized, yellowish-white mass in contact with the posterior surface of the lens. The left eye appeared to be normal, but without general anesthesia a satisfactory ophthalmoscopic examination could not be made. Immediate enucleation of the right eye was advised, to be followed by x-ray treatment of the right orbit and careful observation of the left eye.

November 24, 1917, the right eye was removed by Dr. Kerrigan and sent to me for pathologic examination. Soon afterward the right orbit was given five severe x-ray treatments by Dr. William Liebman at the Massachusetts Charitable Eye and Ear Infirmary.

May 2, 1918, the patient was again referred to me by Dr.

Kerrigan for observation. I now found in the retina of the left eye in the lower outer quadrant a white, opaque, elevated mass, irregularly oval in shape, and about 4 P.D. in greatest diameter. It did not reach to the limit of the ophthalmoscopic field. Near this mass, but entirely separate from it, were two small white spots, each about ¼ P.D. in size. The patient was immediately referred to Dr. Liebman for *x*-ray treatment of the left eye, with instruction for suberythema dosage to be employed and the exposures to be made through a perforated lead plate so as to protect the lens and anterior part of the eye. Dr. Liebman gave the first treatment on the same day, a suberythema dose through a 5 mm. aluminum filter. After this, similar treatment was given once a week for three weeks, and on June 6, June 27, August 1, November 1, 1918, and on January 17, 1919.

The patient was seen by me at intervals of one or two months, but without general anesthesia it was impossible to make a careful study of the ophthalmoscopic appearances, only glimpses of the tumor, as a rule, being obtained. On May 23, 1918, I noted that the tumor appeared less white. On August 1, the tumor appeared translucent and smaller in size. October 19, 1919, the patient was examined under ether narcosis. The tumor appeared translucent, somewhat smaller and less elevated. The white spots near it had completely disappeared. April 4, 1921, a good view of the tumor was obtained. It appeared only slightly elevated, gray, and translucent, and somewhat smaller than the original tumor. Its outline was fairly sharp in places, but not easily seen. No traces of the white spots could be found. A few small vessels traversed it. The retinal vessels became extremely tortuous as they approached the tumor.

On June 8, 1921, another good view of the tumor was obtained. This time there was seen, just below its center, a circular depressed area, about ⅓ P.D. in size, slightly pink in color in contrast to the rest of the tumor. Its margin was sharply defined. My attention was called to this area by Dr. Schoenberg, who examined the patient with me on this date. No doubt I had previously overlooked it. It suggested to me a shallow hole in the tumor, perhaps due to rupture of the retinal surface at some time. There was no pigmentation either within or around the tumor. The lens was still clear, and the vitreous remained free from opacities. Owing to the youth of the patient it was impossible to obtain an accurate idea of the visual acuity, but by the use of a chart with pictures it was determined as certainly better than 20/30. The mother said that, according to her observation, the vision of the child was excellent. Since the macula was uninvolved there is no reason to believe that the child's vision was not perfectly normal.

PATHOLOGIC EXAMINATION OF RIGHT EYE.

No. 3403. The globe is normal in size and shape. On section, after fixation in 10 per cent. formalin, the retina is found to be completely separated by serous coagulum and to inclose a tumor mass which takes up about three-quarters of the globe. The tumor extends from the optic disc to the posterior surface of the lens, to which it is closely applied. It thus completely replaces the vitreous body. The anterior chamber is shallow, but not obliterated.

Microscopic Examination.—The tumor is found to be a typical so-called glioma retinæ. Perivascular arrangement of the tumor cells is well marked, and the occurrence of intervening areas of necrosis is, as usual, a conspicuous feature. Some of the areas of necrosis show calcification. Typical rosettes are extremely abundant in almost every portion of the tumor. The cells not taking part in the rosette formations have round, ovoid, or pear-shaped nuclei, and often show indistinct bipolar processes. Cells in mitosis are numerous. On one side the tumor has entirely destroyed the retina, and on the other side it is in contact with the latter and in places has invaded or penetrated it. The tumor extends up to, but has not invaded, the optic disc or nerve. Small metastatic nodules of tumor cells are found on the surface of the pigment epithelium, and on both surfaces of the retina, where the latter is reflected over the ciliary body and has not yet been invaded by direct extension of the growth. No nodules are found in the anterior chamber or in the iris. The growth is nowhere in direct contact with the choroid and has not invaded the latter either by direct extension or metastases.

The ciliary body is compressed by the retina. There is no peripheral anterior synechia. The iris, cornea, and lens are normal.

Pathologic Diagnosis.—So-called glioma retinæ endophytum.

REMARKS.—While the tumor in the right eye was comparatively large, and had given rise to intra-ocular metastases, it had not invaded the optic nerve or choroid, so that the probability of a recurrence in the orbit was less than is often the case. It is, therefore, impossible to say whether or not the absence of tumor recurrence in the orbit was due to the x-ray treatment.

That the tumor found in the left eye was also a so-called glioma there can be no doubt. It was certainly not an inflammatory condition, because it was not associated with vitreous opacities or other evidence of inflammation, and there is no other known non-inflammatory condition of the retina which resembles it. The treatment with x-ray caused little apparent reduction in size of the main tumor, but did cause complete disappearance of the two small white nodules situated near it. It also caused a marked change in the appearance of the main tumor, the latter losing its original opaque white appearance and becoming gray and translucent.

In Axenfeld's case, in which, for a time, the treatment was regarded as successful, and also in Schoenberg's case, cataract developed, while in my case the lens has remained perfectly clear.

In my case the lens was carefully protected from exposure by means of a lead plate. The situation of the tumor just behind the equator in the lower outer quadrant rendered this an easy matter, but it would seem that in any case in which the tumor could be recognized with the ophthalmoscope and in which there was still useful vision, it should be possible to make the exposure through the sclera, first on one side and then the other, and thus avoid possible injury to the lens. I am not, however, convinced that the cataracts in the cases of Axenfeld and Schoenberg were certainly due to radiation, because it seems possible that they might have resulted from toxins given off by the necrosed tumor masses. It is, of course, well known that all degenerative conditions affecting the posterior part of the globe are apt to cause posterior cortical cataract.

While in my case the results of the treatment have thus far been remarkably successful, it is possible the growth may yet resume its activity, or that another tumor may develop. In this connection Maghy's[3] case of bilateral glioma, in which the second eye did not become obviously involved until the patient reached the age of fifteen years, is suggestive. As Knapp points out, a few cases of bilateral glioma have been recorded in which a small tumor in the second eye has undergone retrogression, with preservation of vision, but these are so exceedingly rare that they scarcely need to be taken into account.

Judging by the large number of cases of glioma retinæ that have now been unsuccessfully treated by radiation, it may seem that this form of treatment does not offer much hope of success. It is to be noted, however, that the tumors in these cases were all large, whereas in Schoenberg's case, and especially in my case, the tumor was very small.

The results so far obtained, therefore, seem to render unjustifiable attempts to treat an eye by this means when the tumor is so large that useful vision cannot be expected. It is possible that even a relatively small tumor, if rendered completely necrotic by the radiation, would cause degenerative changes in the eye, which would ultimately destroy all of its vision. As a matter of fact, a child affected with retinal glioma is practically never brought to the ophthalmologist until in one eye at least the tumor is so far advanced that immediate enucleation is imperative. In general, therefore, treatment of retinal glioma by radiation must be restricted to the second eye, after removal of the first, and to the after-treatment of the socket to prevent recurrences.

At the time of the enucleation of the first eye advantage should always be taken of the ether narcosis to make a thorough ophthalmoscopic examination of the other eye.

REFERENCES.

1. Axenfeld: Doppleseitiges Glioma Retinæ und intraocular Strahlentherapie, Klin. M. f. Augenh., 1914, 426. Also Deutsch. Ophth. Gesellsch., Heidelberg, 1919.
2. Kusama: The *x*-ray Treatment of Retinal Glioma, Amer. Jour. Ophth., 1919, 636.
3. Janeway: The Therapeutic Use of Radium in Diseases of the Eye, Arch. Ophth., 1920, 163.
4. Knapp: Bilateral Glioma. Report of a Case Unsuccessfully Treated with Radium, Trans. Amer. Ophth. Soc., 1920, 207.
5. O'Connor: Glioma Retinæ and Atrophia Bulbi, Arch. Ophth., 1917, 312.
6. Duncan: Glioma of Retina with Report of Three Cases Treated with Radium, Amer. Jour. Ophth., 1918, 715.
7. Schoenberg: A Case of Bilateral Glioma of Retina Apparently Arrested in the Non-enucleated Eye, Arch. Ophth., 1919, 485.
8. Maghy: Bilateral Glioma of Retina. Second Eye Excised After Interval of Nearly Eighteen Years. Brit. Jour. Ophth., 1919, 337.

THE USE OF RADIUM PLUGS IN THE DISSOLUTION OF ORBITAL GLIOMATOUS MASSES DEVELOPING AFTER EXCISION OF THE GLOBE.

BURTON CHANCE, M.D.,
Philadelphia.

At the meeting of this Society, in June, 1920, in commenting on the reports of cases of bilateral glioma, I cited an instance of that malady occurring in a child under three years of age who was succumbing, appaiently, to the effects of the disease. The case was spoken of then because it was my desire to record an instance of the bilateral manifestation of the affection, and because it was feared the little sufferer could not survive, even until I could visit him again, and therefore no further note of his case might be made. The child is alive to-day; in the autumn I excised his two eyes. Following the excision of the left globe the orbit became filled with a tumor mass. The orbit is now empty, and it is the manner by which the orbit was relieved, especially, that I desire to speak.

In August the profoundly cachectic child was brought to me suffering much pain, the two eyes being filled with the yellowish masses so commonly seen, which, by the middle of September, seemed ready to burst the globes. At the middle of October the enormously distended right globe protruded between the lids. It had ruptured, and, projecting through the anterior segment, was a dove-colored granular and pultaceous mass which became blood stained at the slightest touch. Not until November 3 would the parents give consent for the removal of the globe; they could no longer endure his agonized crying, and I was entreated to relieve the child. The eye was excised the next day.

The globe was freely movable; the tumor mass seemed not to have perforated the sclera, although there was a small heaping of tissues, as though a mass were surrounding the nerve for a few millimeters up to the line of the cut across the nerve-trunk. The orbit proved to be quite free from nodules, and although for several days the lids were blood-stained and edematous, a clean, healthy socket has resulted. In the meantime the progress of the disease in the left had begun to distend the lids and the globe protruded through the fissure. I expected, or at least hoped for, rupture of the anterior segment of the globe, as had happened in the right. But on November 20 the whole orbital swelling suddenly subsided, and the globe positively sunk into the depth of the orbit—it was clear that it had ruptured posteriorly. By November 25 the contents had begun to distend the globe again; already the intra-ocular growth had pushed the lens forward, abolishing the anterior chamber, and the orbit and the lids were edematous.

On November 27 this globe was removed, but with difficulty, because of nodular enlargement. An examination showed that masses extended from protrusions through the sclera which had burst out at the temporal aspect of the globe and filled the apex of the orbit. The nerve did not seem to be involved, as was apparently the case with the right eye, although the stalk was edematous and thick.

The reaction which followed was severe; the lids continued

ecchymotic and edematous for ten days, yet after the excision, the vitality of the child revived remarkably. Almost immediately he became stronger, his skin pliant, his hair glossy, his cheeks plump and rosy, and he had ceased his fitful crying.

His case went along uneventfully until about the middle of January, 1921, when it was discovered that the left orbit was filling up. Early in February the mass extended beyond the ridges, pushing the lids forward. On the tenth I requested Dr. W. L. Clark to employ radium for the dissolution of the mass, in the manner I had known him to have used in neoplastic growths which were unfit for surgical excision, as I did not wish to attempt the exenteration of the orbit. Into the mass on the left he inserted deeply nine large plugs, or "needles," containing radium, and, into the presumably unaffected tissues on the right, as a matter of precaution, he inserted five smaller and one large needle. These were retained for twenty hours. On the twelfth of February the child was taken home from the hospital, as he could be cared for well enough at home.

The immediate reaction was intense. There was distinct erythema of all the lids, which lasted a number of days. For several weeks the lids on the left were puffed; a more or less ichorous discharge, which at no time was ever offensive, came from the left orbit; yet while the right lids were much irritated, there was no discharge from that orbit. By May 1 the swelling of the lids of the right had subsided entirely, and the socket appeared to be free from any irritation; the left were still faintly edematous, and a thin discharge continued to flow; the cavity, however, was as deep as that of the right. In neither cavity is there now anything unusual; the mucous surfaces have assumed the smoothness commonly supervening on the healing after excision of the globe. There appeared to have been only a dissolution; or, might one speak of it as an involution of the orbital mass? Once the child was brought because of great distention of the lids which had been caused by the retention of the fluid, which immediately subsided when drainage was reëstablished by the daily separation of the lids and the more frequent use of lotions.

There have been thus far no signs of metastases. The

cervical; the parotid, and the submaxillary glands are not enlarged, indurated, nor painful.

The child has gained in weight and grown in height. His intelligence and interest in his toys and play and in the events of the day as read to him out of the newspaper by his father evince a somewhat extraordinary precocity. He has an elder brother and a sister, and a younger sister, born since he came under my observation; the eyes of all are healthy.

I regret that I cannot make a report of the pathologic study of the excised globes. On the day a few sections were cut of one segment of the right globe, the specimens were lost in the laboratory. A week ago one-half of each globe was recovered, too late for me to prepare them for exhibition. The stained sections show typical glioma-cells, with numerous rosettes in the fields.

The plugs, or "needles," as they are called, which were used are hollow, non-corrosive, nickel steel cases, each 20 to 25 mm. long and 2 mm. thick, roundish, with a tapering point, and an "eye" through which thread can be passed and knotted for easy withdrawal and to prevent loss of the costly implement. Each contained 10 mgm. of radium sulphate, a half mm. space existing between the radium and the casing. The parts of the implement are carefully welded and polished, so that no leaking nor corrosion with resultant loss of the radium can occur. Broken "eyes" can be replaced without damage to the radium.

The needles were forcibly inserted their full length directly into the soft tissues, separated a few millimeters from each other, and one transfixed the mass. A special forceps-like applicator was used, although a small pointed hemostat might have served.

Radium emanations were employed in this manner a few years ago, but their use was abandoned because of the uncertainty of their power and the violence of their effects. It is well known that there are present in the radium substance particles which emit what are called beta-rays and others which send out gamma-rays, and on living tissues these different rays have different effects. And further, there are variations in the powers of the qualities of the individual classes of rays. The hardest of the gamma rays are very penetrating, and they exert a powerful action on malignant cells, while the softer rays are effective where slow, prolonged cell inhibition is desired. The difficulties attending the use of radium in metal containers have been greatly overcome by the composition of the metal employed in the hollow slender plugs which Dr. Clark has used for a number of practitioners in Philadelphia. These, as already stated, are composed of nickel steel, which besides being non-corrosive, filters out the harder and the more deeply penetrative rays.

By the deep insertion of these "needles," containing from 5 to 10 mgm. of radium sulphate, into malignant growths such as the orbital masses spoken of in this report, the actions are more efficacious than can be obtained by capsules or plaques. The emanations can be used more accurately, and in a smaller quantity than by the employment of a larger quantity applied to the outside or inserted in capsule form into the tissues through an incision. Moreover, in the use of such metallic needles the entire quantity of radium is utilized in the tissues, whereas when radium is applied from the outside in capsules or plaques, more than one-half of the radioactivity is dissipated in the air.

It has been the experience of all of us frequently to find rapid proliferation and metastasis after surgical removal of masses in the orbit following excision of a gliomatous globe. I have not seen a child recover, nor one live so long as this child has when the orbit had been invaded; and in my experience wide extension of the disease and painful death only too soon have always followed exenteration of the orbital cavity.

This history is not in any way more striking than what, perhaps, might have been repeated in the experience of any one of the Fellows of this Society. I have used the details only as a text upon which to build up a plea for the prompt employment of a remedy which can be used with every hope that the extension of so deadly a disease as that which follows the proliferation of the neuroepitheliomata shall be checked.

DISCUSSION OF PAPERS OF DRS. VERHOEFF AND CHANCE.

DR. E. TERRY SMITH, Hartford, Conn.: We have been fortunate in Hartford in having radium at our disposal for many years. Dr. Heublein has acquired a large amount of this substance, and has been liberal in allowing us to have it for the treatment of poor patients as well as for those who can pay. The most satisfactory way I have ever seen radium used in tumor masses is in the form of emanations. The dosage can be accurately ascertained, and the applications made exactly where wanted with little discomfort to the patient. About eight months ago I saw a child with a large round-cell sarcoma of the orbit. We first applied pre-operative radiations, and at the end of three weeks eviscerated the orbit. At the time of operation the tumor had already penetrated the antrum. Four weeks after the operation the tumor had recurred, and emanations of radium were injected. These emanations are contained in a small glass pearl which is applied to the end of a hollow needle. The needle penetrates the mass, and when you reach the spot where you want to leave the emanations you press a little thumb plug and the emanations are ejected into the mass. It is entirely painless, and the reaction is no greater than when radium is directly applied. In my experience it is exactly the same. The emanations produce the same result as the radium. The applications last eight, ten, or twenty-four hours, depending upon the amount of capsule emanations. In the case mentioned, the tumor of the orbit promptly disappeared, but the child died in a few months from secondary involvement, as these cases usually do. I have had the opportunity to see the radium applied directly to tumors and to see the emanations tried in smaller tumors. The results are very much more satisfactory when the emanations are used, and the reaction is no greater than with the direct application of the radium.

DR. VERHOEFF (closing): In the paper I did not discuss the question of which is preferable in the treatment of tumors, x-rays or radium. I think it is pretty well established that the actions of x-rays and radium are exactly the same. Radium has the advantage only when the tumor is relatively inaccessible, for instance, when it is in the orbit. In this case I do not believe radium would have been nearly as successful. Radium as generally used requires very long exposures, while the x-ray treatment required only about five minutes each time. If you get the dosage right, the x-ray will achieve the same result as radium. Of course, there is a certain fascination about radium, and I think a great many are inclined to overlook the fact that the x-ray will do just as well.

COATS' DISEASE OF THE RETINA.
REPORT OF TWO CASES.

A. EDWARD DAVIS, A.M., M.D.,

New York.

The two cases represent two types of massive exudation into the retina: (1) With extensive vascular changes; (2) without extensive vascular changes. A brief review of the etiology and treatment of the disease is given.

CASE 1.—Leonard L., aged ten years, came to the clinic at the Post-Graduate Hospital September 18, 1920. Father and mother living and in good health. Family history negative. The first knowledge of any trouble was when the school physician reported the right eye defective in December, 1919. The right eye diverged and the patient was advised to have it straightened. The eye has never pained or been inflamed. The patient has had measles, whooping-cough, scarlet fever, and has had swollen glands removed from the neck. At the present time he is in perfect health, excepting the eye trouble. V.R.E., 4/200 eccentric; L.E., 20/30 with + .75 cyl. ax. 75° = 20/20.

Ophthalmoscope: The left eye is normal. In the right fundus there is a large mass of white exudate, yellowish in some spots, under the retina, extending from the temporal half of the optic disc, upon which it encroaches, to the extreme periphery of the temporal half of the fundus. The highest point of this mass measures plus 8.00 D. about 1½ disc-widths to the temporal side of the disc. There are numerous hemorrhages on the surface of the mass near the macula, especially to the temporal side; some of the vessels are dilated into a fusiform shape, as described by Coats in certain cases.

There are numerous cholesterin crystals scattered throughout the mass, especially frequent at the lower and upper margins of the exudate. There are also several round pigment spots in the mass, from 1 to 3 mm. in diameter. (As seen by the ophthalmoscope.) The exudate is about 3 disc-widths wide at its broadest part near the macula. There are no light-streaks on the retinal vessels which run over the mass. One of the unusual features in this case is that one of the retinal vessels is veiled over a short distance in the lower portion of the mass. The vitreous and anterior portions of the eye are clear. The pupils are normal in size and reaction.

The von Pirquet test was positive; this was confirmed a week later by a subcutaneous injection of 1 mgm. of O. T., which was followed by a marked reaction—local, focal, and general. The arm was swollen and red, the vision more clouded, and a decided rise in temperature occurred. The patient was placed on therapeutic doses of O. T., beginning with a 2 minim O. T. (H. K. Mulford) Vial No. 1 (1/1000 mgm.), and gradually increased 2 minims a dose, at week intervals, until 14 minims of Vial No. 1 (7/1000 mgm.) was reached, when the patient had a severe local and general reaction, pains in the stomach, legs, and back, great *malaise*, temperature 101° F. The arm was sore and swollen, but no focal reaction, either subjective or objective, was manifested.

The injections were discontinued for a few weeks and then begun again with a 1/1000 mgm. O. T., and gradually increased as before, until the dose (April 9, 1921) had reached 16 minims of Vial No. 2 (8/100 mgm.) without reactions of any kind. However, on April 9, 16, and 23, the Schick test was given the patient by his school physician, and immediately following this Schick test the eye became slightly red, numerous retinal hemorrhages occurred, the retinal exudate was increased, and the temperature rose to 102° F. Needless to say, all T.B. injections were discontinued. The patient, who had gained eight pounds under the tuberculin treatment, lost three pounds following the Schick tests.

After an interval of three weeks, when the temperature was again normal, the eye white and the retinal hemorrhages absorbing, the O. T. injections were again resumed, beginning with 1/1000 mgm., and this has been carried up gradually to 10 minims (5/1000 mgm.) without reactions. The patient has regained the three pounds lost following the Schick test and is feeling well.

An examination of the fundus (June 10, one month after the first Schick injection) shows the mass of exudate subsiding, the retinal hemorrhages almost cleared, and the eye quiet. Figure 1.

CASE 2.—Molly K., aged nineteen years. First seen September 29, 1920, when her temperature by mouth was 99.2° F. In the last few days the patient noticed that she cannot see well. Family history negative and the patient seemingly in perfect health.

Ophthalmoscopic appearance of the left eye is entirely normal, as are also the cornea, iris, and ciliary body. Right eye: In the temporal half of the fundus the retina is elevated by a whitish, yellowish mass, plus 2.00 D. at the highest point. This mass extends from near the optic disc to the extreme periphery of the fundus, as far as can be seen with the ophthalmoscope. It is about 3 disc-widths at its broadest point, near the macula, which area is affected.

The retinal blood-vessels are normal, except perhaps for almost complete disappearance of the light-streak on the vessels that run on the mass. There are no hemorrhages or cholesterin crystals. Eccentric vision to the temporal side. A large central oval scotoma corresponds to the mass of exudation under the retina. (Fig. 2.)

This patient did not return to the clinic, but we trust she came under other care and will be reported. She gave an assumed name (Molly Kron) and a false address, as we found out when we tried to follow up the case. Wassermann was negative.

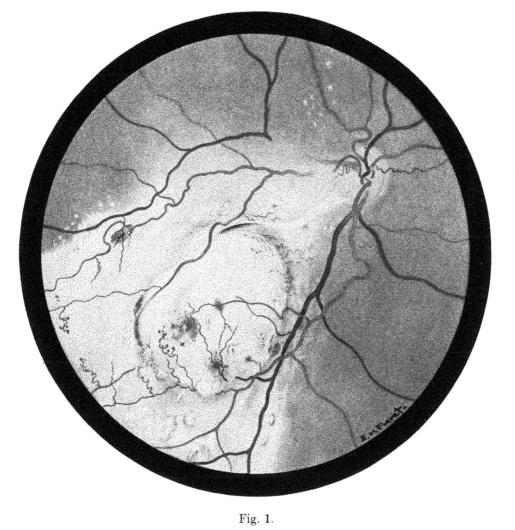

Fig. 1.

There is one feature in each of these cases that heretofore has not been noted, as far as I can find out from the literature, that is, the absence of the light-streak on the retinal vessels over the massive exudate, or, if present, the streak is but very faintly to be seen and then only where the exudate

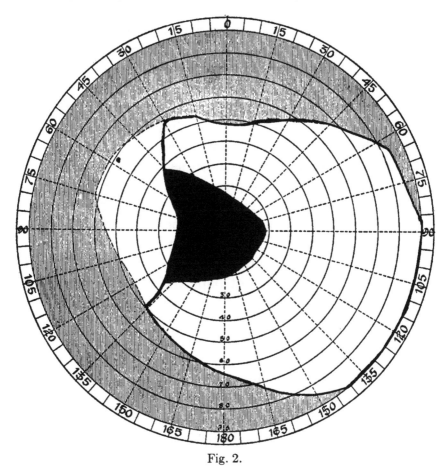

Fig. 2.

is shallow. This corresponds to cases of ordinary marked detachment of the retina where no light-streak is seen upon the retinal vessels; and incidentally it goes to confirm the theory that the light-streak produced on the retinal vessels is due to refraction, and not to the reflection of light, a point

15

that both Loring and myself contended for many years and in which I confirmed the experiments of Loring by vivisection in deciding that refraction and not reflection was the cause of the light-streak as seen upon the retinal vessels.

Another feature unusual in these cases was veiling of one of the retinal vessels in the lower part of the mass in Case 1. Coats claims that this is a very rare condition. The tension in each of these cases here observed was normal.

Coats in 1909 and again in 1911 reported a number of such cases and classified them into two groups: (1) Those without gross vascular changes; and (2) those with gross vascular changes. A third group which he included in his first series of cases, where there were arteriovenous communications, he excluded in his second classification as he came to the conclusion that they should be placed in a separate group and regarded as cases of "angiomatosis" (as described by v. Hippel). No hard and fast rules can be followed in classifying these cases of massive exudation into the retina, as there are many modifications, with probably varying etiology and pathology. Holm[1] in a recent paper (1917) on the subject, "Exudative Retinitis," reports ten cases, with two excellent colored plates and seventeen illustrations. Holm, as does Coats, notes a relationship to retinitis circinata, and Jervey,[2] who reports four cases of hyperplastic exudative retinitis (non-hæmorrhagica), suggests that with these cases (exudative retinitis) it would seem proper to classify, clinically, those conditions of exudative, non-hemorrhagic retinitis which are typified by the so-called retinitis proliferans of non-hemorrhagic origin, and the hyperplastic retinitis of syphilitic and traumatic origin which are not of hemorrhagic formation. Holm cites the investigations of Goldzier and Fuchs on retinitis circinata, as early as 1893, and also notes the papers of v. Hippel, 1905; Coats, 1909 and 1911, and Leber's paper of 1915, the last-named author citing 61 cases from the literature up to that date, 1915.

Etiology.—In most cases, as pointed out by Coats and others, the cause is quite obscure. The family and personal history, as a rule, throw but little light on the subject. Syphilis has been excluded in most cases. Tuberculosis is undoubtedly at the bottom of some cases. The pathologic reports, except for showing that the retina is chiefly affected and that the choroid is not affected, or only in the slightest degree, have not materially aided in clearing up the etiology.

Hajano[3] reports the history of a case occurring in a child of two years of age. In this a glioma was suspected and the eye removed. From the pathologic report he considered that the primary lesion was an arteriosclerosis, even in a child of so tender age.

E. von Hippel[4] referred to a patient forty-nine years of age in which the choroid was involved. In this case the tuberculin and Wassermann tests were negative. The eye came to section, and the presence of recent round-cell infiltration showed that the process was distinctly inflammatory and not due solely to the organization of retinal hemorrhages.

The consensus of opinion, however, is that the disease is a degenerative process and not inflammatory. Holm, in his excellent paper, quoted above, states that the etiology and pathogenesis are quite unknown. Coats claims that it is due to subretinal hemorrhages, while Leber maintains it is a degenerative process affecting the retina and pigment cells, with serofibrous exudation. Coats' idea was that it was a local vascular disease, but to what the hemorrhages were due was in doubt.

Pathologic reports of such cases are extremely rare. Dr. L. W. Crigler, of New York, has been fortunate enough to secure the eye in one case for microscopic examination because of secondary glaucoma. His case differed materially from those described by Coats in that there was very slight deposition of connective tissue beneath the retina, with a progressive atrophy of its inner layers. A coagulum filled the space between the retina and the choroid, in which there were deposits of cholesterin and clouds of "ghost cells." In every other respect the case presented the identical changes described by Coats, classified under Group 2.

Treatment: As the etiology is usually doubtful, the treatment is more or less empirical and unsatisfactory.

The first case here presented had a negative history, and the physical examination revealed nothing abnormal, no clinical symptoms outside of the eye being manifested. He reacted sharply to the diagnostic tuberculin tests, however, both the von Pirquet and the subcutaneous, also to the therapeutic doses of tuberculin. The patient is still under tuberculin treatment, gaining weight, and the eye has steadily gained, as shown by the steady shrinkage of the mass of exudation and the absorption of the hemorrhages; except at the time of the Schick test, which latter caused an acute exacerbation of the trouble.

Differential Diagnosis.—Such cases may be confused with tubercle of the choroid or with pseudoglioma; however, I think myself that careful study of the case, with diagnostic tuberculin tests, that tuberculosis of the choroid should be differentiated. Although, it is possible, in a conglomerate tubercle of the choroid, to be mistaken in the diagnosis.

Pseudoglioma: Here there is a history of exanthemata, and, furthermore, there are always masses of exudation *into the vitreous,* together with mild inflammation of the anterior portion of the eye, usually a circumcorneal flush, which would easily distinguish it from the massive exudate under the retina. In the milder cases of this trouble, Coats' disease, the patients may go for years without any active trouble whatsoever, conditions becoming quiescent. On the other hand, in those cases with vascular changes, retinitis proliferans may supervene, with detachment of the retina, and not infrequently there is a secondary glaucoma and iritis, which may necessitate the removal of the eye.

REFERENCES.

1. Klin. M. f. Augenh., v, 1917, p. 319, et seq.
2. Amer. Jour. Ophth., February, 1919, 127.
3. Cited in Amer. Encyclopedia of Ophthalmology, 11354.
4. Cited in Amer. Encyclopedia of Ophthalmology, xv, 11354.

DISCUSSION.

DR. WILLIAM ZENTMAYER, Philadelphia: Just one point in reference to the differential diagnosis. In cases I have seen, and most of those reported in literature, the presence of cholesterin in Coats' disease is of value in differential diagnosis.

DR. DAVIS (closing): In extenuation I would say that I did not attempt to put in all the literature. I simply reported two cases, and I supposed we were all familiar with the literature of these cases. I recited incidentally Dr. Crigler's case in New York because the eye had come to section.

LIPÆMIA RETINALIS.

WM. F. HARDY, M.D.,
St. Louis, Mo.

The following history is placed on record for two reasons, first, because there are but few authentic cases of lipæmia retinalis in recorded literature, and second, because a complete metabolic study was made which I believe has not been done before.*

The first case of lipæmia retinalis was reported by Heyl before this Society in 1880, under the title of "Intra-ocular Lipæmia." Reports then followed by Hale White, 1903; Fraser, 1903; Reis, 1903; Turney and Dudgeon, 1906; Heine, 1906; Hertel, 1909; Köllner, 1912; Darling, 1912; Foster Moore, 1915 (two cases); Cohen, 1921; and the present report. Lipemia, as has been pointed out by others, occurs in

* This was written before Martin Cohen's report of a case of lipæmia retinalis with hypotony.

pregnancy, chronic alcoholism, diseases of the liver, nephritis, malaria, tuberculosis, cholera, and phosphorus-poisoning. The most marked instances are met, however, in diabetes. Lipemia in diabetes is an old observation, having been noted by Mariet, of Edinburgh, in 1799. Fat in normal blood varies from 1.00 to 3.25 parts per 1000 of blood. Hoppe-Seyler advanced the idea that lipemia in diabetes represented a physiologic phenomenon due to the fact that digestion is continuous, the result of abnormal ingestion of food. This has been disproved by Nanyu and by Ebstein. Lipemia above the normal limits is now generally looked upon as a pathologic process. The amount of blood fat present before lipæmia retinalis can be observed must be considerable— most probably in the neighborhood of 10 per cent. In Fraser's case it amounted to 16.5 per cent.; in Reis' case, 18.1 per cent.; and in Köllner's case, to 26.25 per cent., with 2.16 per cent. of cholesterin. These high figures must be accepted with some mental reservation. A pathologic lipemia is not rare in diabetes; in fact, all the severe cases show an increased fat content in the blood.

Hale White does not think lipæmia retinalis is extremely rare. In the report of his case he stated that he knew of at least one other patient in Guy's Hospital in which this condition was observed. This is not the opinion of others, and many keen observers have never met with a single case. A search through the Index Medicus, from Foster Moore's report in 1915 to the present, did not reveal any reference.

E. C., white, male, aged twenty-nine years, entered Barnes Hospital February 9, 1921.

History: He complained of an eruption over the arms and legs, especially at the joints; some weakness and polyuria and loss of weight.

Family History: Negative.

Past History: Curvature of spine present since two years of age. Accident (?). He had gonorrhea in 1915, and a sore on the scrotum six months ago. His physician advised anti-luetic treatment.

Present Illness: Six months ago the patient weighed 158, now 128 pounds. Gradually increasing appetite and thirst has been noted for past six months. Nocturia four or five times each night. Gradually became weaker. Eruption appeared two months before entrance, first at elbow-joints, then at hips and knees. Bleed easily.

Present Symptoms: Cough; expectoration; epigastric distress, unassociated with meals; weakness and loss of weight; thirst and hunger; skin lesions.

Status Præsens: Fairly well-nourished young male. Spine showed marked scoliosis to the right. Bones showed slight tenderness on pressure; the skin, a papular eruption in the region of the elbows, knees and ankles, and this extended upward and downward a varying distance from these joints. The lesions varied in size from a pin-head to a pea, were yellow in color, umbilicated, and some had bloody crusts; they were mostly on the extensor surfaces.

The face was asymmetric (due to ulcerated tooth); the teeth carious and showed pyorrhea. Neck, negative. The chest presented a marked deformity due to scoliosis, otherwise negative. Heart, negative. Examination of the abdomen revealed a double inguinal hernia, which extended into the scrotum, and an old operative scar; otherwise negative. Extremities: The deep reflexes were obtained only with reënforcement. Sensory examination showed an anesthetic area over the abdomen and down the right leg to below the knee; probably due to the old scoliosis, as patient had noticed it for some time.

Urine: On entrance, sp. gr. = 1028. Acetone and diacetic acid strongly positive; six-hour output = 1560 c.c.; sugar = 43.3 gm.

Description of Lesions by Dr. Weiss (Dermatologist): The patient presents lemon yellow to red yellow nodules, deeply set in skin for most part, and localized to particular areas. These areas may be roughly stated to be the parts of the skin which are subjected to most trauma and motion. Scattered over the arms and forearms from a point about four inches below axilla, and extending to wrists are about 60 typically colored nodules, varying in size from 2 mm. to

1 cm.; raised above the surface from 1 to 4 mm.; they are mostly orange to lemon yellow in color and are rather deeply set.

The skin over a few of them has ulcerated, and slight superficial infection is present. The eruption on the arms is practically confined to the extensor surface. Over right iliac crest is a group of lesions of the same character. The posterior surface of the right thigh and the entire area included in the anterior surface of knees are thickly studded with active lesions of the same type. The wrists and palms show only a few deeply seated lesions. Over the dorsum of the feet a few small similar lesions are noted.

Laboratory Findings: Urine: Benedict's, strongly positive; very faint trace of albumin; no casts; ferric chlorid test strongly positive.

Blood: Red blood cells, 4,400,000; white blood cells, 8,250; hemoglobin, 70–80 per cent. Differential count showed a normal proportion, except for increase in the lymphocytes to 35 per cent. P.S.P., 63 per cent. in two hours. Wassermann; 4 +, both antigens. Blood sugar, 0.278 mgm. per 100 c.c.; plasma, CO_2 vol. per cent., 34.3. Quantitative urine showed: 5,215 c.c. output in twenty-four hours; sugar, 123.2 gm.; $FeCl_3$, 4 +; NH_3, 2.96 mgm. Total N, 13.46 mgm. Creatinin, 2.08 mgm. Blood-serum showed marked lipemia. Serum, a creamy color. Blood cholesterol, 780 mgm. per 100 c.c. (blood control, about 200 mgm.).

February 10, 1921: Fat estimation (Bloor's method) = 9.5 per cent.

February 16: Biopsy; microscopic report of skin lesions. Diagnosis: Xanthoma.

In the two sections which showed the yellow nodule there is an abundance of fibrous tissue in the midst of which are large cells. These cells are oval or polygonal, and have vesicular nuclei which are round or oval. Sudan III shows the presence of fat in large quantities in the corium and subcutaneous tissue.

Course in Hospital and Treatment.—The patient was placed on a diet of about 60 gm. of carbohydrates and thrice cooked food for six days. Given 160 gr. sodium bicarbonate by mouth in five hours.

February 10, 1921: Films of teeth showed abscessed tooth,

which was later extracted. Blood plasma, CO_2 vol. per cent., 46.

February 10, 1921: Eye consultation (Dr. Hardy): "Vessels appear as if filled with an emulsion. Evidence of a lipemia. No areas of retinitis or hemorrhage. Media clear.

February 12: CO_2 vol. per cent., 56. Eyes showed no change.

February 14: $FeCl_3$, negative for first time (urine).

February 16: Diet, proteid 74; fat 0; carbohydrates, 22 gm.

February 21: Urine, sugar free; blood sugar, 0.183 mgm.

February 25: Blood-sugar, 0.125. Fundus examination, normal appearance.

February 27: Diet, proteid, 100; fat 0; carbohydrates, 25 gm.

March 2: Diet, proteid, 100; fat 50; carbohydrates, 50 gm.

March 6: Diet, proteid, 100; fat 75; carbohydrates, 50 gm.

March 9: Diet, proteid, 100; fat 100; carbohydrates, 50 gm.

Patient's lesions were gradually disappearing during stay until almost absent at time of leaving.

February 16: Another complete blood fat done and showed 2.9 per cent. fat.

The patient had ulcerated tooth extracted and two furuncles opened.

Lumbar puncture was thought inadvisable, due to the furuncles. He was discharged March 10, 1921, after receiving one dose of arsphenamin. Further treatment in skin clinic.

Diagnoses: Diabetes mellitus; xanthoma; furunculosis; syphilis—Wassermann, 4 +; scoliosis; hernia, double inguinal; lipemia; acidosis; sebaceous cyst; dental abscess.

Hale White contended that the term lipemia is not strictly correct, "for the turbidity is not entirely due to fat globules—indeed, they may be absent when the turbidity is marked, and that then, in addition to a precipitated proteid, there is present a substance which, although allied to fats, is not a true fat." Futschner previously advanced a similar view. However, their opinions were based to a large extent on the fact that osmic acid did not stain as is usually expected of it, or else did so very poorly. Scharlach R was found by Turney and Dudgeon to impart its stain to the minute globules. These observers stained film preparations with Scharlach R, and were able to demonstrate large numbers of fat-droplets of all sizes. They laid emphasis on the point that Scharlach R and Sudan III gave excellent fat-staining, whereas osmic acid failed to stain satisfactorily. This probably gave rise to Hale White's opinion that the substance in the blood was not true fat. With Turney and Dudgeon unsatisfactory results only were obtained with Busch's osmic acid preparation, and no fat could be demonstrated in red and white corpuscles by any method.

TABLE OF RECORDED CASES.

Observer	Age	Sex	Result	Pathologic Examination	Vision
1880 Heyl..............	20	M	Fatal	Yes	(?) Vision impaired by cataract.
1903 Reis..............	28	M	Fatal (coma)	Of eyes	(?) Retrobulbar neuritis.
1903 Hale White........	26	M	Alive at time of report	....	(?) Not mentioned.
1903 Fraser............	17	M	Fatal (coma)	Yes	(?) Presumably good.
1906 Heine.............	17	M	Fatal (coma)	Yes	Good.
1906 Turney and Dudgeon	35	F	Fatal (coma)	Yes	Good.
1909 Hertel*......... ...	?	?	Fatal	Of eyes	?
1912 Kollner..........	25	M	Fatal (coma?)	Of eyes	Good.
1912 Darling...........	48	M	Fatal	No	V.R.E., 6/200, c.c. 20/200 V.L.E., 20/200, c.c. 20/30
1915 R. Foster Moore ...	(1) 23	M	Fatal (coma)	No	Good.
	(2) 25	F	Fatal (coma)	No	Good.
1921 Cohen	14	M	Fatal (coma)	No	(?) Patient in coma, no tests possible.
1921 Hardy	29	M	Alive at time of report	...	V.R.E. = 20/15 V.L.E. = 20/38

* Hertel showed microscopic specimens of his case, but furnished no history of the patient (as to age, sex, vision, etc.), except that the patient was a young diabetic. He referred to the seven other previously described cases, not including his case. As I have but six references previous to Hertel's, one has evidently been overlooked.

The color of the retinal vessels as described by Heyl and others was that of a light salmon. In my case the color was more of grayish white, likened by me at the time of observation to the color of malted milk. Possibly the amount of retinal pigment present has a bearing on this point. Differences in background probably give rise to different color impressions. Heyl's case was examined by gaslight: the present case with an electric ophthalmoscope. In my case the retinal vessels in no wise resembled normal vessels either in size or in shape. The impression gained was that of looking at *flat* ribbons twice the width of normal veins, filled with malted milk. Possibly only an American familiar with soda-fountain beverages can appreciate this simile, therefore it may be better to say that such an appearance is best described as a flat toned grayish white, the pure milk white being toned down by the admixture of a darker substance. I failed to be impressed with a salmon-pink color which has been the color description in the majority of the recorded cases.

The colored drawing of Hale White's case, while no doubt an excellent likeness, because done by Head, would not serve as a good representation of the fundus picture in the case observed by me. The picture accompanying Darling's article likewise inadequately depicts the fundus picture of my case. I am led to believe that the picture varies in different cases, due to the amount of fat in the blood and the pigmentation of the fundus. In some of the recorded cases the patients were quite blonde, with thin retinal pigment. In the illustrations of Hale White, Darling, and of Köllner, the suggestion of rotundity of the vessels still remains. Unfortunately in the present case no drawing was made, but the most striking feature next to the color of the vessels was the impression of flatness or ribbon-like character of the veins and arteries which were indistinguishable one from the other and absolutely devoid of the light-streak. In but two of the reports (Hale White's and the present one) was there an observation of the disappearance of the fundus picture and a return to normal appearance. With a betterment in the general condition the fundus picture returned to normal in two months in Hale White's case. In the present case the return to normal appearance was much more rapid, due to the modern energetic methods in bringing about a sugar-free state and the combating of acidosis. The fat in the blood steadily and rapidly declined with the general improvement. The fundus picture returned to normal in two weeks.

With reference to the disappearance of the fat in the blood shortly before death (which has been noted), Turney and Dudgeon suggest that this is probably to be regarded as a vital phenomenon conditioned possibly by the febrile state of the last few days of the patient's life. A relation between acidosis and lipemia seems substantiated, which is not surprising inasmuch as marked instances of both conditions occur only in severe cases of diabetes.

According to Stitt, in plasma CO_2 determinations the following findings will serve as a guide to acidosis: 80–53 normal; 53–40 mild acidosis: no symptoms; 40–30 moderate to severe acidosis: symptoms present; below 30 severe acidosis: symptoms of acid intoxication will be present. These figures would indicate only a moderate acidosis in the case under consideration.

I think it can be stated with certainty that lipæmia retinalis of itself produces no pathologic changes in the eye. Sight must not be lost of the fact that the underlying condition, diabetes, may produce retinal, nerve, and lens changes. So far as I know, retinal changes have not been observed,* but retrobulbar neuritis was noted by Reis and lens changes by Heyl. Hypotony was noted by Heine, Hertel, and Cohen, but was not present in my case. Hypotony is occasionally met with in diabetic coma, but its association with lipemia is casual.

There has been considerable speculation as to why the

* Cohen noted several small retinal hemorrhages in one eye.

veins and arteries appear alike in lipæmia retinalis. From Heyl to Moore nearly every contributor has had an explanation or offered a suggestion.

Heyl's explanation of the width of the vessels was based upon the supposition that in health the visible part of the blood in the vessels comprises the axial stream, consisting of corpuscles, whereas the peripheral part of the current is invisible plasma. In lipemia the plasma becomes opaque and hence visible, consequently the vessel appears double its usual caliber. With regard to the fundus picture, R. Foster Moore explains it in this manner. "(1) The ground-glass effect of the opaque plasma does away with the central light-streak seen in normal retinal vessels, as a consequence of which the cylindric contour is lost and the vessels have the appearance of flat bands or ribbons, as is seen in normal choroidal vessels. (2) The color of the retinal vessels in lipemia, where the salmon tint is moderately saturated, is almost exactly that of normal choroidal vessels. (3) In both instances there is the difficulty of distinguishing arteries from veins. It is probable, therefore, that the marked change in color of the retinal vessels is due entirely to the condition of the plasma, and does not imply a change in the blood pigment." This last statement is undoubtedly true, as the red cell count and percentage of hemoglobin have been little below normal limits in most instances.* In the present case the blood in the centrifugal tube was a port-wine color filling half the tube, with the upper half creamy in color and consisting for a great part of fat.

I wish to express my thanks to Dr. Kudner for his assistance in furnishing clinical and laboratory data, and to Professor Shaffer, of the Washington University Medical School, for making the fat and cholesterol estimations.

---

* In Cohen's case the hemoglobin was only 30 per cent., but the patient was *in extremis* at the time of observation.

REFERENCES.

A. G. Heyl: Trans. Amer. Ophth. Soc., 1880, iii, 54–56.
Louis Starr: N. Y. Med. Record, 1880, xvii, 477–481.
Futschner: Jour. Amer. Med. Assn., October 21, 1899.
Hale White: Lancet, October 10, 1903, 1007–1008.
W. Reis: Arch. f. Augenh., lv, 3d pt., 347–368. Abst. Ophthalmoscope,
    August, 1903.
Thos. R. Fraser: Scottish Med. and Surg. Jour., September, 1903, 200–221.
    Brit. Med. Jour., May 23, 1903.
L. Heine: Klin. M. f. Augenh., December, 1906, 451–460.
Turney and Dudgeon: Jour. Pathology, 1906, xi, 50.
E. Hertel: Zeit. f. Augenh., 1909, xxi, 551.
K. Köllner: Cent. f. p. Augenh., July, 1910, 212.
K. Köllner: Klin. M. f. Augenh., July, 1911, 109.
K. Köllner: Zeit. f. Augenh., May, 1912. Also Abst. Ophthalmoscope, 1912,
    535.
C. G. Darling: Arch. Ophth., 1912, xli, 355.
R. Foster Moore: Lancet, 1915, 366.
Martin Cohen: Arch. Ophth., 1921, l, 247–251.

SOME IMPRESSIONS DERIVED FROM THE STUDY OF RECURRENT HEMORRHAGES INTO THE RETINA AND VITREOUS OF YOUNG PERSONS.

WILLIAM C. FINNOFF, M.D.,

Denver, Col.

The symptom-complex of recurring hemorrhages into the retina and vitreous, followed by retinitis proliferans in young persons, has been well understood by ophthalmologists for many years. The predisposition of some young men to spontaneous hemorrhages into the eye was first described by von Graefe[1] in 1854. Modern text-books refer to this condition, and considerable space is allotted to it in the American Encyclopedia of Ophthalmology.[2] The etiology of this condition, however, has not yet emerged from the realm of speculation.

Forty years ago Eales[3] accurately described the symptoms and course of recurrent retinal hemorrhages. His cases occurred in males between the age of fourteen and twenty years. The left eye was first affected. There had been a history of epistaxis and constipation in most of the cases, and the author attributed the condition to a neurosis which affected the digestive and circulatory systems. Eales believed that the disease did not occur in women, and that menstruation acted as a safeguard.

Panas called the condition "Ocular Epistaxis," and noted that in the young the hemorrhage was from the veins, whereas in the old the bleeding was from the arteries. Beaumont[4] and others have reported cases associated with epistaxis.

In 1882 Hutchinson[5] advanced the theory that some cases of recurrent retinal hemorrhages occurring during adolescence were due to congenital gout. Leber suggested oxaluria as a cause, and Jacqueau[6] reported a case which he thought was due to a phosphaturia and excess of urea. The hemorrhages in this case recurred over a period of sixteen years. Syphilis, both congenital and acquired, has been advanced as an etiologic factor.

Noll,[7] in 1908, was the first to suggest tuberculosis as a cause of recurrent hemorrhages into the retina and vitreous.

In 1909 Kipp[8] described a case of recurrent hemorrhage into the retina and vitreous of both eyes in a young man with tuberculosis of the hip and chronic otitis media. The hemorrhages were followed by retinitis proliferans. A second case, which he had reported before this Society in 1895,[9] occurred in a young man who had a cough and lost weight shortly after the occurrence of the retinal hemorrhages, but who later regained perfect health. Kipp suggested that these cases were of a possible tuberculous nature. Axenfeld's[10] article in 1910 called attention to the fact that recurrent retinal and vitreous hemorrhages were often due to tuberculosis, even though no apparent tuberculous changes had occurred elsewhere in the eye. This author reported 3 cases to support his view. He believed that the lesions were due either to the tubercle bacilli or to the actions of their toxins, and that the individuals suffering from the disease were frequently robust and apparently in good health. Improvement followed the administration of tuberculin in Axenfeld's cases, and he advised its use as a diagnostic and therapeutic measure. Since Axenfeld's observations, Igersheimer,[11] Harms,[12] Jackson,[13] and many others have reported cases due to tuberculosis. (See tables.)

Toxemia has been suggested by Moissonier[14] as a cause; and recently Zentmayer[15] has called attention to the possibility of derangements of the endocrine organs, especially the adrenals, as a contributing factor.

Hemophilia, disorders of menstruation, indicanuria, excessively high or low blood-pressure, the anemias, nephritis, exercise, and other conditions have been mentioned as possible causative factors in the production of recurrent intraocular hemorrhage in the young.

In the past six months there have come under my care three young men with recurrent massive hemorrhages into the retina and vitreous. I have been impressed by the similarity of the symptoms in these and other cases that I have seen. In attempting to determine the basic etiology of the hemorrhages, my interest in this disease was sufficiently aroused to search the literature to see what had been written on this subject.

The following reports are of cases which have come under my care since 1916:

CASE 1.—A farmer, aged twenty-eight years, had massive recurrent hemorrhages into the retina and vitreous of the right eye, following a periphlebitis of the retinal veins. A focal reaction to tuberculin was obtained. The hemorrhages remained confined to the right eye. Jackson reported this case with other cases of tuberculosis of the retina before this Society in 1919, and I will refer you to the Transactions for the details of this case.

Case 2.—W. P. B., aged forty-two years, seen first May 16, 1919. Three years before he had developed pulmonary tuberculosis, and had come to Colorado, where he rapidly regained his health. For three years he had felt well and had not coughed. The vision of the left eye always had been poor, probably from an amblyopia exanopsia. History otherwise negative. One year prior to consultation the vision of both eyes had blurred suddenly; it gradually improved, but did not regain its former acuity and floaters have been present ever since. May 12, 1919, the vision became suddenly clouded. There had been no pain nor discomfort in the eyes at the time of the blurring nor since. When first seen, V.R.E., 0.05; L.E., 0.2. The right vitreous contained small masses of blood; these were more numerous in the lower half. The remainder of the vitreous was uniformly hazy. A hammock-shaped subhyaloid hemorrhage, with its convexity downward, was noted, extending from the lower temporal vein to the lower nasal vein. The veins were uniformly distended and tortuous. A perivascular, yellowish exudate, covering one of the terminal branches of the upper temporal vein, was seen. The Wassermann reaction and urine were negative. There was no history or evidence of infection in the tonsils or nasal sinuses; and x-rays and examinations of the teeth and jaws were negative. The systolic blood pressure was 122 mm. of mercury. Upon physical examination a small cavity was found in the apex of the right lung. It was thought advisable not to use tuberculin in this case, because of the danger of lighting up a latent tuberculous focus in the lung, so the patient was sent to a sanatorium for general hygienic treatment. In a letter from the patient, received six months later, he stated that he had gained greatly in general health, and that his vision had improved.

Case 3.—This case was reported also by Dr. Edward Jackson (13, case 3) in the same paper as Case 1. In 1915 the patient, a male, aged twenty-five years, had the first hemorrhage in the right vitreous. Six months after the onset he consulted Dr. Arnold Knapp, of New York, who pronounced the condition tuberculosis and put him on tuberculin. There was temporary improvement, but later a recurrence of activity, with great loss of vision in the right eye. In December, 1916, when he was first seen by Dr. Jackson, V.R.E., moving fingers at 1 foot; L.E., with correction, 1.1. The right vitreous was cloudy; no fundus details were visible. There was a grayish-red reflex in all directions and floating masses, which in the lower temporal vitreous looked almost like detached retina, but no vessels were found. Left eye, slight haziness of vitreous. Choroid rather patchy and "moth eaten," otherwise the fundus was normal. Infiltration of the apices of the lungs, especially the right, was found. Two hemorrhages occurred into the vitreous of the right eye—one in February and the other in April of 1917. The eyes then remained quiet until November 10, 1920, when the vision of the left eye was suddenly obscured in the upper field. He had been free from trouble for so long that he had disregarded his general health and was run down because of overwork indoors. Dr. Jackson referred the patient to me, and I found, V.R.E., light perception; L.E., 0.8. The fundus of the right eye was the same as reported in 1917. The vitreous of the left eye was uniformly hazy. A large, hammock-shaped subhyaloid hemorrhage was noted in the lower portion of the eye, extending from a mass of retinitis proliferans on the temporal side, near one of the terminal branches of the lower temporal vein, to a second similar mass along the first branch of the lower nasal vein (Fig. 1). A smaller subhyaloid hemorrhage was seen about 4 dd. above the nerve head, in the region of a scar which covered a vertical vein. There were hemorrhages into the retina surrounding the masses of scar tissue. The blood absorbed slowly and was replaced, in part, by bands of scar tissue. Tuberculin in small doses (1/500,000 mgm.) was given and gradually increased. December 23d, twenty-four hours after the administration of a dose of 1/100,000 mgm. of tuberculin, new retinal hemorrhages occurred. This was a focal reaction, and the size of the dose was diminished. January 13, 1921, V.L.E., 1.1. January 19, during the excitement of making a political speech, contrary to instructions, the vision suddenly became obscured, due to a hemorrhage into the lower vitreous in about the same location as the former one. The blood absorbed more slowly, and when last seen March 8, there was still some haziness of the lower

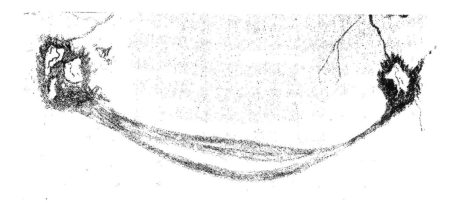

Fig. 1.—Retinitis proliferans. Subhyaloid hemorrhages. Hemorrhages into
the retina.

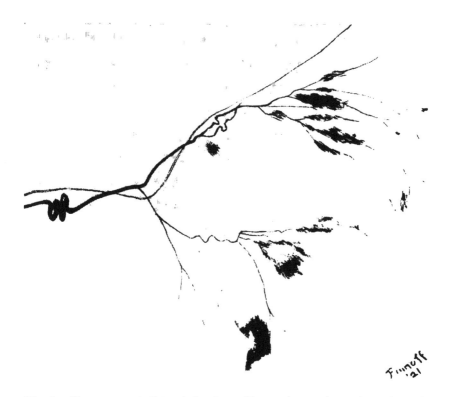

Fig. 2.—Tortuous and distended veins. Venous hemorrhages into the retina.
Perivascular exudates and exudates into the retina.

vitreous and dark blood in the retina around the scar tissue. The patient was ordered to stop work and was sent to a sanatorium, where he could be under supervision. He reported a few weeks ago that he had improved greatly in general health, and that there had been no new hemorrhages.

CASE 4.—K. E. F., aged thirty-five years, first seen April 2, 1921. Two weeks before, while walking, the vision of the right eye suddenly became hazy, but gradually improved, until April 1, when the vision was almost completely lost. The second attack occurred while he was sitting at his desk writing.

There was no history of tuberculosis or hemophilia in his family. He had the usual diseases of childhood without complications. Four years ago he had severe articular rheumatism, which cleared up, and he gained 40 pounds after the extraction of six decayed teeth. About two and one-half years ago he had a severe attack of influenza, but recovered without complications. In December, 1920, he had acute tonsillitis. Since childhood he has had frequent attacks of epistaxis, but has not had bleeding from the nose for several months. He has never suffered from constipation. V.R.E., 0.08; L.E., 1.1. Ophthalmoscope: Cornea and lens clear; vitreous clouded, due to the presence of blood. Only the extreme nasal side of the fundus could be seen. In this portion the upper nasal vein was found to be distended and tortuous, and did not diminish in size toward the periphery, distally to the entrance of good-sized contributing branches. In the peripheral portion, two veins were distended and tortuous. They were bordered, for a short distance, by a fine white exudate into which one of the veins finally disappeared. The accompanying artery was obscured by exudate in this region. A small retinal hemorrhage was seen slightly below the area of exudation. Further to the periphery numerous hemorrhages of venous origin were seen in the retina. In the extreme periphery, as far forward as one could see, the retina contained a silvery-white exudate. The vessels were visible over this portion of the retina, and several small areas of hemorrhage were noted in it (Fig. 2). In the lower portion of the eye, large subhyaloid and vitreous hemorrhages were seen. Left eye: the media were clear   The veins were slightly distended, but showed no signs of disease, otherwise the fundus was normal.

Blood Wassermann, blood counts, and urine were negative. Systolic blood pressure, 118 mm. of mercury. Coagulation time of blood (capillary tube method), four minutes, twenty seconds. Two apical abscesses were found in x-ray pictures of the teeth. The involved teeth were removed, and the abscesses drained. The surgeon thought the tonsils did not show pathology enough for removal. April 12, V.R.E., 0.1; L.E., 1.1. The vitreous had cleared slightly, but no further details could be made out. Old tuberculin, 0.005 mgm., was given subcutaneously, with no local, constitutional, or focal reaction. Increasing doses of tuberculin were injected every forty-eight hours until a 5 mgm. dose had been given; no reaction was obtained, and tuberculosis was excluded as the etiology. It was insisted upon that the tonsils be removed, to exclude every possible focus of infection, and potassium iodid and thyroid extract were prescribed.

May 16, the vitreous had cleared considerably since the last examination. The outline of the disc could be seen. A number of small retinal hemorrhages had absorbed. V.R.E., 0.6; L.E., 1.1.

CASE 5.—G. L., aged thirty years. Family history for tuberculosis and hemophilia negative. He had the usual diseases of childhood and always had suffered from a severe form of constipation. When fourteen or fifteen years of age, the muscles of his legs became weak, and he developed a toe-drop; later this weakness progressed upward, and finally he lost the use of his legs. For a time he had incontinence of urine and feces, but has regained control of the bladder and bowels. X-ray examination of the spine was negative. Tonsils were removed five years ago. About seven years previously he was told that he had some weakness of the eye muscles, and a partial tenotomy of both external recti was done.

About nine months before examination the vision of both eyes blurred rather suddenly, and he consulted an optician, who gave him glasses (0.50 spheres for each eye) and assured him that his vision would improve if he wore them. The

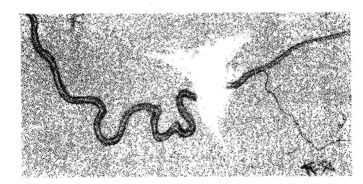

Fig. 3.—Retinitis proliferans and tortuous vein.

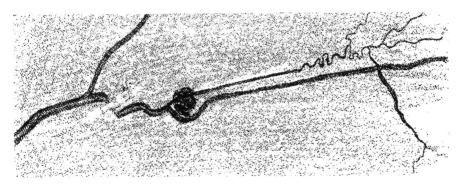

Fig. 4.—Irregular and tortuous veins.   Retinitis proliferans.   Area of retinal
pigment changes.

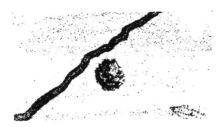

Fig. 5 —Mass of retinal pigment near tortuous vein.

vision gradually improved and almost regained its former acuity. About the same time that the vision began to fail he had a severe intestinal disturbance which confined him to his bed for several weeks.

The patient had been feeling well, and his eyes had been comfortable until two weeks before consultation, when the vision of the right eye suddenly failed. When first seen, April 15, 1921, V.R.E., 0.03 eccentric; L.E., 1.0. Ophthalmoscope: Right eye; cornea and lens clear; vitreous filled with large masses of blood, which obscured all fundus details. Left eye: Cornea and lens clear; vitreous clear, excepting in lower temporal quadrant, in which location a Y-shaped, white, veil-like mass of retinitis proliferans was detected; it extended forward into the vitreous about 7 D., and slightly obscured the details of a branch of the lower temporal vein (Fig. 3). The veins were all slightly tortuous. The upper temporal vein was apparently obscured over a small area by thickened retina and a thin veil of scar tissue, which was located about 5 dd. from the margin of the nerve (Fig. 4). Beyond the obscured area, the vein was convoluted in the region of a round mass of retinal pigment. A branch of the vein entered the main trunk near the mass of pigment. Following the branch from the main trunk toward the periphery, it was seen to cross the pigmented area, and a portion of it was covered by pigment. The vein then took a straight course and was bordered on both sides by a fine white streak, apparently a scar. It then suddenly thinned to about half of its diameter and became very tortuous. The thinned portion of the vein had several branches: a lower branch of it crossed the main trunk, and its caliber was seen to be very much greater than the vein that it emptied into. Two or three round patches of retinal pigment were seen near veins on the nasal side of fundus (Fig. 5). There were no hemorrhages or exudates. The fundus changes were old, probably the result of inflammation which had occurred nine months before. The blood and spinal Wassermann reactions and the urine were negative. The teeth were negative, and nothing was found in the chest. Blood pressure, 125 mm. of mercury. Old tuberculin was given for diagnostic purposes, and no constitutional or focal reaction was obtained after the administration of 5 mgm. subcutaneously. May 6, V.R.E., 0.2, eccentric. The vitreous had cleared quite decidedly, especially in the upper third of the upper temporal quadrant.

This covers a series of five cases of massive hemorrhages into the vitreous; all occurred in males; their ages ranged, at the time of the first attack, from twenty-five to forty-seven years. In all the cases the right eye was the first involved, and the greatest amount of destruction had taken place in it.

In Cases 1 and 3 a focal reaction occurred following the administration of tuberculin, and in Case 2 the man had pulmonary tuberculosis and lost weight just before the occurrence of the intra-ocular hemorrhage. Cases 1 and 3 improved after the administration of tuberculin, and Case 2 improved with the improvement of his general health. In Cases 1 and 2 there was a visible periphlebitis with patches of white and yellowish exudate in the proximity of the veins; and in Case 1 these patches were seen to spread along the veins and preceded the hemorrhages. Cases 1, 2, and 3 were due to tuberculosis. In all the cases the veins were tortuous and irregular in caliber, and the peripheral branches were frequently relatively larger than normal when compared with the main trunk. In Case 1, and apparently in Cases 3, 4, and 5, the earlier changes were in the periphery of the fundus in the beginning, before the appearance of hemorrhages. In Case 4, the inflammatory process was most marked in the retina, and in Case 5 there were patches of retinal pigment which was secondary to retinal inflammation. In Cases 4 and 5 tuberculosis was excluded: the possible cause of 4 was focal infection from abscesses at the apices of teeth and infected tonsils. In Case 5 the attacks were associated with severe intestinal disturbance, and the possibility of focal infection from the intestines was considered.

The conclusions derived from the study of the literature and the foregoing cases are:

1. Recurrent hemorrhages into retina and vitreous in young persons is probably not a specific disease.

2. Tuberculosis of the retinal vessels, especially the veins, is one of the common etiologic factors.

(*a*) To prove that the cause is tuberculosis, a focal reaction should be obtained.

(*b*) When due to tuberculosis, improvement follows the administration of tuberculin and hygienic treatment.

3. Syphilis is an occasional cause.

4. Focal infection is a possible cause.

5. Hemophilia is not a cause, but might be a contributing factor.

6. The hemorrhages are the result of a localized pathologic weakening of the blood-vessels, and increased blood pressure or exercise are only exciting causes.

7. The veins are usually attacked.

8. In some cases there is involvement of the retina early in the disease.

9. In most cases the earlier changes occur in the periphery of the eye, and if patients were examined in the early stages of the disease, we would learn more about the pathology.

10. Retinitis proliferans occurs in most cases.

11. I believe the disease is primarily in the retina, and that the partial or complete detachment of the retina is due to traction from scar tissue and not to subretinal hemorrhages from the choroidal vessels, as has been suggested.

12. The prognosis is poor; both eyes usually become affected, and in most cases the vision is markedly diminished.

13. The disease is much more frequent in men. When occurring in women, it is usually not so severe.

I have reviewed all the literature that was available and collected 110 cases. This material is arranged in tabular form, giving the sex; age of the patient at the time of the first hemorrhage; the etiology; the first eye to become involved; whether the second eye was attacked; and the bibliography.

BIBLIOGRAPHY.

1. Graefe, v.: Graefe's Arch. f. Ophth., i, 1855.
2. American Encyclopedia of Ophth., viii, 5802.
3. Eales: Birmingham Med. Rev., July, 1880. Ophth. Rev., i, 1882, 41.
4. Beaumont: Ophth. Rev., ii, 1892, 352.
5. Hutchinson: Ophth. Rev., ii, 1882, p. 41.
6. Jacqueau: Ophth. Rev., xviii, 1899, 323.
7. Noll: Arch. f. Augenh., lxiii, 1908, 213.
8. Kipp: Arch. of Ophth., xxxviii, 1909, 349.
9. Kipp: Trans. of Amer. Ophth. Soc., 1895, 423.
10. Axenfeld: Bull. de la Soc. Belge d'Opht., No. 29, 1910–11, 115; also Axenfeld and Stock: Klin. M. f. Augenh., xlvii, I, 146, 1909.
11. Igersheimer: Graefe's Arch. f. Ophth., lxxxii, 215.
12. Harms: Klin. M. f. Augenh., July, 1912, 106.
13. Jackson: Trans. Colorado Ophth. Congress, 1915, 207.
14. Moissonier: Soc. d'Opht. de Paris, 1911, 110.
15. Zentmayer: Amer. Jour. Ophth., 1920, 652.

SYPHILIS

Sex	Age	Etiology	First Eye	Second Eye Involved	References
?	?	Syphilis	?	?	Moissonier: Arch. d'Opht., v. xxiv, p. 438.
M.	25	Syphilis	?	?	Chevalier: Soc. Fran. d'Opht., 1912, p. 444.
M.	21	Syphilis	L.	?	Appleman: Amer. Jour. Ophth., v. i, 1918, p. 24.
M.	18	Syphilis (hereditary)	L.	?	Scheffels: Deutsch. med. Woch., 1897.
M.	33	Syphilis	R.	?	Sulzer: Soc. Fran. d'Opht., 1912, p. 450.

Total syphilis, 5. Sex, M., 4; not specified, 1 Range of age at time of first hemorrhage, 18–33. Eye involved first, R., 1; L., 2; not specified, 2.

GASTRO-INTESTINAL, VIZ., CONSTIPATION, ETC.

Sex	Age	Etiology	First Eye	Second Eye Involved	References
M.	Ranged from 14–20	Constipation	L.	+	Eales: Ophth. Rev., v. i, 1882, p. 41.
M.		Constipation	L.	+	
M.		Constipation	L.	+	
M.		Constipation	L.	+	
M.		Constipation	L.	+	
M.	24	Constipation	L.	?	Hutchinson: Trans. Ophth. Soc U. K., 1880–81
M.	21	Constipation	?	?	Walker: Trans. Ophth. Soc. U. K., 1921, p 181
M.	30	Gout and constipation	?	?	Carpenter: Jour. A. M. A., July 29, 1911, p. 376.

Total gastro-intestinal, 8 Sex, M., 8. Range of ages at time of first hemorrhage, 14 to 30. Eye involved first, L., 6; not specified, 2.

TUBERCULOSIS

Sex	Age	Etiology	First Eye	Second Eye Involved	References
F.	30	Tuberculosis	R.	+	Axenfeld and Stock: Klin. M. f. Augenh , 1911, v. 1, p 28.
M.	21	Tuberculosis	R.	+	Kipp: Arch. of Ophth., 1909, v. xxxviii, p. 349.
M.	10	Tuberculosis	R.	+	Kipp: Trans. Amer. Ophth. Soc., 1895, p. 423.
M.	22	Tuberculosis	R.	+	Noll: Arch f. Augenh., v. xliii, 1909, p. 213.
M.	20	Tuberculosis	L.	+	Cords: Zeit. f. Augenh , v.
M.	23	Tuberculosis ?	L.	?	xxvi, p 441.
F.	20	Tuberculosis	L.	?	Axenfeld: Soc. Belge d'Opht ,
F.	30	Tuberculosis	R.	+	No. 29, 1910–11, p. 115.
F.	20	Tuberculosis ?	R.	?	Knapp: Arch. Ophth , v. xlii,
M.	16	Tuberculosis ?	R.	+	p. 1.
M.	15	Tuberculosis ?	R.	?	Woods: Jour. A. M. A , July 29, 1911, p. 375.
M.	20	Tuberculosis	?	..	de Schweinitz and Holloway: Univ. Penn. Bull., March, 1910.
M.	20	Tuberculosis ? Low coagulation time	L.	?	Roberts: Jour A. M. A , July 29, 1911, p 380.
M.	23	Tuberculosis ?	R.	+	Bordley: Jour A. M. A., July
M.	20	Tuberculosis ?	R.	+	29, 1911, p. 376.
M.	23	Tuberculosis	L.	?	
M.	19	Tuberculosis	L.	+	Igersheimer: Graefe's Arch. f.
M.	20	Tuberculosis	R.	?	Ophth., v. lxxxii, 1912, p 215.
F.	17	Tuberculosis	L.	?	
M.	22	Tuberculosis (with chorioretinitis disseminata)	R.	+	
?	19	Tuberculosis	?	?	Harms: Klin. M. f. Augenh., v. ii, 1912, p. 106.
M.	19	Tuberculosis	R.	?	Wilder: Trans. Ophth. Sec. A. M. A., 1907, p. 159.
M.	37	Tuberculosis	?	?	Fleischer: Klin. M. f. Augenh , 1912, v. ii, p. 245.
M.	24	Tuberculosis	Both	..	Davis: Trans. Amer. Ophth. Soc., 1912, Part I.
M.	30	Tuberculosis	R.	+	Taylor: Trans Ophth Soc. U. K , v. xxxiii, 1913, p. 1.
M.	18	Tuberculosis all retinal	L.	?	Oloff: Munch. med. Woch., 1914, p. 1103.
M.	21	Tuberculosis	L.	?	Jackson: Trans. Colo. Ophth.
F.	20	Tuberculosis	R.	−	Cong , 1915, p. 198.
F.	27	Tuberculosis	L	+	Spencer: Trans. Amer. Ophth.
M.	20	Tuberculosis	L.	?	and Oto-Laryn. Soc , 1916, p.
F.	27	Tuberculosis	L.	?	60.
M.	32	Tuberculosis	L.	?	
F.	Adult	Tuberculosis	L.	−12 years later	Stieren: Penn. Med. Jour , v. xxii, 1919, p. 187.
M.	21	Tuberculosis	Both	..	Buck: Amer. Jour. Ophth , v. iii, 1919, p 731.
M.*	19	Tuberculosis (possible apical abscess of tooth)	L.	+	Fisher: Trans Amer. Ophth. Soc , v. xiv, 1915–16, p 583.

* Possible focal infection from teeth.

Total tuberculosis, 27.. Sex, M. 20; F., 7. Range of age at time of first hemorrhage, 10 to 37 years. Eye involved first—R., 9; L., 13; both, 2; not specified, 3.

Total probable tuberculosis, 9. Sex, M., 8; F., 1. Range of age at time of first hemorrhage, 15 to 23. Eye first involved, R., 5; L., 4.

FOCAL INFECTION

SEX	AGE	ETIOLOGY	FIRST EYE	SECOND EYE IN-VOLVED	REFERENCES
F.	40	Source not specified	L.	..	Appleman: Amer Jour. Ophth., v. i, 1918, p. 24.
?	?	Buccal	?	?	Moissonier: Arch. d'Opht , v. xxiv, p 438.
M.	23	Bronchus and pleura	R.	+	Fromaget: Ann. d'Oculist., 1903, p. 165.
F.	29	Possibly due to buccal infection	L.	?	Woods: Jour A M. A., June 29, 1911, p. 375.

Total focal infection, 4. Sex, M , 1; F., 2, not specified, 1. Range of age at time of first hemorrhage, 23 to 40. Eye involved first, R., 1; L., 2; not specified, 1.

MENSTRUAL DISTURBANCE

SEX	AGE	ETIOLOGY	FIRST EYE	SECOND EYE IN-VOLVED	REFERENCES
F.	28	Hemorrhages recurred 9 times at time of menstrual period	R. and L.	..	Landolt: Soc. d'Opht. de Paris, March, 1908
F.	26	Menstrual disturbance	R.	+	Weeks: Trans. Amer. Ophth. Soc , 1897, p. 158.

Total menstrual disturbance, 2. Range of age at time of first hemorrhage, 26 to 28. Eye involved first, R., 1; both, 1.

DISTURBANCE OF BLOOD AND CIRCULATION

SEX	AGE	ETIOLOGY	FIRST EYE	SECOND EYE IN-VOLVED	REFERENCES
M.	22	Hemophilia	R.	+	Noll: Arch. f. Augenh., v. lxiii, p. 213.
F.	29	High blood pressure and nephritis	?	?	Woods: Jour. A. M. A , July 29, 1911, p. 375.
?	?	Inequality of circulation. 2 cases	?	?	Hutchinson: Trans. Ophth. Soc. U. K., 1880–81.

Total disturbance of blood and circulation, 4. Sex, M., 1; F., 1; not specified, 2. Range of age at time of first hemorrhage, 22 to 29. Eye involved first, R., 1; not specified, 3.

CAUSE UNDETERMINED

SEX	AGE	ETIOLOGY	FIRST EYE	SECOND EYE IN-VOLVED	REFERENCES
F.	24	Healthy	R.	+	Axenfeld: Münch. med. Woch., 1905.
M.	Young	..	R.	?	Batier: Echo Med. du Nord, 1909, p. 234.
F.	23	Improved under thyroid extract	L.	+	Bennett: Ophthalmoscope, v. xi, 1913.
F.	27	..	?	?	Black: Ophth. Y. B., 1910, p. 217.
M.	23		R.	?	Bordley: Jour A. M A., July 29, 1911, p. 376.
M.	17		?	?	Bulson: Jour. A. M A., July 29, 1911, p. 376.
M.	?		?	?	
M.	?	..	L.	+	Carmalt: Ophth. Rev , 1887, p. 299.

Cause Undetermined—*(Continued)*

Sex	Age	Etiology	Fi Eʀsт	Second Eye Involved	References
M.		..	?	?	Chandler: Jour. A. M A., July
M.	Between 25-34	..	?	?	29, 1911, p 376.
M.			?	?	
M.			?	?	
M.	25		L.	?	Clegg: Ophthalmoscope, v,
M.	29		L.	?	xiv, 1916, p. 583.
F.	32		R.	+	
M.	20		R.	+	Cunningham: Trans. Ophth. Soc. U. K., 1912, p. 177.
M.	19		L.	+	Davies: Trans. Ophth. Soc. U. K., 1912, p. 182.
F.	22		R.	?	Davis: Jour. A. M. A., July 29,
M.	30		?	?	1911, p. 377.
M.	?	..	L.	+	Doyne: Ophth. Rev., v. xxii, 1903, p. 144
M.	34	.. .	L.	+	Elschnig: Arch. Ophth., 1906, p. 33.
M.	?		L.	?	Friedenwald: Amer. Jour. of Ophth., March, 1920, p. 224.
M.	24	..	L.	+	Fromaget: Ann. d'Oculist, 1903, p 165.
M.	29		R.	?	Gunn: 1891, From Cord's article. Zeit. f. Augenh., v. 26, p. 441.
M.	22	..	?	?	Kennon: Jour. A. M. A., July 29, 1911, p. 377.
M.	18		L.	..	Knapp: Arch. Ophth., v. xlii,
M.	23		R.	+	p. 1.
M.	26		Both	..	Koening: Rec. d'Opht., 1898.
M.	26		R.	—	Krauss: Ann. Ophth., 1908, p. 58.
M.	19		L.	+	Kyrieleis: Klin. M. f. Augenh., May, 1908.
F.	15	..	?	?	Lewis: Jour. A. M. A., July 29, 1911, p. 377.
M.	16		?	?	May: Jour. A. M. A., July 29,
M.	20	..	?	?	1911, p. 377.
M.	36		?	?	
M.	17		L.	+	Mayweg: Bericht der Ophth. Gesell. Heidelberg, 1889, p. 92.
M.	28		L.	+	Morton: Trans. Ophth. Soc. U. K., v. xxv, 1905, p. 185.
M.			Both	..	Nieden: Bericht der Ophth.
M.			Both	..	Gesell. Heidelberg, 1882.
M.			Both	..	
M.	Mostly in young		R.	..	
M.			R.	..	
M.			R.	..	
M.	Young and ro-bust		?	?	Panas: Maladie des Yeux.
M.			?	?	
M.	21	..	L.	?	Schneideman: Trans. Amer. Acad. of Ophth. and Oto-Laryn., 1905, p 109.
M.	27		R.	L.	Simon: Cent. f. p. Augenh., 1896, p. 325.
M.	43	..	L.	?	Stilwill: Ann. Ophth., v. xxv, 1906, p. 401.
M.	23		?	?	Wadsworth: Ophth. Rev.,
M.	30		?	?	1887, p 299.
F.	17		R.	?	Weeks: Jour. A. M. A., July 29, 1911, p. 38.
M.	29	..	R.	+	Weeks: Trans. Amer. Ophth. Soc., 1897, p. 158.

Total undetermined, 51. Sex, M., 44; F., 7. Range of age at time of first hemorrhage, 16 to 43. Eye affected first, R., 15; L., 15; both, 4; not specified, 17.

Total number of cases found, 110. Total number of males affected, 86; females, 20; not specified, 4. Range of ages, 10 to 43 years. Total right eye affected first, 33; total left, 43; both, 7; not specified, 27.

DISCUSSION.

DR. T. B. HOLLOWAY, Philadelphia: Some of you may recall that at the last meeting I referred to certain cases of this type that had been placed on record from my clinic, and in at least one of these the underlying factor was regarded as a focal infection. At the present time I have three of these cases under observation, and they have been put through the most exhaustive medical examinations; all have shown positive tuberculin tests. What I desire particularly to refer to is that in some of these cases, although the lesions are essentially peripheral, macular changes of a proliferative type develop. When these are first noted you will question whether it is a reflex or beginning pathologic change. You will be uncertain whether you use the ordinary reflecting scope or the electric, and whether the illumination be intense or reduced.

As the process slowly increases, delicate fenestrations of varying sizes and shapes will be noted and delicate strands will be seen to override the vessels at certain points. I am perfectly free to confess that I do not know the pathology and have never seen the condition described in these cases, but I have observed it in two instances, and in one case watched its progress for one and a half years.

DR. WILLIAM H. WILMER, Washington, D. C.: I have had the misfortune to see several of these cases, and, unfortunately, I usually see them late when the beginning fundus changes are not visible. I have noted some points in this disease. There seem to be two types, for which the old terminology, sthenic and asthenic, might be appropriately used. In my experience, the cases occurring in robust, athletic young men do better than those in young men of the so-called feminine type. In the latter type I have seen some very disastrous results—practically blindness in both eyes. In the last few years the majority of the cases seen have shown a positive tuberculin reaction, getting very marked general, local, and focal reaction from doses of O.T. under 2.5 mgm. In addition, most cases have had bad tonsils and constipation. The last patient seen, a few weeks since, showed a positive tuberculin reaction, a seemingly normal thyroid but a pancreatic disturbance. This condition occurs so frequently in youths of about nineteen years of age, when the function of puberty is being established, that one feels that there may be a close relation between this phase of development and some obscure disturbance of the endocrine organs. The study of the organs of internal secretion in their relation to recurrent hemorrhages into the retina in adolescents is very important, because in the light of our present knowledge they afford a great field for speculative philosophy. Everything should be done to remove the etiology of these cases from the realms of alluring speculation to those of scientific medicine.

DR. HARRY FRIEDENWALD, Baltimore, Md.: I should like to emphasize the importance of vascular changes, which are chiefly seen in the finer vessels, and which show marked enlargement and great tortuosity, and frequently the appearance of varicosities, but what I want especially to mention is the fact that the prognosis is not so universally bad as was pointed out. The cases have sometimes a tendency to recur frequently for some time, and then cease entirely. I have had an opportunity to follow certainly two cases for a great many years after these hemorrhages had finally ceased, with the retention of excellent vision as the final outcome.

DR. GEORGE S. DERBY, Boston, Mass.: Following Dr. Friedenwald's lead, I would like to say a word on diagnosis. I think we see these cases occurring later on in life, perhaps from forty to fifty-five, and certainly these particular cases I am referring to are not due to cardiorenal disease and general changes in the vessels. In regard to prognosis, I reported, some ten years ago, a woman aged fifty-one years who lost vision in each eye from repeated recurrent hemorrhages into the vitreous; she became blind—had only light perception in one eye. She remained blind five years; at the end of that time she walked into my office with vision in one eye, so she was able to go around by herself and do her own work. The etiology of the case was entirely in doubt.

DR. ARNOLD KNAPP, New York: I think in most of these cases a tuberculous origin is probably the most likely. The characteristic feature is, as has been mentioned, the perivascular alterations in the little veins, and it seems to me it is this perivascular character which gives rise to the proliferative changes which we find in the later pictures. So far as I understand, the recognition that it is the small veins which are the cause of the hemorrhage came from Hirschberg's clinic, and I think was made by our member, Dr. Friedenwald. The cases are striking and usually mean the loss of one eye, and, curiously enough, the second eye has done well. The consideration of these cases brings up a word in regard to the interpretation of the tuberculin test. We have been giving that test and following results for a number of years, and are coming to the conclusion that the interpretation is not always an easy one, and that there is probably a non-specific reaction in a great number of these cases. Furthermore, the interpretation of the local reaction is also a difficult one, and many of the reactions are simply an expression of the hyperpyrexia. I think, of course, that tuberculin treatment can be regarded not necessarily as specific, but tonic, which applies to a great many of your patients, whether they are tuberculous or not.

DR. A. E. DAVIS, New York: I want to call attention to one point Dr. Finnoff spoke of, that is, he regarded a diagnostic test of 5 mgm. as final. I found in some of these cases, if you will let them rest two months or longer, and go back and give a diagnostic test of tuberculin, you get a reaction, and I do not think we should regard all these tests given at once, even going to 5 mgm., as excluding tuberculosis.

DR. H. M. LANGDON, Philadelphia: I wonder whether the retinal detachment, mentioned by Dr. Finnoff, was due to choroidal hemorrhage? I had a case where a massive hemorrhage into the vitreous brought the vision down to light perception; with treatment there was a complete return of vision. He was discharged from the hospital, and in three days returned saying he had another hemorrhage. He had a complete detachment of the retina, and since there were no adhesions or proliferative retinitis, I think it was due undoubtedly to choroidal hemorrhage.

DR. EMORY HILL. Richmond, Va.: I should like to ask Dr. Finnoff to go into some detail as to his method of using tuberculin. We are all aware of the apparent safety and great efficacy of tuberculin in tuberculosis of the uveal tract and cornea, but it would seem that there are possibilities of damage where the retinal vessels are involved. Dr. Jackson has called attention to this in a recent article. The question is, how far may we go in using tuberculin in cases in which a focal reaction in a vessel-wall might produce massive hemorrhage into the vitreous?

DR. W. L. BENEDICT, Rochester, Minn.: I should like to speak of the non-specific action of salvarsan, and recommend its use in the treatment of hemorrhagic lesions of the character under discussion. I would mention two or three instances of hemorrhage into the vitreous in young persons whom we have studied carefully. We examined these patients for foci of infection, eliminated every discovered focus without changing the course of the disease. We have attempted to produce hemorrhages in the eyes of animals by inoculating strains of organisms cultivated from foci of infection of persons having recurrent hemorrhages into the vitreous without positive results. A few years ago Dr. Stokes, of the Mayo Clinic, reported some cases of tuberculids of the skin, lesions which closely resemble lesions of syphilis, and demonstrated the value of salvarsan in these cases. They all did badly with tuberculin, but responded particularly well to salvarsan. Syphilis had been eliminated by every known means. Following this experience we began the treatment of patients having recurrent hemorrhages into the retina and vitreous, with excellent results. A young man, twenty-two years of age, came under my observation with a history of having had recurrent hemorrhages into the vitreous and retina of both eyes for several years. While undergoing examination he suffered an extensive hemorrhage in the eyes, which made him practically blind. He was placed under treatment with salvarsan, and within three months the vitreous became clear and has remained clear since—nine months afterward. Patients having tuberculous lesions about the eyes often respond much better to salvarsan than to tuberculin—even though there is no evidence of lues present.

DR. EDWARD JACKSON, Denver, Col.: In reference to

causation, it is probable that with the number of tuberculous cases which have been reported in recent years, a new set of statistics, from this time on, would show rather a larger proportion of cases from tuberculosis. Another point is that, among cases that are probably of tuberculous origin, a very large proportion occur in women. The proportion is much larger than of the cases in general. The third point is that the tuberculous cases—all I think that I have seen—and in large measure the mass of those that are reported, show the perivascular lesions. The cases like those of Dr. Finnoff, that seem to be due to focal infection, and perhaps some other classes of cases, do not show the lesions in the peripheral veins particularly. In the cases presented undoubtedly we have several groups of entirely distinct origins. One, perhaps, may be the group occurring in young men, non-tuberculous, and Dr. Wilmer's suggestion is very interesting as to the share of the endocrines at this time of life. But perhaps the tuberculous group is the largest, and we now have the best clinical picture of cases of that kind.

DR. F. H. VERHOEFF, Boston, Mass.: I do not think syphilis is the cause of the class of cases of which Dr. Finnoff was speaking, but it does sometimes cause hemorrhage into the vitreous and retinitis proliferans. In these syphilitic cases the retinitis proliferans does not follow hemorrhages recurring over a long period, but the whole thing happens within a relatively short time. I think every one has seen, in cases of syphilitic chorioretinitis, a few vessels extend from one of the lesions into the vitreous, but I am referring now to cases in which well-marked retinitis proliferans is produced. I recall two recent cases, in each of which the condition followed salvarsan treatment. These patients had each received six doses intravenously, had a negative Wassermann, and was apparently well, but a few weeks afterward developed a most intense chorioretinitis with hemorrhages into the vitreous, shortly followed by marked retinitis proliferans. It would seem that when salvarsan fails to cure the patient completely, the spirochætes, when they resume their activity, are apt to produce choroidal lesions more severe than if no treatment had been employed.

I have seen, in fact, so many cases of severe chorioretinitis following salvarsan treatment that I have entirely abandoned its use.

DR. W. R. PARKER, Detroit, Mich.: It seems to me that we are on the verge of knowing much more about the general effects of foreign proteins, and it appears to make very little difference how administered, whether we give egg-albumen, old TB, or antisyphilitic or anti-typhoid vaccine. These cases do well whether they are tuberculous in origin or not. If this be true, it is not right to conclude that a suspected case of tuberculosis that does well under the use of tuberculin is necessarily tuberculous in origin, nor is it necessary to prove that we have a tuberculous lesion before we give a foreign protein. My experience in this line is still very limited. We have been working with it two years now and have nothing definite to report. We have gone only far enough to know there is a big field before us, and doubt is to be thrown on some cases thought to be tuberculous because they got well under the use of old tuberculin.

DR. FINNOFF (closing): In discussing Dr. Wilmer's interesting suggestion, I think possibly the endocrines have something to do in some of these cases, although there has been nothing definite in that as yet. As to Dr. Davis' method of using tuberculin as a diagnostic, I think it would be rather dangerous, because we can give the tuberculin in the doses, bringing it up to 5 mgm. or possibly 10 mgm., and not get a reaction, but if we wait a month or two months that patient has become sensitized to that particular protein and might react to it in a so-called anaphylactic way and give us a false impression. The reaction might not be due to tuberculin, but to anaphylaxis. I do not believe tuberculin is a cure-all for all of our cases of tuberculosis, but I do believe that it is of great therapeutic value, and I think that some cases improve very decidedly when it is used. I think enough cases have been reported in the literature to prove that. The improvement might be due to a foreign protein, as Dr. Parker has brought out. Foreign protein therapy is new—it has been only the last four or five years that we have injected diphtheritic antitoxin and a number of other types of foreign protein. That, of course, must be studied

17

carefully, and five or ten years from now we might know more about its value. In answer to Dr. Hill's question, I think we must be extremely cautious in using tuberculin both as a diagnostic and therapeutic agent. The two cases I used tuberculin in justified the risk. In the one case only one eye was involved. I saw him shortly after the beginning of the disease, and I felt it was of enough scientific interest and value to the patient to determine absolutely whether it was due to tuberculosis or some other condition. I said, "You have one bad eye and the other is not involved, and if we get a reaction we are quite sure that it is due to tuberculosis." I ran him through, and I got absolutely no reaction with 5 mgm. of tuberculin. In these cases I use smaller doses of tuberculin than we ordinarily employ for diagnostic purposes. The first dose is 1/500,000 mgm.; if there is no reaction, I double it and rapidly increase. If both eyes are involved, I do not think we are justified in trying to make a diagnosis of tuberculosis with tuberculin, because if we get a reaction, we have a massive hemorrhage with increased exudate and the formation of bands of scar tissue, and we possibly will be responsible for loss of the patient's eye. In cases where there is a good eye I think we are justified. In searching literature I find many cases have an involvement of only one eye, where slight involvement of the second eye and vision remains good over a prolonged period of time. In these cases we might learn the pathology. In the extreme periphery in many cases we will find some involvement of the vessels. I believe the disease begins in the extreme periphery of the retina in most cases. The five cases I reported were men, and I have seen other similar cases in women in which this has occurred. The purpose of the paper was to stimulate interest in this subject. The literature is scanty, and it is difficult to find reports of the cases. Some cases have been mentioned in the discussion that I had overlooked.

THE OCULAR SYMPTOMS OF EPIDEMIC ENCEPHALITIS.

MATTHIAS LANCKTON FOSTER, M.D.,
New Rochelle, N. Y.

The ocular symptoms met with in encephalitis are sufficiently striking to have attracted attention from the first. In the earlier reports of cases frequent references can be found to ptosis, diplopia, so-called strabismus, and mydriasis, with an occasional note concerning the pupillary reactions, but very often the record is rather vague. Even in otherwise well-worked-out case reports the writers too often have been content with indefinite statements as to the conditions of the muscles supplied by the third nerve, without making clear the exact branches involved and the degree of involvement of each. Yet the pareses and paralyses of the ocular muscles met with in this disease present some curious features which seem to me to deserve careful study. These features are brought out thus in Tilney and Howe's summary of the ocular findings: Rarely clear-cut complete paralysis of any one oculomotor nerve. The paresis is usually partial and involves more than one, or only part of one neuromuscular group. Ptosis is the most common isolated ocular finding. The disturbances are very frequently bilateral. Unilateral or bilateral paralysis of accommodation, dissociated from pupillary involvement, may occur. The palsies frequently are not stationary, but may change from day to day. I would add to this that the change may be even more frequent. Lesions of the fundus are usually absent, but there may be a slight degree of papilledema.

It seems to me that, for the purpose of gaining what assist-

259

ance we can from the ocular symptoms in making the diagnosis of this disease, the clinical pictures presented need to
be studied with reference to the grouping of the symptoms in
the individual cases in which ocular symptoms are present.
It seems pertinent to inquire whether the successive pareses
of muscles supplied by the third nerve do or do not follow any
order, whether any one of these muscles is apt to suffer first,
whether any one of them is more likely to suffer a greater degree of paresis than the others. The onset of the paresis
appears to be gradual in some muscles, sudden in others; the
palsy of one muscle may be fleeting, while that of another,
perhaps supplied by the same nerve, is comparatively stationary; whether any constant relation between these peculiar facts can be discovered seems worth consideration; so
do the relations of the pupillary reactions, and of the condition of the accommodation, to the other symptoms.

Dr. Holden has recently made a very valuable contribution
to this subject in his masterly analysis of the ocular manifestations in 100 cases of this disease. No one can say that
these cases were not carefully and accurately observed and
recorded. As a statistical study of the frequency with which
the optic disc, the levator palpebræ, the individual extrinsic
muscles of the eyeball, the pupils, the accommodation, and
the facial nerve are affected, nothing better could be asked.
As a study of the possible explanations of the conditions observed, the paper is excellent. But there is lacking information as to the clinical grouping of these symptoms in the
individuals affected which might act as a guide to the clini-
cian and help him recognize the disease in an early stage.
Yet the importance of such information is recognized in the
final sentence, which reads: "Since the eye disturbances of
encephalitis are sometimes of early onset and then the most
annoying of the patient's symptoms, the ophthalmologist
may be the first physician to be consulted, and in times of
epidemic he may, from the eye symptoms alone, if lues can

be excluded, make the diagnosis." Apropos of this it may be remembered that in two of the seven cases reported to this Society by Dr. Woods in 1919 the ocular symptoms were the first to appear.

Such a study as the one indicated above can be made profitably only after the symptoms presented in a great many cases have been accurately observed, recorded, and published. Reliable data must be accumulated first of all, and it is for the purpose of making a slight contribution to the collection of such data that I wish to record my observations in the two following cases:

Case I.—Male, aged forty-six years. Dr. Fairfax Hall, who had the care of the patient, has kindly placed his notes at my disposal, and it has seemed wise to quote rather liberally from them. When first seen, January 19, 1921, the patient said that for four days he had been dizzy, unable to sleep, troubled with diplopia, and suffering constant pain, with exacerbations down the outside of his right arm. Some months before he had received a blow on the head which rendered him unconscious, and since then he had not perfectly regained his strength, consequently a progressive lesion in the brain resulting from that blow had to be excluded before a diagnosis of epidemic encephalitis could be made.

Large doses of bromid, chloral, and codein failed to give him any sleep the following night. In the morning his temperature was 102° F.; systolic blood-pressure, 140; diastolic, 100; neck slightly stiff; pupils contracted; some reflexes diminished, others increased, others normal; no paralysis, but the right arm was weak, stiff, tremulous, and painful; the left eye turned in, but moved past the middle line in looking to the left. The left arm also was somewhat painful. Lumbar puncture showed a very slight increase in pressure; clear fluid; 4 cells per c.c.; 100 per cent. lymphocytes; moderate increase in albumin; moderate amount of globulin; moderate reduction by Fehling's solution; negative Wassermann with both cholesterinized and plain alcoholic extract antigen. The white blood count was about 8000; 68 per cent. polynuclears; 25 per cent. lymphocytes; 4 per cent. mononnclears; 2 per cent. eosinophiles; 1 per cent. basophiles. Blood Wassermann, negative. The urine contained a faint trace of albumin and a few hyaline and small, finely granular casts.

I saw the patient on the afternoon of the twenty-second. He seemed to be rational and willing to help, but sleepy. The sleepiness was ascribed to the large amount of hypnotics which had been administered. The pupils were very small,—about the size ordinarily seen after instillation of pilocarpin,—approximately 1 mm. in diameter. They reacted quickly though slightly to light, but did not respond to accommodation. The left externus was paretic, but not paralyzed. The eye turned in distinctly while at rest, but when the patient looked to the extreme left, it would pass the middle line and then lag along more and more slowly to a point about midway between the median plane and the outer canthus. Both inferior recti were paralyzed; neither eye could turn down below the horizontal plane. This paralysis had appeared since the morning visit of Dr. Hall on the same day, as he had tested the rotations of the eyes at that time and observed both eyes turn downward. The upward rotations of both eyes,—the lateral movements of the right, and the inward movement of the left,—were normal. The patient had a myopia of 18 to 20 D., and was not inclined to open either eye widely until after he put on his correcting glasses; then a slight ptosis of the left upper lid was evident. Its margin was lower than that of the right, but did not encroach on the pupil. Thus there appeared to be a partial loss of function of the left abducens, and, to a less degree, of the left levator palpebræ, with a total loss of function of both inferior recti, the appearance of which was sudden.

The response of the contracted pupils to homatropin seemed to be a little more prompt than usual. There was no haziness over the left retina or papilla, and the vessels seemed to be normal, except that they all bent at the margin of the papilla and then ran smoothly to the center, as though either rising to the summit of an elevation or passing down the gradual incline of an excavation. No markings of the lamina cribrosa could be seen, while the vessels at the point where they turned to enter the nerve seemed to me a trifle more distinct with a lens one diopter weaker than was needed to render the vessels in the retina clear. I do not pretend to be able to measure accurately with the ophthalmoscope slight differences of level in high myopia. Had the case been one of emmetropia or hypermetropia, a positive statement that the center of the disc was above the level of the surrounding retina would have been justified, but as the case was one of high myopia, and as there was no confirmatory haziness, I can only record the observation as made. The right papilla showed no such change in the courses of the vessels; the fundus appeared to be normal except for an ordinary myopic conus.

The next day the patient slept almost continuously, and was somewhat irrational when aroused. The paresis of the ocular muscles had become more marked. The left eye had almost no power of movement except inward, while in the right the only muscle which seemed to function properly was the externus. The relative degrees of paresis of the individual muscles could not be determined. The skin was cyanosed. There was no paralysis of the muscles of the limbs, but the hands and arms were weak, with a constant tremor which was increased by movement. A careful study of the reflexes showed some to be increased and others diminished, in a confusing manner which suggested multiple lesions in the cortex, corpus striatum, and nuclei. Any single progressive lesion referable to the blow on the head was excluded and the diagnosis of encephalitis made.

The patient lay in a lethargic state for five days, and then began to recover. On the twenty-eighth his pupils were moderately dilated, reacted sluggishly to light, but not at all to accommodation. The movements of the eyeballs were limited in all directions except to the right.

On February 2d the ptosis was almost gone, and all of the other extrinsic muscles appeared to have wholly regained their functions, with the exception of the left externus. The left eyeball no longer deviated, but its outward movement was slightly restricted. The pupils were of medium size and reacted promptly to light, but not to accommodation. The general condition was improved. As convalescence progressed the patient learned that he could not read with his glasses, as had been his habit; this difficulty gradually became less.

The myosis in this case may be ascribed reasonably to the large doses of hypnotics, including codein, but it may be susceptible of some other explanation, as it does not appear to be uncommon in this disease. The pupils reacted to light promptly at all times, except when under the influence of homatropin, but at no time did they respond to accommodation. Convergence was present, for the eyes seemed to fix on the finger held near them, although the pupils did not contract. Later the accommodation proved to be paralyzed. Several cases have been reported in which the pupils responded, although the accommodation was said to be paretic or paralyzed; this case differs, as the loss of function was accompanied by the usual loss of pupillary response. Yet, as Dr. Holden has suggested to me, an absence of the pupillary response to convergence is not uncommon in high myopia.

CASE II.—Italian, aged forty-four years, admitted to the New Rochelle Hospital February 28, 1921. He had been suffering fifteen days from dizziness, headache, and pain in the back of the neck. On admission he lay apparently asleep, responding when spoken to sharply, but dozing off again at once, not restless, and seeming to have no pain. The intern noted that his pupils reacted to light and accommodation, and that his left upper lid drooped.

On March 4th there was slight ptosis of the left upper lid, not encroaching on the pupil, paresis of the left superior and inferior recti, causing the eye to lag behind when the patient looked either up or down, with all other movements of both eyes normal. The pupils were of normal size, reacting promptly to both light and accommodation. The patient was very restless and made much resistance to the examination.

The next day the ptosis of the left upper lid was more marked, the paresis of the left superior and inferior recti was unchanged, but the left internus was totally paralyzed. The left eye stopped at the midplane when the patient looked to the right. The functions of the other muscles appeared to be intact. No pathologic change in the fundus.

On the following day the paralysis of the left internus and the pareses of the inferior and superior recti had completely disappeared. The movements of the eyes in all directions seemed to be normal, and the ptosis of the left upper lid was less.

Three days later there was no ptosis and no limitations of the movements of the eyeballs in any direction. The patient looked and felt much better. After an uninterrupted convalescence he was discharged from the hospital apparently well.

About ten days later he was readmitted with the history that since discharge he had had several spells of drowsiness. Several more days elapsed before I was summoned again to his side. The patient was then awake, rational, apparently in good condition, with no signs of ocular trouble. The bedside notes showed that an inequality of the pupils and a ptosis had been noticed three days after readmission, both of which had quickly disappeared, and the nurse said that she had frequently observed a ptosis, which was sometimes partial, sometimes total, and disappeared in a short time. The occurrence of the ptosis seemed to be a precursor to an attack of drowsiness. Nothing else was noted about the eyes, while the patient gradually sank into a state of complete lethargy.

On April 16th he could not be roused, but lay apparently asleep with both eyes closed. When the lids were raised the eyes were seen to be looking straight forward, not turned upward as is usual in sleep, and not deviating in any direction. Whether this position was due to an absence of any paresis, or to total paralysis of all the muscles, could not be determined. A wisp of cotton drawn across the left cornea caused the patient to try hard to close the eye and to turn his head; when drawn across the right, a much less effect was produced. The pupils were of medium size and responded, by dilatation, to pricking of the skin over the malar bone. There was little reaction to light.

On the following day the pupils were dilated, did not respond to light, and the dilatation was only slightly increased by pricking the skin over the malar bone. The right cornea was almost if not quite insensitive, while the left was clearly sensitive. Nothing wrong was observed in the fundus. No further change was observed until the patient's death a few days later.

The very fleeting nature of all the ocular symptoms in this case is most striking. The observation of the nurse that the appearance of a ptosis seemed to be a precuisor of an onset of drowsiness seems to me to be worthy of note. The other symptoms seem to have been of a like fleeting character, as they disappeared so completely, and the patient felt so well, that he was discharged from hospital as cured of a disease which soon reasserted its presence and then went on to a fatal termination. Insensitiveness of the cornea may have been observed before, but if recorded, it has been overlooked. In this case it seems to have been a late symptom, and its probable diagnostic value cannot be said to be great.

DISCUSSION.

DR. HIRAM WOODS, Baltimore, Md.: Dr. Foster asks an important question: whether it is or is not possible to determine logical and consistent sequence in ocular symptoms. It seems to me the most consistent thing about the ocular symptoms of lethargic encephalitis is inconsistency. It is illustrated in Dr. Foster's cases. Let me present hastily the order of symptoms in some of these cases I saw and reported here two years ago: Diplopia due to paralysis of the inferior rectus, cycloplegia, partial ptosis varying in degree, nystagmoid movements, and optic neuritis. Optic neuritis is rare. In another case there was no ocular but a facial paralysis. In another there was diplopia due to paralysis of the external rectus. Case 5 had transient facial paralysis and prolonged paralysis of accommodation; Case 6 showed only a paralysis of the external rectus in the morning, and of the inferior rectus and ciliary muscle of the other eye the same afternoon. As far as my own experience shows, we cannot fix any definite order of eye symptoms. They depend on the nuclei involved. The paresis may be gradual and slow in recovery, or sudden in onset and recovery. They have a tendency to relapse. The ciliary muscle seems the slowest to recover. Something that Dr.

Foster has not spoken of is a peculiar jerking or nystagmoid motion when the eyes change position. You will be making an ophthalmoscopic examination, and while the patient is endeavoring to keep the eyes still there will be a jerking up or in. As Dr. Wilder has pointed out, if you go to extreme lateral motion you often get a wobbly movement that passes off if the patient closes his eyes. Any attempt at fixation seems to bring out these nystagmoid movements. The absence of optic neuritis and the long time in which accommodation takes to recover as compared to the other muscular functions, seem to me the most characteristic symptoms of lethargic encephalitis. Then we may be helped by extraocular symptoms, such as lethargy and spinal fluid examination. Dr. Foster spoke of syphilis being excluded by blood examination. In this class of cases I would not myself be satisfied that I had gone as far as I ought to go in excluding syphilis without examination of the spinal fluid itself.

DR. WILLIAM C. FINNOFF, Denver, Col.: Rosenow has found in the majority of cases of lethargic encephalitis that he can obtain a specific Gram-positive diplococcus from the nasopharynx and from plugs in the tonsils. He has reproduced these organisms and injected them into animals, and has gotten all the types of lethargic encephalitis in these animals, even to the Parksonian type. He also has produced an antitoxin by the injection of these organisms into animals, and this antitoxin has cured animals which have developed the disease and has cured some humans. I think that we can look to Rosenow for a specific cure in this disease.

DR. H. FRIEDENWALD, Baltimore, Md.: I should like to ask a question. I have been impressed by the mild character of some of the cases both from the general and eye points of view. One of my cases was that of a young man of about 28, who came with a marked paresis of the externus. I sent him to have a Wassermann made, and about the time the Wassermann report came, two days later, the paralysis had disappeared. At that time the patient felt perfectly well. The disappearance of the paresis and good general condition made me think the patient was well, and I allowed him to go to Chicago from Baltimore on a business trip. While out there he passed into lethargy, returned to his home, and recovered rapidly and completely. A short time after this a patient with a similar history exhibited paresis of the ocular muscles, which lasted for some time, but there were no lethargic symptoms at all; negative Wassermann. I would inquire, in these epidemics, does the speaker not find cases with these ocular symptoms not only the earliest, but the only signs that are seen; the diagnosis is therefore an exceedingly difficult one, and in some will always be in doubt?

DR. FOSTER (closing): I did not speak of nystagmoid movements because they were absent in both of these cases. As far as the Wassermann test is concerned, this was made of both the spinal fluid and the blood. The spinal fluid was tested with both cholesterinized and plain antigen. The cases of encephalitis are divided into fourteen varieties of which lethargic is only one, so I have avoided the term lethargic encephalitis.

The most important features of my second case were the mildness of the symptoms, and the fatal result. The eye symptoms were slight, the general symptoms were slight, and the patient apparently got absolutely well in the hospital and was discharged, to be readmitted a few days later, the symptoms still slight, yet to sink steadily until he died in lethargy. This case proves that mild symptoms do not necessarily indicate a favorable prognosis. I am inclined to believe that there are cases in which the ocular symptoms may be the only ones observable, and therefore I wish to emphasize the need of so grouping, or of learning how to group, the symptoms of this disease, which is a dangerous one, that epidemic encephalitis can be recognized with a fair degree of certainty by the ophthalmologist, who is apt to be the first physician to be consulted.

THE EFFECT OF VARIATIONS IN INTENSITY OF ILLUMINATION ON ACUITY, SPEED OF DISCRIMINATION, SPEED OF ACCOMMODATION, AND OTHER IMPORTANT EYE FUNCTIONS.

C. E. FERREE, PH.D., AND G. RAND, PH.D.,

Bryn Mawr College.

(By Invitation.)

This work was begun as a war study. There was a need to speed up the industrial output, and it was thought that an increase in intensity of illumination might help to accomplish this result through a possible benefit to ocular functions. While perhaps of primary interest to the lighting specialist, results have been obtained which may be of interest also to the ophthalmologist.

Intensity is only one of the lighting factors which influence the functional powers of the eye. In a former paper* we have shown that one effect may be gotten for increase of intensity for a good lighting installation, and another, quite different, for an installation where the increase of intensity is accompanied by an increase in the number or brilliancy of the bright surfaces in the field of view. In the case of the present study we have worked only under conditions in which the increase of intensity did not result in the introduction of harmful glares into the field of view. We have also used much wider ranges of intensity and have tested the effect on other functions of importance to the working eye.

Some of the beneficial effects of increase of intensity may be summarized in the following statements:

(1) There is a slow but substantial gain in *acuity* for all

---

* "Further Experiments on the Efficiency of the Eye Under Different Conditions of Lighting," Trans. Illum. Eng. Soc., 1915, x, pp. 448–502.

but low intensities, where the gain is rapid. This gain, moreover, is greater in case of small uncorrected errors in refraction than for the normal eye. Such errors in refraction are very common. Even the corrected eye, more particularly in cases of astigmatism, is rarely corrected with such precision as not to be considerably benefited by an increase in the intensity of the illumination under which it works. The principle underlying the benefit of increase of illumination is not hard to understand. With reference to the object seen, or the work, clear seeing is affected by two conditions, an increase in its size or the visual angle subtended, and an increase in the amount of light which it receives. An increase in either is of benefit, more particularly when acuity is subnormal through an uncorrected astigmatism or some other defect. In case of all of the functions which we have tested,—acuity, power to sustain acuity, speed of discrimination and speed of adjustment for clear seeing at different distances,—the subnormal eye approaches more nearly to the normal eye in functional power as the intensity of the illumination is increased. There is a strong probability also that the middle-aged and old eye benefit more by an increase of illumination than the young eye.

The fact that the acuity of the eye with a small defect in refraction approximates more nearly to that of the normal eye with increase of illumination should be of interest to the ophthalmologist, as well as to the lighting specialist, inasmuch as it indicates that small errors in refraction or in their correction cannot be picked up as readily at high as at low illuminations by the acuity test. Apparently the effect of small differences in the resolving power of the refracting media on clearness of seeing tends to be obscured or obliterated at high illuminations by the greater power of the retina to discriminate the slightly blurred detail at these illuminations. That is, there are three factors in acuity or the power of the eye to see clearly: the resolving power of the refracting media, the space discrimination of the retina, and its sensitivity to light. To put it in another way, there are the resolving power of the refracting media, or the power to form clear images on the retina; and the resolving power of the retina itself, or the power to discriminate detail in the physical image formed. The resolving power of the retina increases with increase of illumination and compensates for slight defects in the resolving power of the refracting media.

(2) There is a gain in the *speed of discrimination*. This gain is very great from low to high illuminations when the object is small. As might be expected, the effect of increase of intensity of illumination on the speed of discrimination grows less as the visual angle increases. However, at a value of angle of 3.45 minutes of arc the effect is still great. With an angle of 1.15 minutes of arc the increase in speed produced by changing the illumination from 0.4 to 12 foot-candles amounted to 603 per cent.; with an angle of 2.49 minutes of arc, a value roughly approximating the details in 10-point type at the conventional reading distance of 33 cm., the increase was 331 per cent.; and with a value of 3.45 minutes of arc, the increase was 309 per cent.

(3) There is a gain in the *speed of adjustment* for clear seeing at different distances. The adjustment for seeing at different distances involves changes in both convergence and accommodation. Clearness of seeing is both the incentive for these changes and the check on their accurate accomplishment. It is only natural to suppose, therefore, that whatever leads to quick and accurate seeing favors quick and accurate changes in adjustment. With increase of the intensity of light the eye with defective refraction gains in its speed of making these adjustments more than the normal eye.

(4) There is a gain in the *power to sustain clear seeing* when the size of the test-object or the visual angle is kept the same for the different illuminations. Since we cannot

at will change the size of the work or the object seen, this is obviously the more significant test condition. This gain is very great when a comparatively small visual angle is used. Obviously, a large visual angle could not be used to measure this function because the acuity or power to see clearly might suffer great loss without blurring the vision of a large angle. Again there is a very marked benefit for the defective eye in increasing the intensity of illumination.

All the functions referred to above are aspects of acuity. They are aspects, however, which are not brought out by the conventional method of testing acuity. The conventional test of acuity takes little account of either speed or power to sustain, two aspects which are not only of great importance to the working efficiency of the eye, but are extremely sensitive indicators of differences in functional power. Add either of these aspects to the method of testing acuity and the effect is very similar, so far as sensitivity is concerned, to that obtained when an amplifier is added to a physical recording instrument.* For example, changes of intensity, which produce comparatively small differences in acuity as ordinarily tested, cause very large changes in the speed of discrimination and the power to sustain acuity. The conventional acuity test is, comparatively speaking, not only insensitive, but it is not sufficiently comprehensive in the range of aspects covered to bring out differentially some of the most important functional powers of the eye †

* The analogy to an amplifier is perhaps misleading. The greater result is obtained by testing the aspects of clear seeing, which are the most strongly affected by any condition which augments or depresses functional power, not by a process of amplifying or magnifying the real effect.

† Further, a consideration of the number of factors on which acuity depends: intensity of illumination; time of exposure of test-object (the effect of time of exposure is enormous at low illuminations); state of adaptation or sensitivity of the retina; number of meridians in which the resolving power is tested simultaneously, or successively if a test-object taxing the resolving power in only one meridian is used (if such a test-object is employed, the determination should be made certainly in no less than four meridians); brightness of preexposure; brightness of surrounding field and evenness of brightness of surrounding field; breadth of pupil, etc., leads one to a realization of how little a statement

(5) A fifth point of importance is whether the eye tends to fatigue more under the high illuminations. Using the method for testing fatigue employed in all of our former work on lighting in its relation to the eye,* no significant difference in effect could be found for reading for three hours from uniform type and paper under well-diffused daylight illumination with 0.4, 2, 4, 6, 8, 12, and 36 foot-candles of light on the reading page when the eye was adapted for fifty minutes to each intensity of illumination prior to beginning the test. The light was received from a skylight covering the entire ceiling, beneath which were swung large diffusion sashes of ground glass filling the entire opening. The control of intensity was secured by an elaborate system of curtains, thin white and light-proof, also covering the entire ceiling. There was also no significant difference at these illuminations in the tendency to produce discomfort, as measured by the method employed for this purpose in our former work, under the conditions of adaptation and with the distribution and control of illumination described above.

In view of the results obtained with the preceding tests for increase of intensity of illumination, this result may cause some surprise. That is, it might seem reasonable to suppose that a benefit should be expected here as well as in case of the former tests. In comparing this result with those of the former tests, the following points should be borne in mind: (1) The visual angle subtended by ordinary print at

of acuity means unless the exact conditions under which the determination is made are given.

When a simple test-object is used, there is in general a tendency to overestimate acuity. The power to see more complex objects is not fairly gauged by a test-object which taxes the resolving power in only one meridian, even when successive tests are made in different meridians, *i. e.*, the effect of the slight distortions present in the refracting action of nearly every eye, which tends to confuse the discrimination of complex objects, is lost on the simple test-object.

* "Test for the Efficiency of the Eye Under Different Systems of Illumination and a Preliminary Study of the Causes of Discomfort," Trans. of the Illum. Eng. Soc., 1913, viii, pp. 40–60; "Some Experiments on the Eye with Inverted Reflectors of Different Densities," *ibid.*, 1915, x, pp. 1097–1129, etc.

18

the reading distance (33 cm.) is large. A different result would doubtless have been obtained if fine print or a smaller visual angle had been used. (2) The visual angle subtended by the test-object used in the three-minute record before and after the three-hour reading period was changed to sustain approximately the same ratio of time clear to time blurred for the fresh eye for each illumination used. This is always done in this test so as to get as nearly as possible the effect of the reading alone. (3) There is no guarantee that the eye read with the same speed and accuracy at the different illuminations, therefore no guarantee that the eye did the same amount and quality of work at the different illuminations. There doubtless would be a tendency for the eye to read more slowly under the more difficult conditions of work, although the intention of the observer was to read at the same speed at all illuminations. Had it been possible to secure a feasible standardization of the features of speed and accuracy of work during the three-hour period, the test would doubtless have been rendered more sensitive for picking up small differences in the favorableness of the lighting conditions employed in this and all of our former work. That is, a strict standardization of the speed and accuracy of performance during the working period would doubtless have given us even a greater difference in result for the different lighting conditions during the past several years of work than were obtained. So far we have not found it feasible to incorporate the testing of the features: speed, accuracy, and power to sustain in one and the same test. We have instead tested speed and accuracy together, and power to sustain and accuracy; there has, however, been no strict standardization of speed and accuracy during the period of work in the fatigue test.

THE EFFECT OF INTENSITY OF LIGHT ON ACUITY.

In one series of experiments four observers were used and the acuity was determined at 0.001, 0.005, 0.01, 0.015, 0.02, 0.05, 0.1, 0.2, 0.4, 1, 2, 3, 5, 10, and 20 foot-candles of light normal to the test-object. The eye was adapted to each illumination by a thirty-minute practice series with proper rest-periods. The broken circle (the international test-object) mounted on a rotating graduated dial was used as test-object. In making the observation all that was required of the observer was to indicate the direction in which the opening pointed. The judgment on which the estimate of acuity was based was thus reduced to very simple terms and an objective check was had on its correctness. In the final series of determinations this opening was turned in haphazard order right, left, up, down, and the four 45-degree positions; and a correct judgment was required in five out of the eight positions. The breadth of the opening was measured on a micrometer comparator and the visual angle computed. The coefficient of reflection of the test surface was 78 per cent. The preëxposure and surrounding field were made in each case as nearly as possible of the same brightness as the test surface. An exposure of one second was allowed for each judgment. The work was done under artificial illumination, the light of frosted type B Mazda lamps. The angle of incidence of the light on the test surface was kept constant throughout the experiments. Constancy of position of the observer's eye was secured by biting a mouthboard in which the impression of his teeth had been previously made and hardened in wax.

A curve showing the average results for the four observers is given in Fig. 1. In this figure acuity is expressed as the reciprocal of the visual angle discriminated, that is, 1 divided by the value of the visual angle. Acuity is plotted against foot-candles. It increases rapidly with increase of illumination up to a value of 1, or what we usually call 6/6 or 20/20. The value of the angle discriminated here is one minute. This acuity is reached at about 0.2 foot-candle of light on the test-object. An acuity of 1½ or 6/4 is reached at about 2 foot-candles of light; at 5 foot-candles the acuity is 1.94; at 10 foot-candles, 1.97; and at 20 foot-candles, about 2.1.

From 0.001 to 0.1 foot-candle the minimum visual angle

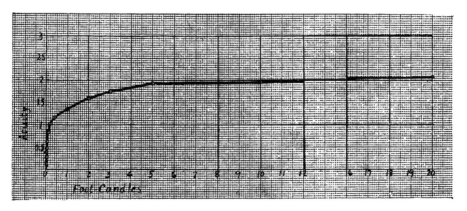

Fig. 1.—Showing the effect of increase of intensity of light on acuity (four observers), acuity plotted against foot-candles of light normal to the surface of test-object.

Intensity (foot-candles)	Acuity	Intensity (foot-candles)	Acuity
0.001	0.140	0.40	1.158
0.005	0.2075	1.00	1.350
0.010	0.2655	2.00	1.611
0.015	0.381	3.00	1.743
0.02	0.483	5.00	1.9385
0.05	0.615	10.00	1.973
0.10	0.8245	20.00	2.097
0.20	1.028		

changed from 7.143 to 1.213 minutes of arc, a gain of 488.9 per cent. in acuity; from 0.1 to 1 foot-candle it changed from 1.213 to 0.741 minutes of arc, a gain of 63.7 per cent. in acuity; from 1 to 5 foot-candles it changed from 0.741 to 0.516 minute of arc, a gain of 43.6 per cent. in acuity; and from 5 to 20 foot-candles it changed from 0.516 to 0.477 minute of arc, a gain of 8.2 per cent in acuity.

In another series of experiments the most practised observer was selected for a comparison of the effect of change of intensity of light on the eye with normal refraction and the same eye made slightly astigmatic in the following ways, by a +.12 diopter cylinder; a +.25 diopter cylinder; a +.25 diopter cylinder with a correcting cylinder 5 degrees off axis; and a +.25 diopter cylinder with a correcting cylinder 10 degrees off axis. Refraction defects of this type and magnitude are of very common occurrence. Even in case of the corrected eye the correction for high astigmatisms is frequently off from 0.12–0.25 diopter in amount; and for low astigmatisms, 0.12 diopter in amount and from 5 to 20 degrees in the placement of the correction. Artificial astigmatisms were chosen for this work in order that we might know the exact amount and location of the defect and have a comparison of the effect on the same eye in the normal and defective condition. They were not chosen with the belief that they are the exact functional equivalent of the natural astigmatisms. We are too strongly impressed with the possibility that the astigmatic eye may progressively acquire some power to compensate for its defect to be of this opinion. The eye was presensitized by thirty minutes of adaptation to each illumination. The brightness of preëxposure and surrounding field was the same as that of the test surface. The reflection coefficient of the test surface was 78 per cent. The intensities of illumination were 0.015, 0.05, 0.1, 0.25, 0.5, 1, 1.5, 2, 4, 6, 8, 12, and 36 foot-candles normal to the test surface. The results of these determinations are shown in Fig. 2A and Fig. 2B. In Fig. 2A acuity is plotted against foot-candles, and in Fig. 2B percentage gain in acuity with increase of illumination is plotted against foot-candles. In Fig. 2A it will be observed that the effect of increase of illumination on acuity is greater for the defective than for the normal eye. Because of the greater benefit for the defective eye, the difference in the acuity between the defective and the normal eye is slight at the higher illuminations and considerably greater at the lower illuminations. For ex-

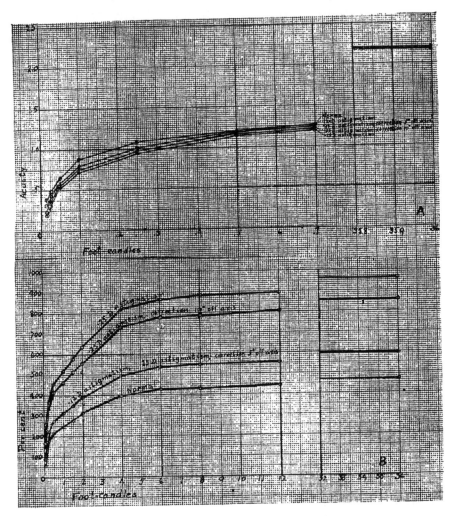

Fig. 2.—Showing the effect of increase of intensity of light on acuity for eye with normal refraction, and same eye made slightly astigmatic: A, Acuity plotted against foot-candles; B, percentage gain in acuity plotted against foot-candles.

ample, at 0.25 foot-candle the difference in acuity between the fully corrected eye and the 0.25 diopter astigmatism with its correction 5 degrees off axis amounts to 7.5 per cent.;

at 12 foot-candles it amounts to only 1 per cent. At 0.25 foot-candle the difference between the normal eye and the same eye given a 0.25 diopter astigmatism amounts to 15 per cent.; at 12 foot-candles it amounts to 3 per cent.

In Chart 2B the comparative benefits experienced by the normal and the defective eye are expressed in per cent. The benefit is shown to be less for the normal eye and to increase with the magnitude of the defect in case of the defective eye.

THE INTENSITY OF ILLUMINATION OF TEST-CHARTS.

The question frequently comes before standardizing committees,—At what intensity of illumination should acuity be tested?* Our answer would be: It depends upon the purpose for which the test is to be made. There are three obvious applications of acuity testing: vocational selection, diagnosis, and hygiene or welfare of the eye.

In the rating of the eyes as to fitness for vocations, the test should be made as nearly as possible at the illumination usually employed in the vocation in question. The study of even a small number of cases shows that eyes cannot be given the same relative rating as to acuity at different intensities of illumination. For example, experience has shown in the Navy that only 20–25 per cent. of the men accepted for the service on the basis of the conventional acuity test at the higher illuminations are able to qualify for the lookout work at night on the bridge of the battleships. Further in a test of 61 observers made by us, all under 25 years of age

* This question should by no means be confused with our former discussions: "Visual Acuity at Low Illuminations: Apparatus and Results," These Transactions, 1919, xvii, pp. 370–395; The Use of the Illumination Scale for the Detection of Small Errors in Refraction and in Their Correction, Amer. Jour. Ophth., 1920, iii, pp. 243–256. In the discussions referred to, the illumination, not the visual angle scale, was employed as the measuring scale for the detection of low astigmatisms and small errors in the amount and placement of their correction. The present discussion refers wholly to the use of the visual angle scale, the question being if we use the visual angle scale to measure acuity, at what intensity of illumination shall the determinations be made.

and rating 6/4 acuity by the conventional test with 5 foot-candles of light on the chart, 13 per cent. rated below 6/6 at 0.55 foot-candle of light and 33 per cent. below 6/6 at 0.2 foot-candle. The acuity of the remainder was 6/6 or better at these illuminations. If speed in the use of the eye at low illuminations be added to the requirement, the scatter is very much greater. The amount of time required just to discriminate 1 minute of visual angle in this group of observers who were all put in the same class by the acuity test at the high illumination, covered a range from slowest to fastest of 1333 per cent. at 0.55 foot-candle of light and of 1443 per cent. at 0.2 foot-candle. It is quite obvious that any attempt to rate eyes for vocational purposes at only one or even one order of intensity of illumination is based on a lack of knowledge of the differential effect for different eyes of intensity of illumination on the power of the eye to see clearly.

Doubtless all will agree that the object in diagnosis is to give the test under the conditions providing the maximum sensitivity for detecting errors in refraction. A glance at the curves given in Fig. 2A is sufficient to show that this maximum degree of sensitivity is not obtained at the higher illuminations. For the smaller uncorrected astigmatic errors represented in this figure, the difference in acuity is scarcely detectable at the higher illuminations; but readily detectable at the lower. The reason for this has already been discussed. The details in the slightly blurred astigmatic image can be discriminated at high illumination but not at low because of the effect of increase of intensity of illumination on the resolving power of the retina. This increase in diagnostic sensitivity was further directly tested as follows: Low artificial astigmatisms were made and corrected. Starting with the proper placement of the correcting cylinder, the axis was shifted from its position by graded changes, ascending and descending series, until the judgment was made of just noticeable difference in the clearness of seeing of the letter B subtending a total visual angle of five minutes. This was done at 15, 10, 5, 3, 0.45 and 0.25 foot-candles of light on the test card. The tests were made very carefully. Seven concordant judgments out of ten were accepted as the criterion of just noticeably different in any one set of trials. The results for six observers are shown in Table 1.

TABLE 1.—SHOWING NUMBER OF DEGREES AT WHICH CYLIN-DER MUST BE PLACED OFF AXIS TO GIVE NOTICEABLE DIFFERENCE OF CLEARNESS OF TEST-OBJECT. RESULTS ARE BASED ON 7 OUT OF 10 JUDGMENTS.

OBSERVER	ASTIGMATISM	DEGREES CYLINDER MUST BE PLACED OFF AXIS TO GIVE JUST NOTICEABLE DIFFERENCE OF CLEARNESS	
		High Illumination (Average of results at 5 and 10 f c.)	Low Illumination (Average of results at 0 25 and 0.45 f.c.)
H.	0.25 cyl. ax. 90°	15.0	2.5
B.	0.25 cyl. ax. 90°	13.5	5.0
L.	0.25 cyl ax. 180°	8.5	6.5
S.	0.37 cyl. ax. 180°	13.5	4.0
C.	0.50 cyl. ax. 90°	20.3	9.5
Bs.	0.75 cyl. ax. 90°	9.0	5.0

In any hygiene or welfare test of the favorableness of working conditions for the eye, the tests should also be made at more than one intensity of illumination. Conditions which apparently are equally acceptable at the higher illuminations are often far from equally acceptable at the lower. In all cases it will be found too that the sensitivity of the acuity test, whether the purpose be vocational, diagnostic or hygienic, is very greatly enhanced when the procedure is made to include speed, power to sustain, and accuracy; instead of accuracy alone, as is the case in the conventional method of testing acuity.

THE EFFECT OF INTENSITY OF LIGHT ON SPEED OF DISCRIMINATION.

For the case of normal refraction this work was done on 13 observers. Two of these observers were selected for a comparison of the effect on the normal eye and the same eye given a slight refraction defect. Slight astigmatisms were produced by a +0.12 diopter cylinder, and by a +0.25 diopter cylinder with a correcting cylinder 5 degrees off axis. Again, the test-object was a broken circle, the opening of which subtended respectively visual angles of 1.15, 1.73, 2.49, and 3.45 minutes of arc at the eye of the observer 6 meters distant. The circle was mounted at the center of a graduated rotating dial. Exposures were made by means of a tachistoscope somewhat similar to that devised by us for the Air Service of the United States Army, later supplied to the Japanese Army, furnished with only one set of exposure discs rotating in front and as close as possible to the test-object. On the front surface of these discs, in line with the observer's eye and the test-object, was placed a fixation cross in order that the exposure might begin with the eye in approximate adjustment for the test-object. The determinations were made at 0.4, 2.0, 4.0, 6.0, 8.0, and 12.0 footcandles of light normal to the surface of the test-object. The reflection coefficient of the test surface was 78 per cent. The angle of incidence of light on the test surface was kept constant for all illuminations. The eye was allowed to adapt to each intensity of light through a thirty-minute practice series provided with proper rest periods. In the final series for the eyes with normal refraction eight positions of the test-object were used—up, down, right, left, and the four 45-degree positions. For the eyes with the refraction defect, the same number of exposures were given to the test-object but only four positions were used for the opening in the circle, those midway between the meridian of the astigmatism and the normal meridian. This was done in order that each position should set as nearly as possible the same task for the resolving power of the eye.

The average results for the thirteen observers of normal refraction for 1.15, 1.73, 2.49 and 3.45 minutes of visual angle are plotted in Fig. 3, A and B, 2.49 minutes of arc is approximately the visual angle subtended by the details of 10-point type at the conventional reading distance, 33 cm. Speed is expressed as the reciprocal of the time in seconds

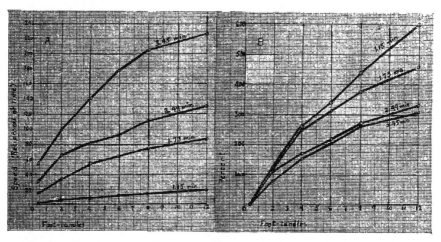

Fig. 3.—Showing the effect of increase of intensity of light on speed of discrimination for eyes with normal refraction (13 observers). In A speed is plotted against foot-candles; in B, per cent. gain in speed is plotted against foot-candles.

required to make the discrimination, *i. e.*, 1 divided by this time. In Fig. 3A speed is plotted against foot-candles.

In Fig. 3B is shown in per cent. the increase in speed produced by increasing the illumination for each of the visual angles. As might be expected, the effect of increase of illumination grows less as the visual angle or size of object is increased. There is good reason to believe, however, that there is considerable effect even for very large visual angles.

The foregoing results show that the speed of discrimination has been obtained for visual angles of the value of 1.15,

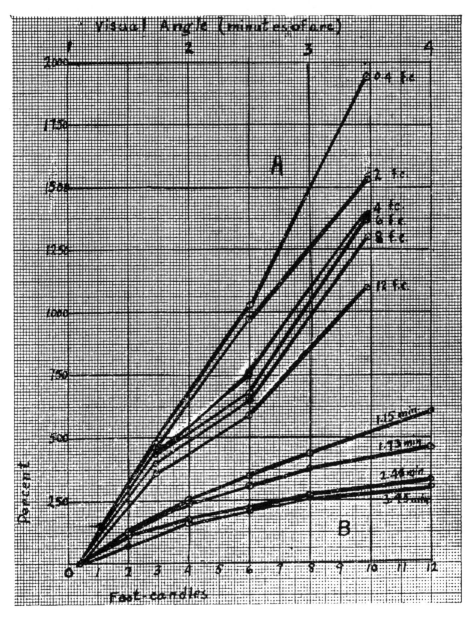

Fig. 4.—Showing the effect on speed of discrimination, both of increase of illumination and increase of visual angle. In A, per cent. increase in speed is plotted against visual angle; in B, per cent. increase in speed is plotted against foot-candles.

1.73, 2.49, and 3.45 minutes of arc at 0.4, 2, 4, 6, 8, and 12 foot-candles of illumination. It is obvious that the data can be plotted to show the effect of increase of illumination over the range specified for each visual angle, or the effect of increase of visual angle for each intensity of illumination. Both types of plotting are given in Fig. 4. Fig. 4A shows in per cent. the effect of increase of visual angle and Fig. 4B,

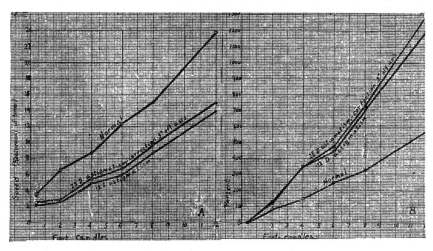

Fig. 5.—Showing the effect of increase of intensity of light on speed of discrimination (two observers) for eyes with normal refraction and same eyes made slightly astigmatic: A, speed of discrimination plotted against foot-candles; B, percentage gain in speed of discrimination plotted against foot-candles.

for comparison, the effect of increase of illumination on speed of discrimination. Both sets of curves are plotted on the same per cent. ordinate. The following points may be noted: (1) The effect of increase of visual angle is greater than the effect of increase of illumination. (2) Just as the effect of increase of illumination on speed grows less as the visual angle is increased, so does the effect of increase of visual angle on speed grow less as the intensity of the illumination is increased. That is, we get a greater benefit of increase of illumination when the work is small, and a greater benefit of increase of the size of the work when the illumination is low.

The results for the two observers with refraction defect are shown in Figs. 5A and B. In Fig. 5A speed is plotted against foot-candles and in Fig. 5B percentage gain in speed with increase of illumination is plotted against foot-candles. In Chart 5A the point of particular interest to the ophthalmologist is how much the speed of discrimination is decreased by such small errors of refraction as a 0.12 diopter astigmatism and a 0.25 diopter astigmatism with its correcting cylinder only 5 degrees off axis. In Chart 5B the point to note is how much more eyes with these small uncorrected defects benefit by the increase of illumination than does the normal eye.

THE EFFECT OF INTENSITY OF LIGHT ON THE SPEED OF ADJUSTING THE EYE FOR CLEAR SEEING AT DIFFERENT DISTANCES.

Determinations were made of the time required to change the eyes from a position of exact adjustment for the clear seeing of the test-object at 20 cm. to one at 6 meters, and back again to 20 cm., at 0.4, 2.0, 6.0, and 12.0 foot-candles of light normal to each of the three test-objects. The process measured included the change of adjustment from one of the near test-objects to the far object, the discrimination of the far object, the change of adjustment back to the other near object, and the discrimination of this object. The determinations were made with the apparatus devised by us for the Air Service of the United States Army for determining the speed of adjustment of the eyes of aviators. For a description of the apparatus and method of using, references are given in the appended footnote.* Larger visual angles were used in these experiments because of the difficulty of

* The Inertia of Adjustment of the Eye for Clear Seeing at Different Distances: "A Study of Ocular Functions with Special Reference to Aviation," Trans. Amer. Ophth. Soc., 1918, xvi, pp. 142–166; Amer. Jour. of Ophth., 1918, i, pp. 764–776. "The Speed of Adjustment of the Eye for Clear Seeing at Different Distances," Amer Jour. Psych., 1919, xxx, pp. 40–61.

getting a test-object small enough to subtend the smaller values of visual angle at the distance of the two near positions, 20 cm. For the near objects the value was 2.6 minutes of arc, and for the far object 1.4 minutes of arc. Again an objective check was had on the correctness of the judgment, *i. e.*, the test-objects were mounted at the center of rotating dials, the task for the observer being to indicate the direction in which the opening was turned.

In making the determinations the test-objects were carefully adjusted to the level of the observer's eyes; the far object, in the median plane between the objects on either side slightly farther apart than the interocular distance, their separation being just great enough not to obscure the view of the far object with either eye. Constancy of position of the observer's eyes was secured by biting a mouthboard in which the impression of his teeth had been previously made and hardened in wax. The far object was illuminated by a 100-watt frosted type B Mazda lamp in a Beehive reflector, the changes in intensity being produced by change of distance and measured with an illuminometer with its test plate in the position of the test-object. The angle of incidence of the light on the test-object was kept the same for all illuminations. The near objects were illuminated by light reflected from the mat white screen which formed the back of the apparatus and through an oblong aperture in which the observer viewed the three test-objects. The source of light was a tubular tungsten lamp installed in the horizontal in a plane midway between the screen and the near test-object so that the center of the filament was about 12 cm. above the two test-objects and equidistant from them.

The lamp was provided with a tubular reflector in the circular wall of which was an oblong aperture equal in breadth to about one-third of the circumference of the tubular reflector. By rotating this reflector the angle of incidence of the light on the reflecting screen could be changed and the intensity of the beam reflected to the near test-objects varied by small amounts. As already stated the intensity of light on the far test-object was measured with an illuminometer with its test plate in the position of the test-object; the near test-objects were matched in brightness to the far object at the different intensities of illumination. Adaptation was allowed for each intensity of illumination during a preliminary practice series of 30 minutes provided with proper rest periods.

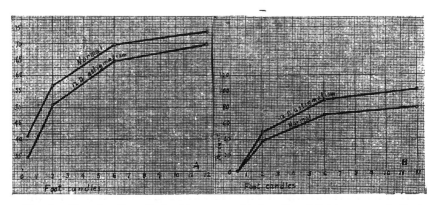

Fig. 6.—Showing the effect of increase of intensity of light on speed of adjustment of eye for clear seeing at different distances for eyes with normal refraction and same eyes made slightly astigmatic (two observers): A, speed plotted against foot-candles; B, percentage gain in speed plotted against foot-candles.

For the case of normal refraction two observers were chosen, normal both as to refraction and muscle balance. The refraction defect was produced by +0.12 diopter cylinders, axes 45 degrees in one eye and 135 degrees in the other. The results of these determinations are shown in Fig. 6A and 6B. In Fig. 6A speed is plotted against foot-candles; and in Fig. 6B percentage gain in speed with increase in illumination is plotted against foot-candles. The points to note in Fig. 6A are the increase in speed of adjustment with increase in intensity of illumination and how much the speed of adjustment is slowed by so small an error in refraction as a 0.12 diopter astigmatism; and in Fig. 6B, how much more the speed of adjustment is increased for the defective than for the normal eye by an increase in the intensity of the illumination. The factors in speed of adjustment are speed of discrimination, the elasticity of the lens, and the speed of coördinated reaction of the muscles of accommodation and convergence. In all probability the effect of small refraction errors and intensity of illumination on speed of adjustment comes largely if not entirely through the effect on speed of discrimination.

Effect of Intensity of Light on Power to Sustain Clear Seeing.

The determinations of power to sustain clear seeing were made at 0.4, 2.0, 4.0, 6.0, 8.0, 12.0 and 36.0 foot-candles of light normal to the test surface. The coefficient of reflection of the test surface was 76.5 per cent. For the case in which the visual angle was kept the same for the different illuminations, a value of visual angle had to be chosen which could be discriminated at all illuminations. A value was selected slightly greater than the minimum visual angle for the lowest illumination, namely, a value of 0.883 minute of arc. The test-object was the same as was always used for the work on power to sustain clear seeing: the printed letters li, the task being to resolve and hold clear the break between the dot and its stem in the letter i. The breadth of the break was 0.159 mm., and the visual angle subtended by the break at the observer's eye was, as already stated, 0.883 minute. A record was made on a kymograph with a key, electromagnetic recorder and a Jacquet chronograph of the time the break could be discriminated in three minutes, the measure of the performance of the eye being expressed as a ratio of time seen clear to time seen blurred. It could also be expressed as time seen clear to total time of observation.

19

There being no objective check on the correctness of the judgment, its precision had to be checked up by the size of the mean variation as it is in photometry and other subjective performances in which an objective check is not possible. As in photometry, carefully tested and practised observers are also needed. The work was done under well-diffused daylight. This light was received from a skylight covering the entire ceiling of the room, beneath which was swung large diffusion sashes of ground glass filling the entire opening. The control of intensity was secured by two systems of thin white curtains running on spring rollers beneath the skylight, and a light-proof curtain. One of the systems of white curtains and the light-proof curtain ran lengthwise of the room; the other system of white curtains ran across the room. By means of the white curtains either small local or general changes could be produced in the illumination of the room, and by means of the light-proof curtain larger changes could be produced ranging from full illumination to the darkness of a moderately good dark room. The breadth of the light-proof curtain was equal to that of the room and it ran in a deep light-tight boxing. The white curtains were narrower and were made to overlap at the edges. These curtains ran on wire guides to prevent sagging or wrinkling. The walls of the room were mat white and the floor a light gray. The eye was presensitized by 50 minutes of adaptation to each illumination. Constancy of position of the eye was secured by having the observer bite a mouthboard on which the impression of his teeth had previously been made and hardened in wax. The tests were made with normal refraction and for the same eyes made slightly astigmatic by a +0.12 diopter cylinder, a +0.25 diopter cylinder, a +0.25 diopter cylinder with a correcting cylinder 5 degrees off axis, and a +0.25 diopter cylinder with a correcting cylinder 10 degrees off axis. The axis of the cylinders used to produce the astigmatism was placed in each case at 90 degrees, the position of minimum effect on the detail to be discriminated.

The results of these determinations are shown in Figs. 7A and 7B. In Fig. 7A ratio time clear to time blurred is plotted against foot-candles, and in Fig. 7B the percentage gain in the ratio time clear to time blurred with increase of illumination is plotted against foot-candles. The points to be noted in Fig. 7A are the increase in the eye's power to sustain clear seeing with increase of intensity of illumination, and how much this power to sustain is decreased at all illuminations by these very small defects in refraction; and in Fig. 7B, how much more the power to sustain clear seeing is increased with increase of intensity of illumination for the defective eye than for the normal eye.

For various obvious reasons the foregoing curves were not all plotted on the same scale, nor was the same number of observers used throughout. In order to make possible a comparison of the effect of change of intensity of illumination on the different functions under the conditions tested, Figs. 8A and 8B are given in which the curves are all plotted on the same scale and represent the results of the same observer. Fig. 8A shows the effect on the eyes with normal refraction, and Fig. 8B, on the same eyes made slightly astigmatic by a 0.12 diopter cylinder.

An inspection of Fig. 8A shows that the functions most affected by increase of illumination are in order from greatest to least the power to sustain acuity, speed of discrimination, speed of adjustment, and lastly acuity. So far as we have been able to tell from all of our work up to the present time, this order of ranking holds in general for whatever affects the functional powers of the eye: errors of refraction, favorableness or unfavorableness of working conditions, bodily health and fatigue, etc. From the standpoint of testing, therefore, the power to sustain acuity affords the most sensitive, and the conventional acuity test the least sensitive

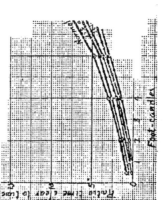

Fig. 7.—Showing the effect of increase of intensity of light on the eye's power to sustain the clear seeing of the test-object for three with normal refraction and for same eye made slightly astigmatic, visual angle (0.88′) constant for all intensities of illumination: A, time blurred plotted against foot-candles; B, percentage gain in ratio time clear to time blurred plotted against foot-candles.

basis for detecting small functional disturbances in the eye whether they be due to errors in refraction or any of the causes mentioned above. Speed of discrimination, however, is a very sensitive test and more feasible for general laboratory purposes than power to sustain. In Fig. 8B the effect of increase of illumination on all the functions tested is given for the 0.12 diopter astigmatism. The order of ranking from greatest to least is the same as for the normal eye, but the

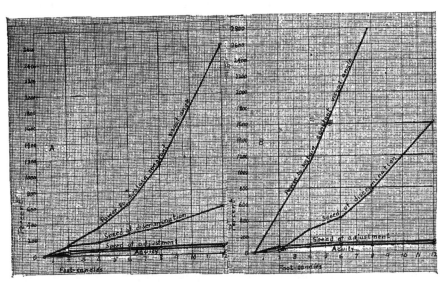

Fig. 8.—Showing percentage gain in all of the functions tested, plotted to the same scale: A, Eyes with normal refraction; B, same eyes made slightly astigmatic.

effect is much enhanced particularly in case of the power to sustain and the speed of discrimination.

It has been popularly supposed that the eye by adaptation changes its sensitivity to compensate for changes of illumination over a very wide range. So it does, but the compensation is by no means complete so far as the effect on clear seeing is concerned, more particularly with regard to the very important aspects: speed of discrimination, speed of change of adjustment for clear seeing at different distances, and power to sustain clear seeing. The eye has developed its functional powers under the higher intensities which characterize daylight illumination. It is perhaps not surprising, therefore, that it should have its highest functional efficiency under these intensities.

With reference to the difference between the amounts of light to which we are accustomed for daylight and artificial illumination, the writers recall having been asked to measure the daylight illumination of the magazine room of a college library which was about to be condemned because of insufficient intensity of illumination. The measurements showed a range of 5–15 foot-candles, vertical component, in various parts of the room on a mediumly bright day. Another striking illustration of the difference of intensity in daylighting and artificial lighting, as it impresses itself by experience, is to pass suddenly from daylight to artificial illumination while reading on a train as it enters a tunnel. Experiences of this sort help us to realize how much we rely on adaptation to bring the eye up to daylight efficiency when working under artificial illumination of the intensities ordinarily employed.

There is danger also of being misled by results and curves showing the change in retinal sensitivity by adaptation. Acuity changes slowly with change in retinal sensitivity. For data showing the change in acuity with adaptation, the reader is referred to these Transactions, 1919, xvii, pp. 370–395, and to the American Journal of Ophthalmology, 1920, iii, pp. 408–417.

DISCUSSION.

DR. C. F. CLARK, Columbus, Ohio: I would inquire if the authors of this paper have a fully developed outfit that may be found in the market for accurately determining the degree of illumination and for accurate adjustment during the testing of patients?

DR. M. L. FOSTER, New Rochelle, N. Y.: In regard to the

examination of the Naval men, I would ask to what extent the custom or habit of looking off at long distances affects the power of perceiving a distant object? Years ago, when I first came down to the seashore, I found that other men could see a boat in the distance and recognize correctly not only its rig, but also its nationality, while I could not see a thing. In time, without any change in glasses, I became able to pick up such small objects in the distance, and this I ascribed to a habit I cultivated of looking off on the sea. It seems to me that if you take a man from the interior and put him in the Navy he cannot, with the same visual power, pick up an object at sea as well as a man can who has been brought up by the seashore. Was that taken into consideration in the testing of these men of the Navy?

This reminds me of an interesting case which I would like to have explained. I was consulted by a navigating officer of the Navy; his eye had been wounded, and its vision was decidedly inferior, so much so that a rigid application of the rules would have excluded him from the Navy, but he had testimonials from several captains under whom he had served, stating that he could pick up with that injured eye a light farther away than they were able to see it, and that they had needed binoculars to enable them to see it as well. Tests showed reduced vision of the eye. The testimony of these gentlemen under whom he had served showed increased power to pick up small objects at great distances at sea.

Dr. Ferree (closing): In the experiments for determining what intensity of illumination is most favorable for picking up small errors in refraction, the test chart was illuminated by the acuity lantern, which we demonstrated to this Society two years ago. This lantern will be put on the market in such a form that it can be used simply and conveniently for the illumination of test-charts over a wide range of minutely graded intensities from low to high, without any change in the color value of the light. It will probably be made by the Bausch and Lomb Optical Co. I believe that it would pay the ophthalmologist to give more attention to the relation of illumination to acuity and to the sensitivity and usefulness of the acuity test. The illumination controls needed could be made with very little increase in time and trouble. In the progress that has been made along other lines this factor has been somewhat neglected.

The statistics on the ocular fitness of men in the navy for the look-out work on the bridge of the battleships were based on a trial of the men admitted on examination. Twenty to 30 per cent. of the men who passed the ocular tests for entrance were found by trial to be unfit for this service, which requires keen discrimination at low illuminations. Our tests of a large number of eyes for acuity at low and high illuminations confirm the verdict reached in the navy by experience. That is, a group of eyes having approximately the same acuity at high illuminations, shows a wide scatter at low illuminations. It was for testing the fitness of eyes for this branch of the naval service that the acuity lantern was devised originally, by request.

Two points, as I understand, were raised by Dr. Foster: differences in ability to see objects at a great distance by eyes equally well corrected as to refraction, and differences in ability to sense light. Both of these points are somewhat different from the one just discussed, namely, differences in acuity at low illuminations. The ability to see objects clearly depends on two functions—the resolving power of the refracting media, or the power to form clear images on the retina; and the resolving power of the retina, or the power to discriminate detail in the physical images formed. The resolving power of the retina depends on three factors: sensitivity to light and to color and power to discriminate spatial separations. The difference in the ability of eyes equally well corrected as to refraction to see objects at a great distance is to be explained in terms of differences in the resolving power of the retina, not of the refracting media. Differences in ability to sense light, Dr. Foster's second point, is, of course, a matter primarily of the sensory, not the refracting, mechanism.

It is quite possible, of course, that eyes apparently equally well corrected as to refraction, as judged by the conventional chart tests at six meters, are not actually equally well corrected. The ability to see objects clearly at great distances adds a refinement to our checks on acuity which is not possible in testing with the acuity chart at high illuminations, with its rough gradations of difficulty of task set to the resolving powers of the eye. In short, Dr. Foster has in substance suggested here a refinement on acuity testing—a refinement, however, which cannot be as conveniently, minutely, and precisely applied as the decrease of illumination.

SOME HITHERTO UNRECOGNIZED SIGNS IN SKIASCOPY.

J. HERBERT CLAIBORNE, M.D.,
New York.

Cuignet, of Lille, first described and used for the determination of refractive errors the method of examination known as retinoscopy, skiascopy, etc. Cuignet himself called it keratoscopy. Many other terms have likewise been suggested. The word retinoscopy, which is entirely incorrect, is perhaps more generally used than any other. Of course, keratoscopy is out of the question. I conceive skiascopy to be the best of all, inasmuch as it is based upon the behavior of the shadow when light from the ophthalmoscope is thrown upon the pupil and is then moved in various directions. The method might equally be called photoscopy, since the light precedes the shadow. I do not think this term has ever been proposed. One term should be agreed upon, and should be used to the exclusion of all others. While skiascopy is the best so far suggested for the method, the word retinoscope has come to stay, probably by reason of euphony.

I consider it interesting to state that the late Dr. Hepburn and myself first taught the use of skiascopy in this country in the clinic of Dr. E. Gruening, New York Polyclinic, in 1884. Dr. Hepburn showed me the method in an imperfect and inconclusive manner. After prolonged study I published a description of it in *New York Medical Record*, November 5,

1887, and likewise incorporated that article in a brochure for students entitled, "The Theory and Practice of the Ophthalmoscope, 1888." I have reason to believe this was the first paper published on this subject in America. The method appealed to me on account of the rapidity and ease with which it could be employed. In those days the concave mirror of the ophthalmoscope was used by Hepburn and myself, a habit to which I have consistently clung. The use of the plane mirror was introduced many years later, and became popular doubtless on account of the more or less parallelism of the rays of the light reflected from it, whereby the observer can stand at a greater distance and estimate smaller errors than with the concave mirror. As is well known, the movement of the shadow with the plane mirror is the reverse of that with the concave mirror.

Of recent years skiascopy has been developed as a fine art, and it is taught with great success in the post-graduate colleges and in the hospitals. As now taught, it is a method which requires expenditure of considerable time and nervous energy, but the element of time has been somewhat modified through the invention of several devices for the rapid placing of lenses in front of the eye in the act of correction. Whatever may be the value of these devices, they are more or less clumsy, and one or two have fortunately been relegated to the lumber room of antiquity. As stated, it has always been my custom to use the concave mirror, and I desire to say frankly that I never have gone into the exquisite refinements of skiascopy with the plane mirror as some of my colleagues have. I do not see how any busy surgeon could employ that method thoroughly in the determination of refractive errors in his office. Its value is certainly not to be underestimated, but I think it can only be used profitably in its refinements in large clinics presided over by an expert, the minutiæ being placed in the hands of subordinates for practice or instruction. I have always and I still employ skiascopy for the purpose of qualitative, approximately quantitative estimates of refraction, and for the proving and checking of other methods, particularly the functional examination which I conceive to be the final and decisive one. I am likewise able to determine with satisfactory accuracy the axis of the astigmatism even when it is off the vertical and horizontal meridians. For that purpose I rely upon the observations I have made and the conclusions I have drawn concerning the axis of astigmatism as published in the *Annals of Ophthalmology*, July, 1909, wherein I demonstrated that the angles at which the astigmatic axis occurs varies, as a rule, in multiples of the number 15.

In using skiascopy, ordinarily the observer alternately rotates the mirror upon a vertical and then upon a horizontal axis, or vice versa. When rotated upon the vertical axis, the shadow in the horizontal meridian is determined; when upon the horizontal, that in the vertical. When the astigmatism is oblique, the shadow will always be oblique, it matters not upon what axis the mirror is rotated. This peculiarity of the oblique shadow is caused by the shape of the shadow upon the retina, as shown by Hartridge over twenty-five years ago, by others and by myself in the textbook referred to. The signs to which I refer are to be seen only when the mirror is rotated in a circle, that is to say, upon an anteroposterior axis. The statements presently to be made are based upon the movements of the shadow with the use of the concave mirror.

When the mirror is rotated on the anteroposterior axis, either in spherical myopia or hypermetropia, the shadow moves in a circle, and ultimately always in the same direction with the movement of the mirror. It resembles more than anything that I know of the turning of a wheel upon an axis or a revolving circle. The shadow chases itself around the pupil, so to speak. In hypermetropia, as the circular movement commences, the shadow is observed to creep from the opposite side of the pupil and chase itself in a circle, from left to right when the mirror is moved from right to left, or from right to left when the mirror is moved from left to right. The movement in this case is against the movement of the mirror, and yet the ultimate direction of the shadow is with the movement of the mirror (Fig. 1).

In the case of myopia the shadow moves with the movement of the mirror, and starts from the quadrant in which the circular movement of the mirror starts, and chases itself around the pupil, as in hypermetropia. The movement in both cases, therefore, is circular, and the shadow appears to move always in the same direction, though in the two cases it starts from opposite points (Fig. 2). A little practice will enable one to tell the existence or non-existence of a spherical error. Of course, the degree of the error is indicated by signs which are well known to all those conversant with this method—a gray slow shadow indicating high error, a black, rapid shadow low error.

In the case of astigmatism the appearance described is not found. In short, the shadow does not chase itself around the pupil, but halts at the meridian of division.

It is well to indicate the behavior of the shadow in each form of the astigmatism, and to this end attention is again called to the schematic drawings. Fig. 3 indicates the behavior of the shadow in simple far-sighted astigmatism with the rule. The movement, of course, is against the movement of the mirror, and, as the meridian of division is reached, the shadow ceases and recommences on the opposite side. In Fig. 4 the behavior of the shadow is indicated in simple myopic astigmatism with the rule. The shadow moves from below upward until the meridian of division is met, when it disappears and reappears above. Fig. 5 represents the shadow in compound far-sighted astigmatism with the rule. The long arrow indicates the slow shadow in the horizontal meridian which has the greater refractive error, and the

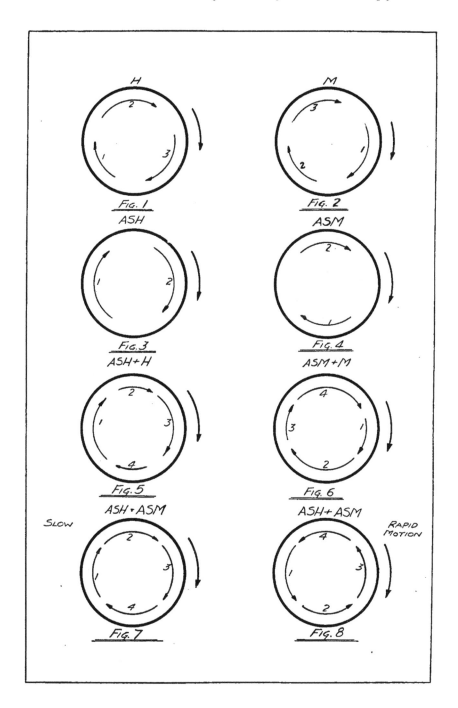

short arrow that in the vertical, the meridian of less error. Fig. 6 represents the shadow in compound myopic astigmatism with the rule. The long arrow indicates the shadow in the vertical meridian which has the greater refractive error, and the short arrow that in the horizontal, the meridian of less error. In mixed astigmatism the behavior of the shadow is different in slow and in rapid movements of the mirror. If the mirror be rotated slowly, the shadow will be seen to behave in its respective meridians exactly as in simple far-sighted and simple near-sighted astigmatism, and the shadow is seen to move with the movement of the mirror (Fig. 7). If, however, the mirror be rotated rapidly, the shadow moves against the movement of the mirror (Fig. 8). This must be its apparent motion and not its real one. I believe the phenomenon is analogous to, if not identical with, the movements of the spokes of the wheels of field guns seen in moving pictures when the horses drawing them are in rapid motion. Most people have noticed that when the guns are moving slowly the spokes of the wheel appear to move from rear to front, but in rapid motion, from front to rear, that is, backward, and the entire wheel seems to have a sliding motion as if the tire were stationary. I believe the cause of the apparent reversal, whatever it may be, is analogous in the two cases. Lippincott, of Pittsburgh, has studied this phenomenon, but his explanation has never been completely clear or satisfactory to me. This behavior of the shadow in skiascopy when the mirror is rapidly rotated was called to my attention by the late Dr. E. B. Coburn, of New York, to whom I had demonstrated the phenomena herein mentioned.

Rotation of the mirror on the anteroposterior axis is of practical value for me, and I always employ it first in using skiascopy. If I find a spherical error to be present, I do not rotate the mirror on the vertical and horizontal axis, but judge the amount of error by this method alone, approximately, of course, by noting the rapidity and blackness of the shadow. If astigmatism be present, I usually rotate the mirror likewise on the vertical and horizontal axis, making the approximate estimate of the degree of error in the same way. In spherical errors and simple astigmatism I rarely miss the amount by more than a half of a diopter. This applies to the meridians of greater error. In compound errors estimate of the meridians of less error is less easy, but, after all, the meridian of greater error is the main one. In the article on skiascopy referred to I described the character of the shadow in emmetropia as "flitting," calling it the "emmetropic flit." In emmetropia the shadow is so rapid I feel quite confident of its character.

I have seen no reference to these phenomena by any writer since I first mentioned them, and I desire to call attention to them again, as I consider they have not only an academic and scientific interest, but also a practical value.

The following explanation of the apparent counter rotary motion of a revolving wheel as projected by a motion picture camera is made by Mr. G. E. Olsen. The explanation of the reverse movement of the shadow in skiascopy in rapid motion of the mirror upon the anteroposterior axis, is without doubt the same as in the motion picture phenomenon.

The assumption is made that the speed of the film through the camera when the pictures are taken is constant, and that the wheel is rotating at a uniform and constant speed in a clockwise direction.

GROUP I.—Consider point A, Group I (the end of a spoke), on the rim of the wheel in the position shown in picture 1. At this instant a picture is made. The point A moves, and the next successive picture is made before A arrives at its original position. Therefore, picture 2 shows A before it has made a complete revolution and, to the observer, it apparently has moved from picture 1 to picture 2 in a *counterclockwise* direction, whereas as assumed, it has actually moved to its position in picture 2 through a clockwise rotation. The third successive picture 3, shows A bearing the same relation to picture 2, as picture 2 bears to picture 1. Successive pictures would be similar, and the wheel would apparently be rotating continuously in a counter-clockwise direction, opposite to its actual direction of rotation.

GROUP II.—Again consider point A in the position shown in picture 4, Group II. If the speed of rotation of the wheel continues constant and unvarying as heretofore, by slowing

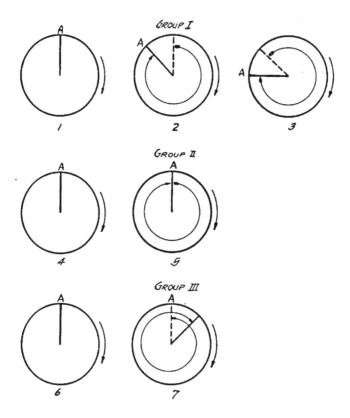

up the camera speed a sufficient amount, picture 5 can be obtained after A has made a complete revolution and again is in its original position. To the observer of the successive pictures, point A apparently will not have moved at all, whereas it actually has made a complete revolution (or any number of complete revolutions) between successive pictures. *When projected by the camera, the observer does not see the motion of a point (as A at the end of a spoke) on the rim of a wheel, which is revolving, but sees only the successive instantaneous positions of the point at intervals along its path.*

GROUP III.—If the speed of the camera film is further reduced, starting again with point A, in picture 6, the next successive picture 7, Group III, will show A as having moved only slightly past its original position, *i. e.*, as having passed over the small arc of the circumference between its position in picture 6 and that in picture 7. To the observer, the wheel this time will apparently, and of course actually, have moved in a clockwise direction. While A has traversed, (apparently) only the length of the small arc, it actually has moved through one *complete* revolution plus the length of the small arc. As before, only the instantaneous results of the motion are visible; not the motion itself.

By proper synchronization of camera and wheel speeds, the wheel may be made to appear to be revolving either rapidly or slowly in either direction, according to the desire of the operator of the camera, regardless of the true velocity and direction of rotation of the wheel.

A mathematical statement could be made as follows: Assume a wheel D feet in diameter revolving about its axis at the rate of R revolutions a minute. Point A would, therefore, rotate through (D × R × 3.1416 −) feet a minute. To make A appear stationary when projected upon the screen, R separate pictures would have to be made each minute. A less number of pictures would show A revolving clockwise; a greater number would show A revolving counter-clockwise. A very slow camera speed would show a very rapid rotary speed of the wheel; a very fast camera speed would show an exceedingly slow speed of rotation of the wheel.

DISCUSSION.

DR. WILLIAM TARUN, Baltimore, Md.: Do you use this method for determining refractive errors in your office?

DR. W. E. LAMBERT, New York: I have been using skiascopy for over thirty years in estimating errors of refraction and regard it the most accurate objective test we have. Dr. Claiborne's observations are extremely interesting, but I fail to see their practical value in aiding us to obtain better results. One can estimate the amount of

20

astigmatism to within a quarter diopter, but I think this only possible in using cylinders as well as sphericals in making the test. With the cylinders we not only are able to estimate a small amount of astigmatism but can also determine the axis.

Dr. Claiborne says that several devices have been made for the practical application of this test. Many years ago I devised an apparatus on the principle of the Loring ophthalmoscope which was satisfactory to me, but as it was somewhat cumbersome and rather expensive, it has never been generally adopted.

DR. CLAIBORNE (closing): I do not know whether Dr. Lambert was in New York in 1884, but I believe he was one of the pioneers in introducing skiascopy into New York. It is certain, however, that Dr. Hepburn demonstrated the method to me in 1884, and that both he and I subsequently taught it in the Polyclinic on the staff of Dr. E. Gruening that year. Dr. Lambert remarks that the signs which I have indicated are of no practical value. They certainly have been of practical value to me. I am enabled by this method of examination to acquire in a few seconds what I conceive to be a considerable information. In a turn of the instrument I can tell whether there is spherical refraction or astigmatism. In the case of astigmatism, whether it is simple, compound, or mixed, and the last with unerring accuracy by reason of the reverse movements of the shadow in rapid rotation of the mirror. I can do this far more rapidly and with as much accuracy as in the old method. I conceive these things to be of importance, academically and practically. The reverse movement of the shadow in mixed astigmatism, when the mirror is rotated more rapidly than is usual, I believe is to be explained in the same way as the apparent reverse movements of the spokes of wheels in rapid motion when the camera in the movies is speeded up, as mentioned in the paper.

Mr. Olsen's explanation of these phenomena is entirely clear and correct, and the explanation of the apparently reverse movement of the wheel in rapid motion is, without a doubt, the explanation of the apparently reverse movement of the shadow in rapid rotation of the mirror on the anteroposterior axis in skiascopy.

THE OCULAR CHANGES IN INFANTILE SCURVY.
REPORT OF A CASE.

EUGENE M. BLAKE, M.D.,
New Haven, Conn.

The infrequency of scorbutus in infants and the scanty literature concerning the ocular changes in this condition make the recording of an additional case seem worth while. Since the ophthalmologist may be consulted before the diagnosis of scurvy has been made, it is well for us to be cognizant of the changes which that disease may bring about in the ocular structures.

Infantile scurvy may be defined as a constitutional disease due to some prolonged error in diet. It is frequently referred to as Barlow's disease, because of the clear demonstration of its clinical and pathologic features described by Sir Thomas Barlow in 1883. The disease is characterized by spongy, bleeding gums, swellings and ecchymoses about joints, especially the knee and ankle, hemorrhages from the nose and other mucous membranes, extreme hyperesthesia, and often pseudoparalysis of the extremities. There is usually a marked general cachexia and anemia.

Age is an important factor, four-fifths of the cases occurring between the sixth and fifteenth months, and one-half between the seventh and tenth months. Previous disease does not appear to be a factor of importance, although derangements of the digestive tract may predispose in certain cases. The only etiologic element known to be constant in the production of scurvy is diet, no specific scorbutic poison being present, but rather an absence of some antiscorbutic element from the food. The cases occur most commonly in

307

infants fed on proprietary foods, on condensed milk or milk which has been too thoroughly boiled. Generally several months elapse before such improper feeding produces the signs of scurvy.

Usually the first symptom observed is tenderness of the legs when handling the affected infant. Associated with this hyperesthesia are fretfulness, pallor, and failing nutrition. The soreness of the legs increases and swellings appear about the joints. Coincidentally with this the gums become purplish, swollen, and bleed easily, and there is loss of color, weight, and appetite. Unless proper treatment is instituted, these symptoms increase and paralysis of the extremities may be simulated, due chiefly to the pain incident to movement of the part. Traumatism may be suspected because of the appearance of ecchymoses in the skin.

The pathologic lesions are most marked in the bones, blood-vessels, and the blood, and the most striking feature is subperiosteal hemorrhage, which may be very extensive. Extravasations may be found between the muscles and beneath the pleura, peritoneum, and pericardium. A rarefying osteitis may be present, and separation of the epiphyses from the shaft of some of the long bones is generally found in fatal cases.

Probably the most frequent and certainly the most striking ocular complication of infantile scurvy is exophthalmos, due to hemorrhage into the orbit. In 1898 the American Pediatric Society conducted a collective investigation of infantile scurvy in North America. In all 379 cases were found, in 49 of which exophthalmos was recorded. This agrees fairly well with the statement of Holt that 10 per cent. of the cases present exophthalmos. In 1912 L. R. DuBuys, of Tulane University, collected 13 cases, including one seen by himself. Huebner reported 4 cases of exophthalmos among 65 cases of infantile scurvy (6.15 per cent.), and Nicolay, 13.17 per cent. A rather careful search of the literature since 1912 revealed one other case of exophthalmos, reported by Brandes in *La Clinique* in May, 1912.

Exophthalmos occurs suddenly, and may be so slight that it is referred to as swelling of the eye, or so marked that the eye is lost from exposure and sepsis, as occurred in the case of Mr. Sutherland, of London. It may be an early sign, but usually appears as a late manifestation. The exophthalmos is often seen for the first time after a fit of crying, and may occur in one or both eyes, either together or separately. There may be recovery followed by recurrence, or the eye may remain stationary and at intervals the symptoms increase. The exophthalmos is due to one of two causes— either a hemorrhage into the areolar tissue of the orbit or hemorrhage beneath the periosteum of one of the orbital bones. The latter corresponds to the condition found in other parts of the body, and was demonstrated at autopsy in the cases of Meyer and Snow. In Snow's case the hemorrhage was found between the periorbita and the bone, and filled almost the entire orbital cavity. The orbital plate of the frontal bone appears to be the most common site of the hemorrhage. When the latter extends in front of the fascia orbitalis, there is generally associated an ecchymosis and suggillation of the upper lid.

Infantile scurvy affects other portions of the ocular structures far less often than the orbit. Subconjunctival hemorrhage has been noted at times, and Hirschberg relates a case in which a large, flame-shaped hemorrhage occurred in the retina, appearing when the orbital hemorrhage was subsiding. Blood in the anterior chamber is reported in one case by Otto Kaltz, and Sidney Stephenson reports a case of ecchymosis in the lower lid, unassociated with orbital hemorrhage.

The practical significance of the orbital hemorrhage and other ocular changes recorded lies in the fact that they may be early symptoms, and therefore be seen first by the ophthalmologist. A suddenly appearing exophthalmos in an infant is most likely due to scurvy, since neoplasms and cysts never grow so rapidly and syphilis can be excluded by other signs and tests. Traumatism is often suspected because of the frequently associated hemorrhage into the lids, and should lead to an examination for the signs of scurvy. Retinal hemorrhage may be more common than reported through failure to use the ophthalmoscope. Subconjunctival hemorrhage in an infant not suffering from pertussis would be a suspicious sign of scurvy.

CASE.—On October 25, 1920, I was requested to examine the eyes of Baby S., aged one year. The history was that he had been well until one month previously, when he developed "rheumatism" in the legs. The child was pale and very irritable, especially when handled. There was no fever and no increase of pulse-rate, and the urine was reported to be normal. The right eyeball began to protrude one week before the examination, the swelling subsiding within a few days, only to recur. After a second subsidence it recurred again.

At the time of the ocular examination the right eye was markedly exophthalmic, but with motility unimpaired, except as due to the proptosis. There were no hemorrhages into the lids or conjunctivæ and no chemosis. There were no pathologic changes in the retina, the eyeball was not tender, and no mass could be felt.

The diagnosis of infantile scurvy did not occur to me, but the suddenly occurring exophthalmos, without inflammatory signs or preceding acute illness, could only be explained as due to an orbital hemorrhage or edema of the orbital tissues, and such was the explanation offered to the attending physician. A few days later the case was seen by an able pediatrician, who telephoned me that the child had all the symptoms of scurvy and that he thought the exophthalmos was due to an orbital hemorrhage.

The previous history of the case was typical of that found in infantile scurvy. The child was born at term, but had never been nursed, having been fed from the beginning on malted milk, which diet was continued to the age of eleven months. Feedings were then changed to Mellen's Food, and pasteurized milk, both, of course, devitalized foods. At the age of ten months the legs became painful and swollen, the swelling being marked and extending from the knees to the ankles. No hemorrhages appeared in the skin, and at no time were the gums swollen. A pseudoparalysis of the legs was present, and a diagnosis of rheumatism was made.

When the correct diagnosis was established, the diet was changed to raw cow's milk and orange-juice, one dram of the latter three times a day. Within four days the exophthalmos had disappeared, the swelling of the legs had gone, and the child appeared greatly improved in every way. There have been no further relapses, and the child to-day is robust and healthy.

DISCUSSION.

DR. E. E. JACK, Boston, Mass.: Dr. Blake's statement that 10 per cent. of infantile scurvy cases have exophthalmos surprises me, because in a service of 15 to 20 years at the Boston Children's Hospital, I remember only one case. That recovered promptly.

THE RELATION OF HEADACHE TO FUNCTIONAL MONOCULARITY.

ALBERT C. SNELL, M.D.,
Rochester, N. Y.

Headache is indisputably the most common symptom for the relief of which patients consult the ophthalmologist. Snydacker found that in 2,000 consecutive patients, 40 per cent. complained of headache. Brav, in 3,000 consecutive cases, found that 30 per cent. asked relief from headache, there being no other symptoms. Approximately three out of every four of our patients (excluding those with acute inflammatory conditions) complain of headache or give a history of having had headache in some form. Yet there are many patients who rather surprise us by stating that they do not have, or that they never have had, headache. Volumes have been written about headache, especially that associated with eye-strain or some form of ocular maladjustment, but scarcely anything has been said about the cephalalgic patient. Therefore I trust that the statistics which I herewith present may have some scientific value and interest. This paper is the study of 1,010 cases of partial or of complete functional monocularity, and the relation of such conditions to the prevalence of headache.

When one considers the class of cases which are relatively less subject to headache, it seems to be quite universally accepted that the higher degrees of hypermetropia are less likely to cause asthenopic symptoms than the lower or the intermediate degrees; and that myopia, corrected and uncorrected, is less likely to cause headache than hypermetropia. One author presents these observations by saying, "Poor vision excludes eye-strain." The question of the prevalence of headache among the blind has been studied by Walton, who found that 66 per cent. of persons blind from infancy were free from headache. Later he investigated the frequency of migrainous headache among the blind and found it only one-half as frequent among the blind as among seeing persons of like age and conditions.

Several years ago I was impressed with the fact that many patients with only one useful eye often have a history of the absence of headache. A search through the literature revealed only a few references relative to this observation. I found the unique and well-known case of Dr. Noyes, in which the removal of a nearly normal eye, having standard vision, afforded complete relief to a patient who had suffered for years almost constant "agonizing headache" and other asthenopic symptoms. Ranney states that "a typical cross-eye is not, as a rule, the cause of serious nervous disturbance —eye-strain is practically absent in extremely cross-eyed subjects." Wilder, in writing of the visual standards in the army, states that persons with congenital amblyopic eyes are "seldom annoyed by asthenopia if the fellow-eye has fairly good vision and no great refractive error, for they do not have binocular single vision." Oliver, in the chapter on Ametropia in Norris and Oliver's "System of Diseases of the Eye," says: "Were the human eye cyclopic, the problem (asthenopia) would be easier of solution, and eye-strain would be less disastrous in its consequences." Donders ("Accommodation and Refraction of the Eye," p. 415), as early as 1864, made the observation that asthenopia was overcome by strabismus convergens or divergens, and expressed the fact in the following striking antitheses: "Hypermetropia causes accommodative asthenopia to be actively overcome by strabismus convergens. Myopia leads to muscular asthenopia, passively yielding to strabismus divergens."

Although all of these references indicate at least a mitigation of asthenopic symptoms in proportion to the loss or absence of single binocular vision, I could find no reference to any statistics to substantiate these opinions or my own belief that the monocular are comparatively free from headache. Therefore I have undertaken a study of a series of cases falling within the class of the functionating monocular, believing that such a study would be interesting and would shed some light on this subject. I have taken from my files 1010 cases having different degrees of monocularity and have tabulated them. In the tabulation I have recorded for each patient the age, occupation, refraction, visual acuity, muscle balance, condition of general health, and the presence or absence of headache or head-pain. For simplicity, the cephalalgias were divided into two classes only— the severe or habitual, and the mild or occasional.

In selecting the cases for tabulation the following were excluded: cases under fifteen years of age; cases in which the vision of the better eye was less than 20/25, and those clearly showing the presence of some active local or constitutional disease. In excluding persons under fifteen years of age we felt that, prior to this age, a sufficient period of time had not elapsed to establish the fact of the presence or absence of habitual headache; that the personal history of these patients in regard to headache would often be unreliable; and, further, that, prior to fifteen, especially with girls, many other factors incident to the beginning of adolescence concern the etiology of headache. Only those cases in which there was present a central visual acuity of 20/20 or 20/25 in the better eye were used, as a perfect, or nearly perfect, vision in one eye was desirable in considering monocularity. The visual test was recorded and considered with the use of glasses when the patient was wearing them, and without glasses when the patient was not using them. The reason for excluding those with active constitutional or local ocular diseases is self-evident, as such conditions would have a direct relationship to the presence of headache.

Considering the different degrees of disturbances of binocular single vision the cases seemed rather naturally to fall into the following four groups: I. The one-eyed; II. The anisometropic; III. The amblyopic; IV. The strabismic. The first group contains all those cases which had lost one eye, considering only those in which the monocularity had existed for five years or more, and those having only one good eye, the other eye having an acuity of less than 10/250; the second group includes those cases of anisometropia in which binocular single vision was not present or in actual use, also a limited number of cases presenting a very marked dominance of one eye, although in these latter cases single binocular vision was present and visual acuity was standard in each eye; the third group includes all cases of monocular amblyopia; the fourth group includes all cases of strabismus, both convergent and divergent, constant or intermittent.

Group I. Complete Monocularity.—In this group there were 96 cases. Of these, 30 had been blind in one eye for five to twenty years; 40 had been blind in one eye for twenty to thirty years; and 26 had been blind for forty years or more. Headache of a severe or habitual type was found in only 2 cases. One case had suffered headache for a period of twenty years, and the other for forty-five years. Six cases gave a history of an occasional or mild headache. Therefore only 2 per cent. of the absolute monocular patients showed habitual or severe headache, and 6.2 per cent. occasional or mild headache, or a total of 8.3 per cent. having any form of headache. In this group there were 8 cases which gave a history of severe or habitual headache before losing an eye, and a complete absence of all headache after the loss of an eye.

TABLE SHOWING THE NUMBER OF CASES AND THE PERCENTAGE OF HEADACHE.

Group	Kind or Degree of Monocularity	Total Number of Cases	Number without Headache	Number Having Habitual Headache	Number Having Occasional Headache	Total Number with Headache	Percentage of Headache
B	Binocular	1010	298	606	106	712	70
I.	One-eyed or absolute monocularity..................	96	88	2	6	8	8.3
II.	Anisometropia or suppressed monocularity..............	120	105	5	7	15	11.4
III.	Amblyopia or relative monocularity.................	546	436	44	66	110	20.1
IV.	Strabismus or functional monocularity.................	248	192	24	32	56	22.6
	Total for Groups I, II, III, and IV..................	1010	821	75	111	189	18.7

Group II. Anisometropia or Suppressed Monocularity.— In this group are included two classes of cases: first, those of unequal vision (anisopia), due to a high degree of anisometropia, so that only one eye was functionating with good central visual acuity; while the other, although having a possible standard visual acuity with proper glasses did not or could not adapt itself to the use of the correction for that eye having the greater refractive error.   Generally there was a difference in the spheric correction of the two eyes of more than four diopters.   Second, those with one very dominant eye, but with equal vision (isopia), the monocular dominance

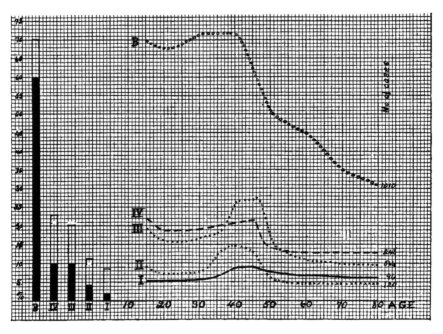

B = binocular cases; I, II, III, IV = groups.   Solid column = percentage habitual headache cases.   Hollow column = percentage occasional headache cases.   Entire column = percentage for all headaches for each group.   Horizontal lines = percentage headache for age period for groups B and I, II, III, and IV.

being determined by the winking test of Rider, and because of an habitual desire or habit almost constantly to close one and the same eye.

In this group there were 120 cases of which 93 had anisopia and 27 isopia.   Of the former, 5, or 5.3 per cent., had severe or habitual headache, and 6, or 6.4 per cent., occasional or mild headache;   and of the latter none had severe or habitual headache, and 1, or 4 per cent., had mild or occasional headache. Taking the group as a whole and including both classes of headache, the total percentage of headache was found to be 11.4 per cent.

In 3 of the cases of anisometropia a persistent attempt had been made to use correcting glasses, but these always caused the recurrence of severe headache. Without the glasses or with only the better eye corrected these patients were perfectly comfortable and free from headache.

Group III. Amblyopia or Relative Monocularity.—This group includes all cases of monocular amblyopia. These cases were divided into four classes, depending on the visual acuity of the amblyopic eye. The best vision with correcting glasses was taken in every case, and the question of cephalalgia was considered with the use of correcting glasses. In each class are included all cases with vision in the amblyopic eye as follows: (Vision in the non-amblyopic eye, with glasses, being 20/25 or better) Class A, 20/33–20/40; Class B, 20/50–20/65; Class C, 20/80–20/160; Class D, 20/200–10/250. In Class A there are 120 cases. Of these, 10, or 8.3 per cent., had severe or habitual headache, and 24, or 20 per cent., had slight or occasional headache. In Class B there were 122 cases. Of these, 4, or 3.2 per cent., had severe or habitual headache, and 14, or 11.6 per cent., had occasional or mild headache. In Class C there were 119 cases. Of these, 8, or 6.7 per cent., had severe or habitual headache, and 10, or 8.3 per cent., had mild or occasional headache. In Class D there were 185 cases. Of these, 18, or 10 per cent., had severe or habitual headache, and 23, or 12 per cent., had mild or occasional headache. Comparing the classes in this group we find that the percentage of headache, considering both classes of headache together, shows a proportionate decrease with the decrease of visual acuity in the amblyopic eye, except in Class D, where the total percentage of headache considerably increased. The percentage for each class was A, 30 per cent.; B, 15 per cent.; C, 14 per cent.; and D, 24 per cent. I find that in Class D I had included 8 cases of migraine associated with severe headache. Had these been omitted, the percentage in this class would have been 17 instead of 24. The total percentage of headache for all classes in this group was 20.1 per cent.

Group IV.—In this class are placed all strabismus cases of every form or degree. There are a total of 248 cases; 7 had vertical deviation, 114 were convergent cases, and 127 were divergent cases. In 6 of the convergent cases, and in 39 of the divergent cases, the squint was not constant. Of the total 114 convergent cases, 12, or 10 per cent., had a history of habitual or severe headache, and 15, or 13 per cent., slight or occasional headache. Of the total 127 divergent cases, 12, or 9 per cent., had habitual or severe headache, and 17, or 13 per cent., slight or occasional. The convergent and the divergent show practically the same percentage of prevalence of headache.

Considering all forms of strabismus together, out of the total of 248 cases, 24, or 10 per cent., had severe or habitual headache, and 32, or 13 per cent., had occasional or mild headache, making a total for all forms of headache of 22.6 per cent. for the strabismus cases. In this group there was one case of isopia with intermittent convergent strabismus who suffered nearly daily with headache, especially after close work, until he learned to cover up one eye. This gave complete relief from the headache.

Considering all four groups together for the purpose of comparing the frequency of headache, we find that Group I (absolute monocularity) shows the lowest percentage of headache, only 2 per cent. having habitual or severe headache. Then comes Group II, in which there was functional suppression of single binocular vision (cases of high anisometropia) with 4.1 per cent. of habitual or severe headache. Next in order follow Group III (amblyopia), 8 per cent., and Group IV (strabismus), 10 per cent., with habitual or severe headache.

Considering both classes of headache, the habitual or severe and the occasional or slight together, the percentages as shown in the graph are for Group I, 8.3 per cent.; for Group II, 11.4 per cent.; for Group III, 20.1 per cent.; and for Group IV, 22.6 per cent. Thus we find that there was a proportionate smaller percentage of headache in proportion to the greater degree or completeness of monocularity.

In a review of the consecutive records of 1010 private cases having good binocular single vision (all cases falling under any of the groups considered in this paper being excluded, as well as all inflammatory cases), I find that the percentage of such cases having headache is 70, the habitual or severe headache being complained of in 60 per cent., and the occasional or mild in 10 per cent. Thus a comparison of an equal number of records of patients having constant binocular single vision with the monocular will show that severe or habitual headache occurs seven times more frequently in the former than in the latter.

There are many illustrative normally monocular patients in this series which demonstrate our premises in a converse way in that, by attempting to produce coördinate use of the eyes, severe and unconquerable asthenopic symptoms were produced. I shall not burden this paper with case histories, but shall insert abbreviated records of two cases, one of which illustrates the above point, and one which seemed to show that, by establishing monocularity, a severe cephalalgia and other asthenopic symptoms were relieved.

CASE I.—Mr. J. P. H., aged fifty-five years, a college graduate, teacher by profession. Has never enjoyed very good health. Usual weight, 125 pounds. Has had recurrent symptoms of fatigue neurosis. Ocular history: Twenty-eight years ago had an operation for a divergent strabismus. Has always been near-sighted, and has worn glasses since boyhood. Refraction at present: R.E. − 6.00 sph. ◯ − .75 cyl. ax. 35° = 20/25;   L.E. − 1.50 sph ◯ − .75 cyl. ax. 180° = 20/20. Has fusion, but maintains it with difficulty; slight convergence. For the past ten years has used full correction for the left eye, and − 3.25 sph. ◯ − .75 cyl. for the right eye. With this latter correction he has enjoyed perfect ocular comfort and has been entirely free from headache, using the left eye for distant vision and the right eye for near. About ten years ago he tried persistently, under the care and direction of a competent oculist, to use the full correction for each eye, but was unable to do so because of severe asthenopic symptoms which this produced.

CASE II.—Mrs. H. R. H., aged thirty-nine years. General health good; has not had any serious illness, but has always had a nervous temperament and describes many recurrent attacks typical of neurasthenia. Ocular history: Has suffered considerable headache over a period of many years, and has never been able to use her eyes without distressing symptoms. While in college was under the care of a well-known specialist, who spent several months in an attempt to give her proper correcting glasses. During this time she was unable to follow her college work, and lost several months' time. Has used glasses for twenty-five years. Without glasses V.R.E., 20/80; L.E., 20/20. Refraction under cycloplegic: R.E. − 1.75 sph. = 20/20; L.E. + .12 cyl. ax. 90° = 20/20.

This is practically the same correction which she used while in college and since. She was told that it was very essential that she wear her glasses, therefore has done so. On April 18, 1919, the writer advised her to go entirely without glasses. Since laying them aside she has been very much more comfortable, has been able to use her eyes for longer periods, and has been entirely free from headache. She states that during the past two years she has not known what a headache was, and that she has never been so comfortable in all her life. With the full correction there is only a very slight muscle imbalance. In 1919, ½ degree of exophoria. March 18, 1921, exophoria, 1½°; right hyperphoria, ½°.

A study of the age epoch in the relation to the frequency of headache reveals a striking similarity both in the binocular and in the monocular, there being a slight peak of greater proportion between the ages of fifteen and twenty years, then a sharp but small decline, the percentage then being maintained at a nearly uniform ratio between twenty and thirty-five. Between thirty-five and forty-five the proportion of headache greatly increases, reaching the highest peak at forty-five or forty-six. From this age the percentage curve is sharply downward, passing below the curve of youth and adolescence at fifty-five. From this age onward there is little fluctuation.

An explanation for the infrequency of headache in the monocular patient as compared with the patient employing single binocular vision is found in the fact that the former, because of his monocularity, must experience less nervous or brain fatigue, the normal monocular visual act being less complex because of the elimination of the fusion sense and of coördinate muscular adjustment which are necessary in maintaining single binocular vision.

REFERENCES.

Snydacker: Klin. f. Augenh., 1909, 629.
Brav: Amer. Medicine, December, 1908.
Walton: Trans. Sec. Ophth., Amer. Med. Asso., 1908. Boston Med. and
    Surg. Jour., 1905.
Hunter: N. Y. Med. Jour. and News, January, 1911.
Ranney: N. Y. Med. Jour., 1892, 50.
Wilder: Jour. Amer. Med. Asso., lxxii, 268.
Oliver: System of Disease of the Eye, Norris and Oliver, 449.
Donders: Accommodation and Refraction, 415.
Rider: Trans. Amer. Ophth. Soc. viii, 434.

21

THREE CASES OF WORD-BLINDNESS.

ELLICE M. ALGER, M.D.,
New York.

The subject of this paper may seem out of place in an ophthalmologic program, since it belongs in the indefinite borderland between ophthalmology, neurology, and psychology. The patients I have seen, however, all consulted an ophthalmologist first, either directly or at the instance of their physician, because the trouble was thought to be an ocular and not a cerebral defect. I do not suppose the condition is such a very rare one, but it might very easily be overlooked or masked by more obtrusive symptoms. Indeed, both my congenital cases had passed through the hands of several ophthalmologists without recognition. This is the more important because the whole future of such children depends on its early recognition.

Acquired word-blindness was first noticed by Kussmaul[1] some fifty years ago, and the congenital type a few years later. Indeed, the latter could hardly have been suspected or diagnosticated without a previous knowledge of the former, and for that reason I have included them both in this paper.

The term "word-blindness" has been severely criticized as unscientific, and various substitutes offered, but it now seems so firmly engrafted in our terminology that criticism is probably superfluous. It implies that a person who can see perfectly, recognize objects and numbers, write correctly, and perform calculations has suddenly become unable to recognize letters or words with which he was previously perfectly familiar, perhaps not even his own name. And yet their meaning is grasped instantly when they are spelled or spoken aloud.

Thomas L., a Greek, aged fifty-nine years, while apparently in robust health, had an attack of dizziness on going to bed one evening, and the next morning was found to have a slight paralysis of the right side, diplopia, and some defect of vision which prevented his reading. The paralysis was apparently an evanescent one, for he was confined to the house only a few days. The nature of the seizure was at once suspected, a strongly positive Wassermann found, and under very active treatment his physical condition improved rapidly. He seemed about as well as usual, except that for a time he was unable to find his way about the small town in which he lived because he did not recognize familiar buildings and landmarks, and as he was still absolutely unable to read his paper he was, a few weeks later in May, 1919, referred to me for an examination of his eyes. By that time he walked and talked perfectly well, his diplopia had disappeared, he had begun to find his way about town again, and that morning was able to recognize the railway stations on his way to New York which he had previously been unable to do.

So far as his eyes were concerned, the media were clear, the fundi normal, the pupils normal except that the right was slightly larger and slower in its light reaction than the left. The red glass test showed some weakness of the left external rectus, but there was no longer any spontaneous diplopia. He apparently had very much reduced central vision, because he could read no letters on the test chart at all, though he was said to be familiar with English. To my great surprise, when I turned his attention to a chart with numbers, his vision was normal in each eye, and with presbyopic correction he read the numeric equivalent of No. 1 Jaeger without hesitation. Of the headlines of a Greek paper, however, he could not read a word. While he could not recognize words or letters either in English or Greek, he was able to write them readily enough, but when they were shown to him a few moments later they meant nothing to him—not even his own name. I noticed that if he watched me write a word he could recognize it if it was a short one, though only for an instant, and then discovered that if allowed to trace a letter or a short word with pencil or match, he could generally recognize it. He recognized objects and their uses readily enough, but occasionally hesitated over their names, to his great vexation.

Numbers he recognized normally and was able to perform correctly various calculations.

He was found to have a right homonymous hemianopsia, quite sharply marked, and not involving the fixation-point in either eye. This hemianopsia was a curious one because, while it seemed complete under the usual tests, he claimed at times to see hand movements if quickly made in the blind field, and did not fall over things or collide with people as much as one would expect.

I saw him again a month later and presented him at the New York Ophthalmological Society, when his condition had improved very materially. He could now recognize Greek letters and words fairly well, and was able to read a little Greek text, which he could not do before, and could recognize his own name but could .do nothing with English. The hemianopsia was unchanged.

In spite of several efforts I have not been able to secure another examination. His family physician tells me that he got perfectly well, of which I am very skeptical. It is, of course, possible that many of his symptoms were "distant" ones.

Every normal individual has the power of storing up and reproducing more or less at will the impressions received through the various senses and this constitutes memory.

For instance, an eye may react to light and show a perfectly clear retinal image, but if the connection between it and the primary visual area about the calcarine fissures is destroyed or blocked, the individual is not conscious that he sees. And unless he can compare what he sees at one instant with previous impressions, every visual impression is absolutely new and valueless from the point of recognition or as a basis for judgment. These visual memories seem to be stored in the cortex about the angular gyrus: in right-handed people, on the left side. Each one of the senses seems to have a similar memory center in the same general neighborhood, and these various centers seem to be connected in very intimate fashion. What little we know about the subject comes from the careful study and comparison of clinical cases and occasional autopsies, and our information is extremely indefinite. In many cases, as in the one reported, where the visual memory center is blocked but not destroyed, the patient is able to get at this area in some roundabout way through the connection with the auditory or tactile memories, so that when he hears the object named or can touch or taste or smell it, he at once remembers how it looked: for instance, he can write, though he cannot afterward read what he has written. But if the area be destroyed or completely isolated, visual memories cannot be got at through the other senses and the so-called "mind blindness"[4] results, in which the patient has not the faintest idea what he is seeing. He has no visual memory to project and, therefore, cannot write.

Apparently this visual memory area is still further divided or specialized. Less complete destruction or blocking has resulted in recorded cases of word-blindness without letter blindness,[5] of letter- without word-blindness,[6] of musical note blindness,[7] of psychic color blindness,[8, 9] of blindness for one language, like French, while ability to read another with similar characters, like English, was preserved, of inability to read English while Greek or Arabic were retained.[8] In almost all these cases a right hemianopsia was present. This of itself would not cause any interference with the visual memory so long as a connection between the memory center and the opposite hemisphere was preserved. If this was interrupted, some form of memory blindness would occur. This is the usual type, the commonest lesion being some vascular changes in the Sylvian artery or its branches which supply the whole region of the angular gyrus and the communicating paths leading to it. It is quite likely that in a good many hemiopic patients word-blindness is overlooked, the inability to read being interpreted as the result of very poor vision. There is no apparent reason why word- or letter-blindness should be any more common than number or note or object blindness.   Probably they are less often detected by routine tests.

The prognosis must of necessity depend on the amount of actual destruction as compared to the amount of temporary pressure or edema or anemia, but hemianopsia notoriously is not likely to disappear.   Younger and more intelligent patients can learn to read by developing roundabout methods of communication through other centers, such as by actually or mentally tracing a letter or word and saying it aloud.   Hinshelwood[3] records one case where a patient, by enormous effort, reacquired the ability to read haltingly, the autopsy showing a very unusual development of the corresponding region in the other hemisphere.   This would naturally be easier in the young and almost impossible in the old.

Congenital word-blindness implies a congenital defect which prevents an otherwise normal child from learning to read, either entirely or after very great difficulty.   It could hardly have been identified clinically without the suggestion derived from knowledge of acquired cases.

At first considered a very rare condition, the pendulum has now swung so far in the other direction that the term is twisted to include all sorts of cases, whether due to organic defect or poor teaching or general stupidity.   The following cases perhaps will serve to outline the clinical picture.

Master B., aged ten years, child of normal, healthy, intellectual parents, who married late in life, was born when his mother was thirty-five years of age, after a labor said to have lasted five days and terminated by forceps.   He was always delicate and sickly, but survived a double pneumonia.   As a small child he complained of seeing things upside down, was sent to school at age of six, was able to learn the letters of the alphabet with the greatest difficulty, and was never able to distinguish "m" from "w."   He has never been able to read or spell, stumbling over the shortest words.   He keenly enjoys having stories read to him, but will not make the slightest effort to read for himself.   He cannot write words readily, but recognizes them at once when read to him or spelled aloud, but he converses unusually well for his age and is exceedingly clever in mathematics. His poor progress in school has been a great trial to his parents. He has been taken to several ophthalmologists in the hope that the trouble was due to some defect in the eyes and has worn glasses from time to time.

Both parents have finally come to regard him as a mental defective, and the father, who had looked forward to seeing his own classic career repeated in his son, can hardly bear the sight of him, while the child has the attitude of a whipped dog and has entirely lost his intellectual morale. Careful examination of his eyes showed them to be absolutely normal except for a low refractive error. There was no hemianopsia.

The probable nature of the trouble was explained to the parents, and particularly to the boy himself, with the suggestion that with individual teaching and great patience he would eventually learn to read fairly, but probably never normally: that he should be educated along the lines of strength rather than of weakness.

I have seen the boy occasionally during ten years. He now reads fairly well, but laboriously and not for pleasure. He has never been able to do much with languages, but has been an exceptionally good mathematician and is acquitting himself creditably enough, being ready to enter Boston Tech.

Even to-day he has to spell long and unfamiliar words aloud to assist himself in reading.

J. G., aged ten years, was brought to me because he could not learn to read and was very backward in school, in the hope that there might be some ocular condition which would account for the trouble. His parents are unusually intelligent, educated people, and his younger brothers have completely outstripped him, so that he is considered by the other children, his parents, and himself as more or less of a fool. He hates to go to school and is too discouraged to try very hard at anything.

He was a bright enough boy when talked to about things that interested him. He could not read common words like "dog" and "cat" well, but recognizes them at once when spoken to him or when he was made to spell them aloud for

himself. He took a keen joy in the funny supplement, and
after looking at the picture could stumble through the cap-
tions, which he could not previously read; did mental arithmetic better than normal; naturally left handed, he had been
made to use his right. He was not definitely right or left
handed, writing his name with either hand, but if he wrote
right handed first, did not afterward use his left so freely unless allowed to write backward, which he did much better
than forward with this hand.

In this case, too, the eyes were normal in every way except
for a low refractive error, and there was no hemianopsia.

Explanation of the difficulty made an entire change in the
attitude of parents and brothers toward him, and did even
more to restore his own morale, while individual teaching
along better psychologic lines resulted in rather remarkable
scholastic progress.

There are very wide variations, within psychologic limits,
of the ability to store up visual memories. There are occasional instances which are almost beyond belief. Binet instances a man who could take in at a glance whole columns of
figures and afterward reproduce them at will in his own
mind, just as though he were looking at a photograph.[10]
Gould has reported a patient who could take in a large part
of a page at a glance.[11] Theodore Roosevelt was supposed to
have had this faculty to an unusual degree. On the other
hand, there are whole groups whose perceptions are distinctly
auditory rather than visual, and it is only when word perception is far below the ordinary physiologic limits that we
are justified in classing a child with the congenital word
blind. It is said to occur much more often in boys than girls.

Most of us learned our letters individually from blocks or
large type, hearing the letters called out loud and calling
them ourselves, and so associating the auditory and visual
centers. Short words followed, being spelled aloud, so that
any child with a visual memory competent to embrace the
letters of the alphabet could with patience learn to read a

passable amount through the auditory association even though the visual memory center was not very good. But with practice we learned to recognize words as entities and not as collections of phonetic letters, and in this way alone could we read as the educated man must read. But the modern educational method tends to skip the first two stages, the child no longer learns letters, and instead of his visual memory center having to become familiar with a half a hundred forms, it is compelled to assimilate the infinite number of combinations of letters first in syllables, finally in whole words, and all this with very little aid from the auditory memory center. Under the modern system it would seem as though the cases of congenital word-blindness ought to be much greater, and the teaching them a modicum of reading much more difficult.

From the clinical cases of acquired word-blindness it would seem that letters, numbers, musical notes, words, etc., occupy perhaps closely contiguous but nevertheless distinct areas in the visual memory center, and that they may be destroyed or more often perhaps isolated by various lesions.

In the congenital cases, however, it is much more likely that the defects are cortical and due to lack of development rather than to destructive lesions. For this reason they are not so likely to be extreme defects (and being limited to the neighborhood of the angula gyrus are not accompanied by hemianopsia, as in the acquired type), and we might expect to find the same variety of clinical types, from what has been called congenital "dyslexia,"[12] a very rapid fatigue of the center, up to absolute letter blindness. In youth, too, if one side of the brain is crippled, there is some chance that the other side may take up its normal function successfully, a thing which can hardly be hoped for in the elderly, but attempts at which have been indicated.

The fact of right or left handedness is interesting, too. Feeble-mindedness is said to be much more frequent in left-than in right-handed children. The right handed always have the visual memory center on the left angular gyrus, and vice versa, and some maintain that the manual center precedes and determines the location of the others. It is quite conceivable that the attempts to change a naturally left-handed boy into a right might have prevented the specialization of one definite visual memory center as it did the writing one.[13]

METHODS OF TREATMENT.—It is important to explain matters carefully to parents, and perhaps to the child, in order to remove the stigma of inferiority which affects adversely the whole morale of childhood. Individual instruction and an understanding teacher are indispensable. It would probably be a mistake to teach the child to substitute auditory and tactile for visual memories entirely, but they can certainly be used to facilitate the storing of those memories. The use of block letters, spelling aloud, and reading aloud will be of great assistance. The prognosis must be a rather uncertain one. There is a possibility in childhood that the corresponding area on the right side of the brain might take up the function of the defective left. The choice of occupation or profession in which success should depend as little as possible on visual memories would also be most important.

REFERENCES.

1. Kussmaul: Ziemssen's Cyclop., vol. xiv, 1877.
2. Claiborne: Symbol. Amblyopia.
3. Jackson: Developmental Alexia, Amer. Jour. Med. Sci., May, 1906.
4. Wilbrand: Die Seelenblindheit, Wiesbaden, 1887.
5. Badal: Arch. f. Ophth., March and April, 1888.
   Hinshelwood: Lancet, February 12, 1898.
6. Hinshelwood: Letter, Word, and Mind Blindness, 1900, 68.
7. Edgren: Deutsch. Zeitschr. f. Nervenhk., December, 1894.
8. Hinshelwood: Congenital Word-blindness, 1917, p. 16, etc.
9. Wilbrand: Ophth. Beitrag zur diagnostic Gehirnkrankheit, Wiesbaden, 1884.
10. Binet: Psychology of Grand Calculations, 1894.
11. Gould: Jour. Amer. Med. Asso., July 6, 1912.
12. Berlin: Ein besondere Art der Wort-Blindheit, Wiesbaden, 1887.
13. Claiborne: Stuttering and Manual Dexterity, New York Med. Jour., March 31, 1917.

DISCUSSION.

DR. E. E. JACK, Boston, Mass.: Some years ago I reported a case of alexia which went on to pure mind blindness. Autopsy revealed a tumor. Its situation, however, made it necessary to infer that the symptoms were caused, not by the tumor itself, but by pressure. The interesting thought was suggested to me then by the late Dr. Putnam, that we were not to think of this area as made up of absolutely definite centers but of interdependent parts having to do with visual and auditory interpretation and memory; a break in any part throwing the whole mechanism out.

DR. J. H. CLAIBORNE, New York: I have been studying this subject for fifteen years or more. In 1906 Dr. A. Schapringer and myself read papers on the same occasion before the Section on Eye Diseases, New York Academy of Medicine, on the condition known as word-blindness. My paper followed that of Dr. Schapringer, and I believe he is the first to have reported a case in this country. Since that time I have had nine or ten cases. Subsequently, I read a paper before the Section on Diseases of Children, American Medical Association, Boston, in June, 1906, on the same subject, and called attention to blindness not only for letters and written words, but for the memory of mathematical symbols, and gave that as a possible explanation of the backwardness or inability of some children to acquire mathematics. I likewise referred to blindness for written musical notes, and subsequently the inability of some people to play cards well, which I attributed to blindness for card symbols. I suggested discarding the "word-blindness" and grouped all these cases under the term symbol amblyopia, because in effect it was not blindness, but amblyopia. I remarked at that time likewise that, among the cases I had seen, the children who had symbol amblyopia for letters or words were generally good in mathematics, and that in my experience I had ever noticed that those who acquired and spoke languages easily were not proficient in mathematics and that mathematicians were notoriously poor linguists. I do not remember ever to have seen any one equally proficient in both mathematics and languages. I believe symbol amblyopia is the explanation.

The question of treatment in this condition opens up a still

more interesting field.   Dr. Alger has vaguely referred to the
cultivation or development of the opposite side of the brain
as a means of relieving this condition.   In the paper referred
to read in Boston, I made the radical suggestion that, when
symbol or auditory amblyopia exists in children, it was reasonable they be taught to be left handed in order that the
hand center, together with the speech center, be transferred
from the left side of the brain to the right, so that the right
should take command instead of the left, and suggested that
experiments be made along those lines.   Subsequently, E. B.
McCready read a paper before the Section in Medicine,
Pennsylvania State Medical Society, on "congenital word-
blindness" as a cause of backwardness in school-children, and
reported the case of a boy who stuttered so badly that the
attempt to speak threw him into a panic.   He had word
amblyopia in its worst form, but seemed to have average
intelligence.   He was right handed and, according to
McCready, "to this end the patient was first taught to use
his left hand, as advised by Bastian in the acquired form, and
later by Claiborne, in the congenital form."   To this was
added frequently repeated impressions of words through
every possible avenue.   In the end, in the words of Mc-
Cready, "his improvement has been most satisfactory.   He
can now read a page of ordinary printed matter composed of
the more common words almost as quickly as a person with
normal visual memory, and is able to read for pleasure, a
thing he was never able to do before."   I had noted ante-
cedently to this that change in dexterity was accompanied in
the case of my own son by the development of stuttering.
My son was originally left handed, but became by practice
completely right handed.   During the process of change he
stuttered badly.   This observation has been made in a variety of directions, and is referred to at length by me in a
paper printed in the *New York Medical Journal*, March 31,
1917.   I later relieved stuttering for a while completely in one
case by reversal of manual dexterity.   McCready's case of
stuttering was almost entirely relieved, so that a youth, a
nuisance to himself and others, was turned into a useful individual.   Several cases of symbol amblyopia have been reported, but most of the work has been done in England, on
the Continent, and in Buenos Ayres.   Some one has stated

that anatomic proof of the lesion in the brain in cases of symbol amblyopia has been found, but I am not acquainted with this and have been unable to get any definite information concerning it.

DR. BURTON CHANCE, Philadelphia: I have reported two cases; the boys were not left handed. Dr. Alger is to be commended for bringing the subject before the Society, as it is as much ophthalmologic as neurologic.

DR. EDWARD STIEREN, Pittsburgh, Pa.: Six or eight years ago I examined a lad who could read only when the print was upside down. He was bright in mental arithmetic, gave the correct answer to four or five columns, and could give the answer almost as fast as you gave him the figures to add. This lad is confined to an institute for feeble minded, as he has distinct criminal tendencies, arson and stealing.

DR. EDWARD JACKSON, Denver, Col.: This paper is of especial interest to ophthalmologists, because these patients are very apt to be brought to the ophthalmologist for a defect of sight. I remember one very striking case. A boy of 12 or 14 was brought to me for his sight, and in getting his history I found that in the preceding season he had shot 200 grouse with a rifle. Of course, he had perfect vision, above the usual standard, but his relatives thought that he must be somewhat defective in sight. Afterwards I talked with the teacher who had him first in his early years. She said she devoted three months with him to teach him the first three letters of the alphabet, and at the end of that time he had not learned one of them; he could not recognize them by sight. He is an apparently bright boy. I do not remember as to whether he was right or left handed.

Most of the cases that I have seen have improved very markedly. The first I saw at 11 or 12 years of age did well in school, good at painting and was a bright girl, but could not read and was kept back grade after grade because of her inferior reading. She subsequently, I think, became a very fair average reader. She is married and has a couple of children, they are 8 or 10 years old, and both of them apparently have normal ability to read letters. It has seemed to me, and I think the mass of case histories bears this out, that it is a delayed or imperfect development of memory centers, or memory power, rather than a permanent mental defect.

DR. H. M. LANGDON, Philadelphia: One case on record throws a certain light on the question of the education of a second word memory center.   It is that of a boy with heart disease who had an attack of aphasia due to embolism, cutting off the blood supply to the left third frontal convolution.   He regained his power of speech by training the right third frontal convolution, only to be permanently silenced by an embolism which also deprived this part of the brain of its blood supply.

A case of Déjérine's was word blind for four years before his death, with right homonymous hemianopsia.   Although word blind, he could copy correctly.   Ten days before his death he became totally agraphic, but with no muscular paralysis.   Autopsy showed an old lesion which had destroyed the cuneus and part of the left occipital lobe, and a recent area of softening of the left angular and supramarginal convolutions, which accounted for the later total agraphia.

THE CHARACTER OF IRITIS CAUSED BY FOCAL INFECTION.*

WILLIAM L. BENEDICT, M.D.,
Rochester, Minnesota.

That inflammatory lesions of the iris may be produced by the introduction of living bacteria into the blood-stream has been demonstrated by several workers. Rosenow, in 1914, injected 35 rabbits with strains of organisms from patients suffering from rheumatism, and 2 of the 35 developed iritis. In 1915 he reported 9 cases of iritis or iridocyclitis among 48 cases of lesions of the eye produced during the course of a long series of experiments in which animals were "injected intravenously under uniform conditions with streptococci from rheumatism, from appendicitis, from ulcer of the stomach, from cholecystitis, from erythema nodosum, from herpes zoster, from parotitis, from pyorrhea, from the tonsils, and from dairy farm products."

Rosenow's experiments demonstrated that iritis occurs in animals as a local bacterial infection following bacteremia artificially produced. The experiments were not intended primarily to produce iritis, but to note what organs are affected when pathogenic bacteria isolated from suppurative foci in human beings are introduced into the blood-stream, and further to test the virulency of various strains of organisms after varying periods of growth on artificial mediums in the laboratory. If the ocular structures are affected by these organisms, such infections, Rosenow believes, may be considered an indication of selective affinity for the ocular tissues. Rosenow found that organisms taken from persons

* Candidate's thesis accepted for membership by the Committee on Theses.

suffering from rheumatism more frequently produce ocular lesions than organisms taken from persons suffering from other diseases.

Brown and Irons, in recent experiments, produced iritis in rabbits by intravenous injections of streptococcus, bacillus mucosus capsulatus (Friedländer), bacillus pyocyaneus, and the gonococcus. They concluded that "bacteria reach the eye by the circulating blood and can be recovered from the eye of animals in which the iritis has been experimentally produced." In order, however, to produce iritis it was necessary to give large doses of the organism so that a condition of sepsis was created, and then it was produced only occasionally. In 1916 Irons, Brown, and Nadler conducted experiments "with the idea of discovering the changes in the power of an organism (streptococcus) which had already given rise to iridocyclitis in the patient, to produce similar lesions in animals, after varying periods of residence in the original host, of residence in animals, tissues, and of growths on culture-mediums." These experiments seem to have indicated "that the invasive power of the organisms for special tissues may change within a short period of time during residences in the original host, during animal passage, and in culture, without pronounced or constant changes in culture characteristics or any general virulence for animals."

Lewis (1919) produced iritis in a rabbit by injecting into the blood-stream a culture of streptococcus viridans grown from a peri-apical infection in a patient suffering from acute iritis; the same organism was recovered later from a culture of a section of the iris of the rabbit. Lewis writes: "This experiment proves absolutely for the first time, as far as I know, the selective affinity of the organism found in dental root abscesses for the special structure which had been affected in the individual from which the tooth was taken."

Many clinical reports demonstrate the close connection

between diseases of the eye and dental infection, tonsillar infection, rheumatism, and other infectious diseases. Since Lang, in 1913, published his opinion on the subject, many published case reports have demonstrated the influence of dental sepsis on the eye. Very few of these reports were based on observations further than improvement of the ocular disease following the removal of diseased teeth and freedom from further attacks of iritis. Levy is reported to have said, in discussing metastatic iritis: "No one, I believe, among all those investigating these metastatic eye infections, has been able to produce bacteriologic culture from tissues taken from one of these eyes, and only once has anybody ever claimed to have produced an experimental iritis by animal inoculation."

It was my purpose in this investigation to determine whether organisms taken from a focus of infection, such as peri-apical infection of the teeth or infection of the tonsils in patients suffering from acute or chronic iritis, have a selective affinity for the iris, and whether the affinity of the organisms is greater when taken from an individual during an acute attack of iritis. The experiments were conducted in the laboratory of experimental bacteriology of the Mayo Foundation. The cultures were made, and the animals injected by Dr. E. C. Rosenow and by Dr. G. J. Meisser. Fourteen patients with iritis were selected as test cases. In order that the patient might definitely be considered a test case it was necessary to eliminate, so far as possible, by the history, the physical examination, and the laboratory tests, other causes of iritis, such as syphilis, gonorrhea, and tuberculosis. The method of collecting material from the focus and the cultural methods employed have been described by Rosenow.[9] If a culture was to be obtained from an infected tooth, the tooth was removed under aseptic precautions, sterilized by flaming, the root cracked in a vise, and the pulp transferred to blood-agar plates and tall tubes

22

of liquid medium. For purposes of animal inoculation the tubes with the growing organisms were shaken in order to insure thorough mixing, and 2 c.c. of the fluid, containing usually 4,000,000,000 bacteria, were injected into a vein of the ear of a rabbit.

REPORT OF CASES.

CASE 1 (267625).—Miss A. E., aged twenty-four years, examined April 14, 1919, had suffered pain and lacrimation three days previously from a foreign body lodged in the left

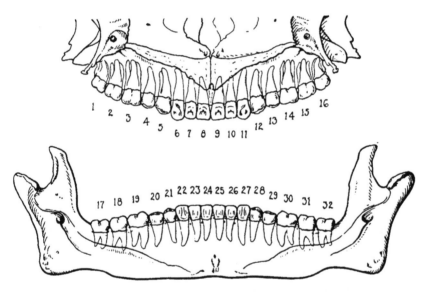

Fig. 1.—Diagram of plan for numbering permanent teeth for clinical references.

eye. The next day the eye became more painful. At the time of examination the palpebral and the ocular conjunctiva were injected. No trace of a foreign body could be found. The injection around the cornea gradually increased, the pupil contracted, and the pain became more intense. Iritis of the left eye developed and local treatment was instituted.

Roentgenograms of the teeth revealed four impacted molars (teeth 1, 16, 17, and 32, Fig. 1) and a fracture of the roots of both upper central incisors (teeth 8 and 9, Fig. 1) sustained eleven years previously. The impacted and fractured teeth were extracted and the sockets of the incisors cureted. The patient made a rapid recovery.

The pulp of the right upper central incisor was calcified; the pulp chamber of the left upper central incisor was enlarged and filled with foul-smelling pus, and there was a small granuloma over its apex. Gram-positive diplococci and a large number of fusiform bacilli and cocci of varying sizes were identified in smears from the pus. A blood-agar plate of the pus produced a moderate number of indifferent colonies of staphylococci, but no green-producing nor hemolytic streptococci. Cultures of the foul pulp in glucose-blood broth produced a diffuse cloud, due to short-chained streptococci. A blood-agar plate of this culture showed green-producing streptococci in pure form. Cultures in glucose-blood broth, of the granuloma of this tooth, of a splinter of bone from between the two teeth, and of the calcified pulp of the right incisor, in twenty-four hours showed a diffuse cloud in the lower two-thirds of the tube, gradually rising to the top. The same type of streptococcus was isolated from blood-agar plates of the glucose-blood broth culture as from the foul pulp. Microscopic sections of the granuloma showed chiefly old dense fibrous tissue containing highly cellular areas of various sizes. The areas of infiltration contained fibroblasts, plasma cells, endothelial cells, arranged in rows resembling capillaries, and a moderate number of leukocytes. Gram stain of the fresh granuloma showed an occasional diplococcus, usually in or adjacent to the cellular areas of blood-vessels. An area at the apex of the granuloma near a blood-vessel contained a number of diplococci.

Primary glucose-blood-broth cultures of the foul pulp, of the calcified pulp, and of the granuloma, were injected intravenously into three rabbits. All had iritis and lesions of the nerve-trunk and one had lesions of the muscles. The first two rabbits (Rabbits 1699 and 1700) had marked lesions of the pulps and contiguous structures of teeth. The culture of streptococcus from the iris of one of the rabbits (Rabbit 1699) was injected into two other rabbits. Both developed lesions of the muscles, lesions around the pulps of the teeth, and in the dental nerves in the jaws. One of the five rabbits died from the injections; the others were anesthetized for examination in from three to six days.

April 30, 1919, 9 A. M.: Rabbit 1699, albino, weighing 1100 gm., was injected intravenously with 3.5 c.c. of the glucose-blood-broth culture of the foul pulp. A small amount of sterile sand was added to a few drops of this culture and placed in the right conjunctival sac. At 8 P. M. the vessels of the iris and surrounding conjunctiva were congested, and both eyes were affected by lacrimation and photophobia. The rabbit seemed well otherwise. May 1st, 7 A. M., the congestion of the vessels of the eyes was more marked (Fig. 2), and the animal appeared to be muscle-sore and inactive, with a tendency to crouch on its abdomen. The fluid in the anterior chambers was cloudy. At noon it appeared to be weaker; the congestion in the eyes had diminished. At 8 P. M. it jumped out of its basket in a convulsive seizure and died in violent convulsions fifteen minutes later. The circumcorneal congestion disappeared with death.

Necropsy was performed immediately. The iris of each eye was opaque and contained focal hemorrhages. The fluid in the anterior chambers was turbid. There were numerous hemorrhages of the posterior aspect of the iris and in the ciliary body (Fig. 3). The base of the appendix and the mesenteric lymph-glands draining the appendix were swollen and hemorrhagic. There were marked degeneration of the myocardium, hemorrhages of the superficial muscles and aponeurosis around the thorax, punctate hemorrhages in the thymus, and numerous subendothelial hemorrhages in the septal wall in the left ventricle and in the papillary muscles. The parathyroid glands were extremely red, edematous, and swollen. The thyroid was hyperemic. In the first centimeter of the duodenum were a few small punctate hemorrhages; the mucous membrane of the cardiac end of the stomach was hyperemic. The lymph-glands beneath the angle of the jaw and ear and along both superior maxillary nerves were edematous and hemorrhagic; those in the axillary and inguinal regions were normal, and those in the popliteal spaces were hemorrhagic and edematous. The posterior tibial nerves were swollen and hemorrhagic. The periosteum opposite the right lower incisor was edematous and separated easily from the bone; the tooth was loose in

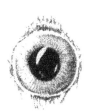

Fig. 2.—Iritis in Rabbit 1699 following injection of a culture from the foul pulp in a case of iritis (Case 1).

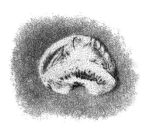

Fig. 3.—Reverse side of the iris shown in Fig. 2.

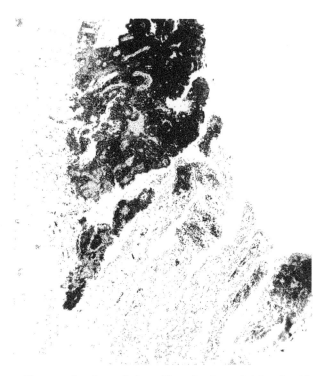

Fig. 4.—Section of the ciliary body and iris of rabb jected with the culture from dental pulp showing marked h rhage and infiltration. Methylene-blue and eosin. × !

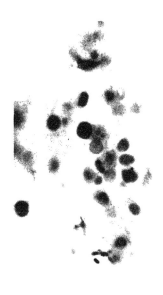

Fig. 5.—Section of the uvea

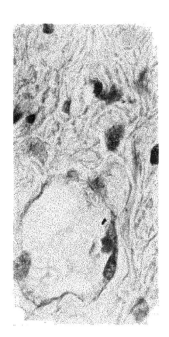

Fig. 6.—Diplococcus in

the socket; the peridental membrane and the pulp were edematous and hemorrhagic. The corresponding inferior dental nerve was hemorrhagic, and the pulps of a number of the molars on the right side were hemorrhagic and edematous. The pulp of the left lower incisor and the left inferior dental nerve were normal. The superior dental nerves were edematous and contained a few punctate hemorrhages. Smears from the hemorrhagic area in the periosteum and from three dental pulps showed Gram-positive diplococci, but no other bacteria. Blood-agar-plate cultures of the blood, of the fluid from the anterior chamber, and of the pulp of the right lower incisor were negative. Glucose-blood-broth cultures of the tissue of the iris and of the pulp of the right lower incisor showed diffuse growth of a short-chained streptococcus, beginning at the bottom of the tube and gradually forcing its way to the top. Sections of the eyes showed marked hemorrhage and leukocytic infiltration of the ciliary body and iris (Fig. 4). Gram stains showed scattered diplococci in and adjacent to areas of hemorrhage (Figs. 5 and 6).

April 30, 1919: Rabbit 1700, a female weighing 1720 gm., was injected intravenously with 5 c.c. of the glucose-blood-broth culture from the calcified pulp of the right upper central incisor. A few drops of the culture were mixed with sterile sand and dropped into the right conjunctival sac. May 1st the animal appeared to be fairly well, but there were lacrimation and moderate congestion of the conjunctival vessels of both eyes. May 2d the eyes appeared to be normal, and the rabbit seemed well generally. It did not use the right hind leg, which it held up as if it were painful. Slight pressure along the sciatic nerve and posterior aspect of the legs seemed to cause pain. The joints were not swollen. May 3d the animal's condition was about the same, and chloroform was administered slowly; the animal went to sleep without a struggle.

The necropsy performed on this animal has been reported in full by Rosenow.[9] No lesions of the iris were found.

CASE 2 (306110).—Mr. S. S., aged thirty-two years, examined February 12, 1920, stated that he had had periodic attacks of inflammation in his eyes, more frequently in the left eye alone, one each year for the past eight years. The attacks seemed to come on when he had a cold and did not leave until the cold disappeared. The last attack began January 1st with itching of the eyelids followed by photophobia. He had had serum vaccine injections. Vision of the right eye was $6/7 + 3$; in the left eye, $6/6$. The left eye was kept closed, and the lids were red. There was a marked ciliary injection. The pupil was moderately dilated and reacted slightly to light and in accommodation. The anterior chamber was normal in depth. Intra-ocular tension was normal to touch. The iris was ragged about the pupillary margin and there were pigment deposits on the lens. Transillumination revealed moderate atrophy of the iris. The fundus was best seen with a -9 lens.

The tonsils were found to be size 3 on a scale of 1 to 4 and to contain plugs. Four teeth (3, 14, 29, 30) showed evidence of peri-apical infection (Fig. 1). Two analyses of urine were negative except for a few pus-cells. The leukocytes numbered 12,000; a differential count of 200 cells revealed polynuclear neutrophils, 73 per cent.; small lymphocytes, 16.5 per cent.; large lymphocytes, 10 per cent.; and basophils, 0.5 per cent.

February 25th, teeth 14, 29, and 30 were extracted. March 3d, teeth 17 and 20 were extracted.

Cultures were made of a granuloma from the upper left first molar. A pure culture was obtained of streptococcus viridans in short chains, as diplococci, and a few long chains. Two cubic centimeters of a broth culture were injected into an ear vein of a rabbit. Two days later the rabbit appeared to be very sick (the day of injection the rabbit was so wild he could hardly be caught); it crouched down low, its head dropped, and its eyes, which were kept half closed, showed some lacrimation and circumcorneal congestion. The following day the iritis was well advanced. The photophobia and lacrimation were increased; the iris of each eye was congested, and the circumcorneal congestion was more intense than on the previous day. The animal appeared to have sore muscles. It died the fourth day after the injection. At necropsy two large hemorrhagic areas in the quadriceps extensor muscles of each hind leg were found, and a periosteal lesion in the region of the lower left incisor. The appendix was highly inflamed. In the stomach were several small hemorrhagic lesions and a few larger ones, about 2 to 3 mm. in diameter, which were beginning to ulcerate. A pure culture of streptococcus viridans was obtained from each eye.

CASE 3 (311972).—Mr. T. M. F., aged thirty-eight years, came for examination April 12, 1920, because of attacks of iritis in the right eye. He stated that he had had attacks of rheumatism on an average of two a year for the past ten years; the first attack followed his being struck in the eye by a small piece of steel and lasted four weeks. The last attack had begun three weeks before examination.

Vision in the right eye was 6/5; in the left eye, 6/4 without glasses. The right pupil was slightly smaller than the left. The intra-ocular tension of both eyes was normal. There was well-marked ciliary injection about the right limbus. The cornea was clear; the anterior chamber, deep. The iris was off color, but not markedly congested. The general examination was practically negative. The adenoids had been removed, but not the tonsils. The urine was negative. The leukocytes numbered 10,200. The serum Wassermann test was negative.

The dental examination revealed two infected teeth, the upper right first bicuspid, tooth 13 (the pulp of which was still slightly vital), and a lower left second bicuspid, which showed evidence of disease in the roentgenogram. Cultures from tooth 13 showed pure colonies of streptococcus viridans. Teeth 20 and 13 were removed by alveolar resection April 15th.

April 16, 1920, at 10 A. M.: Rabbit 83 was injected intravenously with a culture from the upper right first bicuspid. At 8 P. M. the lids of both eyes were stuck together by dried secretion; circumcorneal congestion was marked in both eyes. At 9.30 P.M. the irides of both eyes were extremely congested and contained numerous small hemorrhages; the pupils were contracted, measuring 3.5 by 5 mm.; photophobia was marked. Large periosteal lesions were found on the inner aspect of left tibia and a definite periosteal lesion opposite the apical third of the lower left incisor. Cultures were made from the iris, from the fluid in the anterior chamber of the eyes, and from the joint fluids. Pure culture of streptococcus viridans was obtained from each place.

April 16 at 8 P. M. Rabbit 84 was injected with a culture from the granuloma of the lower second bicuspid, and Rabbit 85 with a culture from the upper right first bicuspid. Both rabbits had slight iritis at 12 midnight and the next morning at 8; it disappeared gradually during the day.

April 17, Rabbit 90 was injected into the anterior chamber of the right eye with a culture made from the fluid from the anterior chambers of the eyes of Rabbit 83. The injection was made with a small pipette. The next day marked lacrimation and congestion of the vessels of the left eye, decided photophobia, and swelling of eyelids were observed. The coat of the right eye was injected deeply and the fluid in the anterior chamber was turbid. The rabbit was chloroformed.

At necropsy the scleral coat of the right eye was quite hemorrhagic and infiltrated; the cornea was much thickened, but the vitreous was clear; the vessels of the iris were markedly congested; the iris was moderately edematous, but it was not covered with exudate; the fluid in the anterior chamber was slightly turbid. Many small hemorrhages were found in the muscles and periosteum, especially on the inner aspect of the right tibia and along the internal popliteal nerves, and a number of hemorrhages in the lower portion of the left tibialis anticus. Opposite the roots of both upper incisors were hemorrhagic, edematous areas. The pulps of both lower incisors were extremely congested and hemorrhagic. Cultures made from the iris, the fluid in the anterior chamber of the eyes, the muscle lesions, the joint fluids, and the pulps of the lower incisors showed pure cultures of streptococcus viridans.

April 17th, a culture made from the iris of Rabbit 90 was injected into the anterior chamber of the left eye of Rabbit 94. The following day the marked lacrimation and congestion of the vessels of the left eye were followed by much swelling, and the fluid in the anterior chamber of the eye was turbid, almost pus-like, in appearance. May 1st the rabbit was killed by chloroforming. Cultures made from the uninjected eye, as well as from the injected eye, showed pure colonies of streptococcus viridans. Cultures from the joint fluid also showed streptococcus viridans in pure culture.

May 2d, Rabbit 104 was injected intravenously with cultures from the iris of Rabbit 94. Two days later the rabbit showed severe iritis in both eyes, marked congestion of the vessels of the conjunctiva, circumcorneal injection, and turbid fluid in the anterior chambers of the eyes. The rabbit was definitely muscle sore. The following day the condition was more marked. The congestion of the vessels and the circumcorneal injection were greater. The fluid in the anterior chamber, especially the lower half, contained a large amount of flaky pus.

Necropsy revealed many muscle lesions, particularly around the joints and the anterior and outer aspects of the left and right tibias. There was a slight area of infiltration over the upper left incisors, but no lesions in the viscera. The knee-joints and the ankle-joints contained a moderate amount of turbid fluid. Cultures from the iris, the fluid of the anterior chambers of the eyes, the muscle lesions, and the joint fluid contained short-chained streptococci and diplococci (streptococcus viridans).

CASE 4 (314223).—Mr. W. L. J., was examined April 30, 1920, because of poor vision, which was reduced to 1/60 in each eye. Because of the deafness of the patient, which followed measles at the age of four, and his speech defect it was difficult to obtain a clear history. About twenty years before examination he had had some difficulty with the eyes, but they recovered and were well until the last four years, when, following an inflammation in both eyes, vision failed gradually. An operation was performed on the right eye at that time. The patient had had rheumatism in the right shoulder and knee for the past year, with swollen and stiff joints.

On examination the right eye was found to have a slight ciliary injection at the limbus, corneal nebulous opacity, and some vascularity, superficial and deep, of the cornea. The anterior chamber was of moderate depth, the iris slightly off color. There was a broad, surgical coloboma of the iris on the nasal side. In the left eye were well-marked nebulous opacities of the cornea and a dull and lusterless iris. Ophthalmoscopically in the right eye there was a red reflex in the coloboma; the fundus details were not made out. In the left eye no red reflex could be seen with the ophthalmoscope, but by transillumination a red reflex was seen through the pupil. The iris was very thin and atrophic.

The patient's tonsils had been cleanly removed. He had a marked eighth-nerve atrophy. The bone conduction was reduced. The urine was negative. The hemoglobin was 85 per cent.; the leukocytes were 7,600. The Wassermann test on the serum and on the spinal fluid was negative. The Nonne reaction was negative. Two lymphocytes were found in 1 c.c. of spinal fluid. Teeth 3, 10, and 19 showed periapical infection. Tooth 32 was impacted (Fig. 1).

May 26, 1920, teeth 3, 10, and 19 were removed.

May 26, 1920, a pure culture of streptococcus viridans was obtained from a granuloma of tooth 19 and injected into a rabbit. Two days later the rabbit showed slight iritis, more definite in the left eye than in the right eye. There was some circumcorneal injection. The following day the rabbit's eyes were again normal. No further injections were made. The rabbit was kept under observation for several weeks, but further symptoms did not develop, and the animal was not sacrificed.

CASE 5 (315836).—Mr. J. R., aged twenty-four years, was examined May 13, 1920. He stated that until the age of twelve his sight had been normal; since then it had gradually failed, more rapidly during the past year. Since the age of three he had had considerable rheumatism, affecting the hands, feet, and hips, but not the eyes. He had had no trouble with his eyes except occasional attacks of soreness for three or four days, but they had no direct relation to his rheumatism. He remembered having measles, but no other children's diseases.

V.R.E. 3/60; L.E., 2/60. The eyes were normal in size, and rotated normally in all directions. Convergence was weak, but under special test this function could be elicited. In the right eye the palpebral conjunctiva showed a moderate injection and there was some injection of the ocular conjunctiva in the palpebral fissure on either side of the cornea. The iris was bluish gray. The pupil was centrally placed,

2 mm. in diameter, and it reacted to direct and consensual light and in accommodation. The left eye showed some conjunctival injection. The cornea was small, barely 11 mm. in diameter. Just inside the limbus, at 9 o'clock, was a greenish, elevated area, 1 mm. wide and 2 mm. long, situated entirely on the cornea, free from the limbus. The entire cornea was hazy. The iris was greenish gray. The pupil was 1.5 mm. in diameter and reacted to direct and consensual light and in accommodation. The tension in both eyes was normal to the finger touch. The right pupil was dilated to 2.5 mm. by the instillation of one drop of cocain solution, and with a +16 lens the iris was seen to be bound down to the lens capsule by numerous synechiæ. There were many pigment deposits on the lens capsule. The fundus could not be seen in the right eye. In the left eye was a fine stippling of the posterior surface of the central portion of the cornea. The balance of the cornea was clear. The iris was bound down to the lens. There were numerous pigment deposits on the lens, and a thin white veil over the pupil. The condition of the media behind the opening could not be ascertained. Atropin solution failed to cause full dilatation of either pupil.

A general examination revealed fibrous tonsils size 2 and chronic tonsillitis. The hemoglobin was 77 per cent.; the erythrocytes were 4,700,000, and the leukocytes 7,100. The Wassermann test on the serum was negative. Peri-apical infection was found of teeth 4, 13, and 40 (Fig. 1). Chronic rheumatism, myocarditis, and endocarditis were found.

May 21st the infected teeth were removed. The tonsils were removed May 24th.

May 30th, V.R.E., 2/15; L.E., 6/100.

May 24th one rabbit was injected intravenously with a culture from the tonsils, and two rabbits with cultures from the granulomata. Symptoms did not appear in the rabbits and they were not sacrificed.

CASE 6 (317695).—Miss L. G., aged eighteen years, was examined in the clinic May 29, 1920. In September, 1918, she had received a rather severe blow on the head, and two days later she saw spots before the left eye. She was told by an oculist that the spots were due to a hemorrhage in the left eye. The vision was very much reduced, but after two weeks of treatment the vision was almost fully restored. She had no further trouble until January, 1920, when she again noticed spots before the left eye and the vision of the left eye gradually failed. She was under treatment by various specialists without improvement.

The right eye was found to be normal. The ocular conjunctiva of the left eye was injected around the cornea. The cornea was staphylomatous. The entire surface of the cornea was finely stippled, like an orange peel. The entire cornea was hazy, the posterior surface covered by small white dots. The anterior chamber was deep; the iris was light brown, muddy, and faded, receded, and funnel shaped. The pupil was 4 mm. in diameter and did not react to stimulus. The eye could be transilluminated clearly in all directions. No definite deposits could be seen on the capsule of the lens.

Wassermann tests on both the blood and spinal fluid were negative. The urine was negative. The blood count and hemoglobin were normal. The sinuses were not infected. The teeth were normal except for a suspected bad root of an upper right incisor shown by a roentgenogram. There was a faint general reaction under 0.3 mgm. of tuberculin, but there was no focal or local reaction. The tonsils were size 2, with plugs which contained green-producing streptococci, staphylococci, and Gram-positive bacilli. The nose and ears were negative. A roentgenogram of the chest was negative. No evidence of infection was discovered except in the tonsils and in teeth 10 and 20 (Fig. 1).

The tonsils were removed June 10, 1920. The infected teeth were removed June 21, 1920. A large growth of green-producing streptococci and a few staphylococci were obtained from the material around the roots of the teeth. Two rabbits were injected with these cultures but no symptoms developed. The rabbits were necropsied a few days after their injection, but only a few muscle lesions were found.

CASE 7 (320901).—Mr. J. G., aged fifty-four years, was examined June 23, 1920. His first attack of iritis had been in the left eye in 1907, and had lasted two weeks. The pain was controlled by aspirin. In 1910 an attack of very painful iritis in the same eye lasted six weeks. A few days after this had subsided the right eye became affected. Since then he had suffered at least 30 attacks—2 very severe and 6 severe. Since 1910 he had had a divergence of the left eye. Since 1911 he had been having pains in the back, more frequently during cold weather. His tonsils had troubled him somewhat. He had had gonorrhea in 1889, followed by cystitis; no venereal infection since.

The vision of both eyes was 6/4. There was a divergent strabismus of 20°. The pupil of the right eye was normal in size and position, but irregular; its margins were free. It reacted to direct and consensual light stimulation. The fundus was normal. The anterior chamber of the left eye was shallow; the iris, steel gray. There were synechiæ below from 5 to 8 o'clock. The upper pupillary margin was free. The pupil dilated upward and reacted to direct and consensual light stimulation. There were large floating opacities in the vitreous; the media was otherwise clear.

The tonsils were size 2; they did not contain pus. The nose appeared to be negative. The urine was negative. A Wassermann test on the serum was negative. A roentgenogram of the teeth showed peri-apical infection of teeth 4, 13, and 19 (Fig. 1). The genito-urinary tract was negative except for a slight enlargement of the prostate.

June 29, 1920, the three infected teeth were removed and cultures made from the infected material around the roots. A large growth of green-producing streptococci and a few staphylococci were obtained. One rabbit was injected with the culture. No symptoms developed, so the animal was not sacrificed.

CASE 8 (322553).—Mr. W. L. C., aged forty-six years, was examined June 30, 1920. His first attack of iritis had occurred fifteen years before in the left eye. Since then he had had seven attacks in the left eye and two in the right eye.

The eyes were quite sensitive to light. Vision of both eyes with correction was 6/4. The right pupil was 4 mm. in diameter, the iris brown, and the markings not obscured. The pupil dilated evenly after the instillation of cocain solution in the conjunctival culdesac. There was an eversion of iris pigment on the pupillary margin corresponding to 3,

7.30, and 8 o'clock. On the anterior surface of the lens, in the pupillary area, was a small ring of pigment deposit. The media was otherwise clear. The fundus was negative. The pupil of the left eye dilated evenly after instillation of cocain solution in the conjunctival culdesac. There was no synechia and no deposit of pigment on the lens.

The general examination was negative except for small tonsils, which contained fluid pus. Two examinations of urine were negative. The hemoglobin was 76 per cent.; the erythrocytes were 4,840,000; the leukocytes, 4,800. The Wassermann test on the serum was negative. All of the patient's teeth had been extracted. A roentgenogram of the chest and colon was negative. Some infection in the upper alveolar process was suspected.

July 6th a radical resection of the upper alveolar process was performed. Cultures were not made. July 15th the tonsils were removed.

Cultures were made from the pus taken from the tonsils before operation and after operation. Green-producing streptococci and a few staphylococci were obtained. Two cubic centimeters of the culture in glucose-brain broth were injected intravenously into each of four rabbits. Symptoms of iritis did not develop in the rabbits. After several days of observation all the rabbits were necropsied. One rabbit had hemorrhagic lesions in the endocardium. Lesions were not found in the other three.

CASE 9 (326969).—Mrs. J. S. W., aged twenty-nine years, was examined July 28, 1920. When she was ten or twelve years old she had an attack of inflammation of the eyes which lasted all summer. She had had no further disease of the eyes until two months ago, May, 1920, when an inflammation of the left eye was followed by ulceration of the cornea. This attack lasted one week. Two weeks later she had another attack in the same eye. Shortly afterward she had a similar attack in the right eye, followed by ulceration of the cornea. The attack from which she was suffering at the time of examination had lasted three or four weeks, during which she had been under constant treatment.

V.R.E., 6/7. Vision of the left eye was not obtained because of photophobia and the patient's objection to attempt to use the eye. A small infiltrated area on the cornea was stained with fluorescein; near by was an ulcerated area with vessels running over the limbus toward it. Local treatment was instituted and a search made for focal infection.

On general examination chronic tonsillitis and dental infection were found. The tonsils were size 3 and contained a small amount of pus. The urine was negative. The hemoglobin was 73 per cent.; the erythrocytes were 4,000,000; the leukocytes, 10,800. The Wassermann test on the serum was negative on three occasions. A roentgenogram of the chest was negative. Evidence of genito-urinary infection could not be found. The cervix was soft, since the patient was five months' pregnant. A roentgenogram of the teeth showed infection of teeth 4, 5, 18, 30, and 31 (Fig. 1).

August 3d, teeth 3 and 5 were removed.

August 8th, the patient was dismissed. The left eye was comfortable. There was a very slight circumcorneal injection. The upper outer quadrant was rather hazy, but well epithelialized.

August 23, 1920, the patient returned to the clinic with another attack of iritis in the left eye. Lacrimation and photophobia were marked. The lids were moderately swollen. The palpebral conjunctiva was congested. Local treatment was instituted, and August 30th the remaining infected teeth were removed under block anesthesia. The patient was discharged August 31, at her own request, to resume treatment with her home physician.

One culture was made from a tooth in which the pulp was dying, and another from a tooth which showed evidence of infection in the roentgenogram. Green-producing streptococci (short chains and diplococci) and staphylococci grew in the cultures. Three rabbits were injected. Twenty-four hours later the eyes of one rabbit were inflamed, and the iris of each eye was congested and contained several small hemorrhages. The following day the rabbit died. The type of organisms injected in pure culture were recovered by culture from the fluid of the anterior chamber of each eye and from culture of bits of tissue of the iris dropped in a tube of medium. The same strains of organisms were also recovered from the blood of the animal immediately after death. The other two rabbits injected with the same cultures failed to show symptoms and were not sacrificed.

CASE 10 (327736).—Mrs. H. C. E., aged forty-nine years, was examined August 3, 1920. In May, 1920, the patient thought there was a foreign body on the cornea of the left eye and an attempt was made to locate and remove it. A foreign body could not be found, but the search for it resulted in irritation of the eye. Both eyes became badly inflamed and painful, requiring the services of an oculist. The patient was referred to me by her physician. She brought a letter from her oculist giving in detail her history and his findings. The examination and treatment before coming to the clinic had been well carried out. She had had a serum Wassermann test, which was negative. Her tonsils had been removed July 15, 1920, and were reported to be septic. Two teeth which had been removed were reported to have had abscesses at their roots. Following the removal of the teeth and tonsils there was an apparent remission of the ocular symptoms, although the patient was unable to use her eyes for her housework because of photophobia and pain.

On the patient's admission to the clinic she had signs and symptoms of chronic iridocyclitis. The vision of the right eye was 6/12; of the left eye, 6/60. Photophobia and lacrimation of the left eye were marked. The lids were swollen, scarred, and wrinkled from applied heat. The palpebral conjunctiva was deeply congested, and there was an injection of the ocular conjunctiva, more marked at the limbus. A well-defined and deep scleral blush completely surrounded the cornea, which was hazy from thickly studded deposits on its posterior surface and infiltration of the middle layers. The anterior chamber was normal in depth; the iris, dark slate gray, with blurring of the finer markings. The pupil was 6 mm. in diameter, round, and with numerous posterior synechiæ. Atropin solution could not be used because of the violent reaction. Neither hemorrhages nor large vessels could be seen on the iris. The lens was covered with small pigment deposits on the pupillary area. The pupil did not react to direct light. Only a dull red reflex from the fundus could be seen with the ophthalmoscope. The intra-ocular tension was normal to touch. The right eye was quiet except for lacrimation and some photophobia when the left eye was exposed. The right cornea was clear, but the iris was thickened; the lens covered with pigment deposits in the pupillary area. The media were otherwise clear and the fundus was normal. The intra-ocular tension of this eye also seemed to be normal to touch. A few Gram-positive streptococci, staphylococci, and Gram-negative bacilli were found.

A general examination was made in order to discover the cause of the iritis. The urine on three occasions was negative except for occasional erythrocytes and occasional pus-cells, an interesting finding in the light of later revelations. The hemoglobin was 75 per cent.; the erythrocytes were 4,680,-000; the leukocytes, 10,000. A Wassermann test on the serum was again negative. The patient had right and left nephrolithiasis, with atrophy of the right kidney. The tonsils had been cleanly removed, and no pus could be found around the ears and nose. The teeth were negative except for three questionable teeth, 3, 6, and 11 (Fig. 1), which were later removed and found to have infection around the roots.

In the belief that the right kidney had something to do with the condition of the eyes, a right nephrectomy was performed October 23, 1920, by Dr. W. J. Mayo, who reported "kidney contains stones, infected." The day following the operation the left eye became very painful and a marked circumcorneal injection with increased haziness of the iris developed. Three days later the inflammation had almost subsided. The patient was very comfortable and the eye quiet until November 8th. Then the eye was not quite so well, and November 10th was very much more uncomfortable than it had been for several days. Local treatment was continued, but the last observation, made December 7th, showed the eye to be irritable, with some photophobia and lacrimation. Healing of the nephrectomy wound was delayed so that the side was draining for more than three months.

Cultures were made from the wound and injected into rabbits several times. Cultures were made from the teeth and from the wound, and one rabbit was inoculated intravenously. In the cultures made from the infected teeth large numbers of green-producing streptococci and a few staphylococci were obtained. The rabbits did not show symptoms so were not sacrificed.

CASE 11 (331185).—Mr. E. A. M., aged forty-three years,

23

was examined August 24, 1920.   He complained of attacks
of iritis for the past thirteen years.   He stated that he had
had attacks in both eyes, more often in the right eye than
in the left, and that only one eye was affected at a time.
The last attack was seven or eight weeks previous to his
examination at the clinic.   He had always had local treatment during the attacks.   His tonsils had been removed
three years before, but attacks of iritis had recurred since
then.   One tooth had been removed three years ago and one
three weeks ago.

V.R.E., 6/60, not improved by glasses; V.L.E., 6/20,
not improved with glasses.   The cornea of the right eye was
clear.   The anterior chamber was normal in depth.   The
iris markings were perhaps slightly muddy, the pupillary
margin slightly irregular.   The pupil was 3 mm. in diameter
and reacted a trifle sluggishly.   By oblique illumination iris
movement was observed around the lower three-fourths of
the pupillary margin, although a rather firm adhesion with
plastic exudate bound the iris to the anterior surface of the
lens.   The vitreous was clear, the fundus negative.   The
cornea of the left eye was clear, the iris of good color; the
pupil was slightly irregular, about 3 mm. in diameter, but
it reacted normally.   By oblique illumination old exudates
and pigment deposits were visible in the pupillary area on
the lens capsule.   The fundus was negative.

A general examination was negative except for evidence
of peri-apical infection in teeth 1, 10, and 30 (Fig. 1).   The
urine was negative; the hemoglobin was 80 per cent.; the
leukocytes were 9,200.   A serum Wassermann test was
negative.   The genito-urinary examination was negative
also.

August 31, 1920, the infected teeth were removed and one
rabbit was injected intravenously with a culture of green-
producing streptococci and staphylococci from the infected
tissue around the roots.   No symptoms were observed in
the rabbit from the injection, and the animal was not
sacrificed.

CASE 12 (333100).—Miss P. H., aged twenty-two years,
was examined September 7, 1920.   For the past six or seven
years she had noticed a gradual loss of vision of both eyes,

unaccompanied by inflammation or pain. She had had the eyes examined a number of times and had been told that she had uveitis. The vision had failed more rapidly during the past three years. Examination of the right eye revealed little change. The iris was of good color, the pupil round, about 3 mm. in diameter, and it reacted normally. In the left eye the iris was decidedly muddy, the pupil eccentric, and the margins irregular and adherent to the anterior surface of the lens in the superior temporal quadrant. The pupillary reactions were sluggish.

By ophthalmoscopic examination of the right eye deposits were found on the posterior surface of the cornea; the pupillary margins were irregular; there was a moderately dense opacity at the posterior pole of the lens, and large floating vitreous opacities. The disc had a rather pronounced pallor, with considerable blurring and loss of detail. In the left eye the pupil was bound down almost completely by a posterior synechia. There was a clover-leaf-shaped opacity in the posterior part of the lens, and floating vitreous opacities. Fundus details were blurred, but the disc appeared to be of normal color. V.L.E., 6/7; R.E., 6/5 with correction. The diagnosis was chronic uveitis of the left eye.

On general physical examination the patient was found to be well developed and well nourished, but with acne vulgaris over the skin of the back. The urine was negative. A serum Wassermann test was negative. The tonsils had been cleanly removed in 1916; the nose had a slight deflection of the septum; the ears were negative. A roentgenogram of the teeth showed apical infection of tooth 4 (Fig. 1).

September 15, 1920, tooth 4 was extracted and cultures made from the infection around the root. Large numbers of green-producing streptococci and a few staphylococci were obtained. One rabbit was injected intravenously with the culture, but it failed to develop symptoms so it was not sacrificed.

January 31, 1921, the patient was again examined at the Mayo Clinic. There was no change in the condition of the left eye.

March 12, 1921, there was a painful superficial keratitis, accompanied by marked photophobia and lacrimation. There was a mild iritis also.

CASE 13 (340150).—Mrs. O. S., aged twenty-six years, was examined November 8, 1920. The previous eye history was negative. The patient had an iritis in the left eye which had started five weeks previous to her examination at the Mayo Clinic. At the time of the examination the vision of the right eye was 6/4; of the left eye, 6/60. A general examination revealed a benign tumor of the left breast. The blood-pressure was normal. Two tests of the urine, made two months apart, were negative. The hemoglobin was 75 per cent.; the leukocytes were 5,000. A roentgenogram of the chest was negative. A serum Wassermann test was negative. The tonsils had been cleanly removed. The nose, sinuses, and ears were negative. A roentgenogram of the teeth showed three teeth (18, 19, and 20) with periapical infection.

November 30, 1920, the infected teeth, 18, 19, and 20, were removed under block anesthesia, and cultures made from infected material about the roots. Green-producing streptococci and a few staphylococci were obtained. Two rabbits were injected intravenously. No symptoms appeared in either rabbit after the inoculation, so they were not sacrificed. December 1, 1920, V.R.E., 6/4; L.E., 6/12. The ciliary injection had disappeared. The pupil, no longer under atropin, was active. R.E. +.75 sph. = 6/4; L.E. +1.00 sph. = 6/10.

DISCUSSION.

Until Lewis published his report demonstrating the selective affinity for the iris of streptococcus viridans from a focus of infection of a person suffering from iritis, there was little direct evidence to prove that organisms may assume an affinity for the iris without being sensitized by passage through eyes. Irons, Brown, and Nadler injected dead organisms into the anterior chamber of the eye of a rabbit, and later injected living organisms into the bloodstream of the rabbit. The eye developed iritis, and they concluded that the previous injection of the killed organism tended to lower the resistance of the eye, making it more susceptible to attack by this particular strain of bacteria.

Thus the iritis simulated recurrent iritis in man. The organism was obtained from a person who had purulent dacryocystitis. It had not produced lesions in the iris of the patient. It is hardly plausible that its development in the lacrimal sac would raise its affinity for the uveal tissue of the eye because of its juxtaposition, or because of the function of the lacrimal apparatus.

Injection of strains of organisms taken from foci of infection of persons suffering from acute or chronic iritis produced other lesions in the animals, but although large doses were given, the rabbits did not develop iritis.

Levy, Steinbugle, and Pease attempted to produce iritis in rabbits by injecting bacteria into the lymph-channels, but all their animals died without showing eye lesions, so they decided they would have to use some other animal in their experiments.

During several years of animal experimentation Rosenow collected and published notes on 48 cases of ocular lesions produced in rabbits by inoculation, but of these only 9 had iritis. The sources of the bacteria used in his experiments were varied, but none, so far as we know, were taken from persons who were subject to attacks of iritis. There were no opportunities for the organism used to be sensitized by passing through a host having eye disease, so we may believe that organisms (streptococci) may develop an affinity for the iris without having lived in a host having lesions of the iris.

The frequency with which bacteria from persons having rheumatism attacked the eye led Rosenow to believe that there is a closer connection between iritis and rheumatism than between iritis and other bacterial diseases. This relationship, however, holds more for cases of infectious arthritis and localized muscular rheumatism than for the acute rheumatic fever. In man the attacks of iritis produced by focal infection may be of any degree of severity. Mild attacks of iritis may occur, "which amount to no more than a transient hyperemia of the conjunctiva or a slightly troublesome photophobia. A rapid succession of mild attacks extending over a period of several years has been demonstrated to be due to peri-apical infection."[1]

One of the experiments (Case 4) seems to show that similar attacks of iritis may occur in the animal, and that the organisms isolated from a focus of infection during an acute attack, or an exacerbation of chronic iritis, are more prone to localize in the iris and produce inflammation than those taken from persons who have not suffered from acute attacks of iritis for a number of years. Some of the patients in these experiments had had low-grade uveitis with punctate keratitis and posterior synechia for years; they had numbers of infected teeth from which streptococci were isolated and cultured, and injected into rabbits without noticeable symptoms in the rabbit. It is possible that the iritis of these patients was not due to focal infection around the teeth, even when the organisms usually found to produce iritis were present, or that the organisms were obtained after they had lost their virulence, or that too small doses were given to the rabbits. In some of the animals the muscle and periosteal lesions indicated a virulency of the organisms injected, but the fact that iritis did not develop could not be interpreted as meaning that the iritis in the patient was not caused by this particular strain of bacteria. It was impossible to secure the results desired except by inoculating with fresh cultures (twenty-four hours or less). Again, other organisms were so attenuated that massive doses failed to produce symptoms in the inoculated animal, even though primary cultures were used. Iritis was produced in the rabbits whenever injected with a culture taken from a person having an acute iritis, but was in no instance produced when inoculated with organisms taken from persons whose eyes were not acutely inflamed.

The symptoms and course of the iritis in the rabbits ran about the same as in the patients. The first sign is hyperemia of the conjunctiva and sclera about the limbus. This is followed by injection of the vessels on the iris, swelling of the iris tissue, discoloration of the iris due to congestion, a slight contraction of the pupil, and turbidity of the fluid of the anterior chamber. The pupil did not contract to less than half its diameter in any case.

That the iritis was produced in the animals by bacteria carried to the eye by the blood-stream was amply demonstrated in these experiments. In one case (Case 3) the culture made from the iris of a rabbit was injected directly into the anterior chamber of the right eye of another rabbit (Rabbit 90). The following day the same organisms, green-producing streptococci, were recovered from the uninoculated left eye. Fluid from the anterior chamber of this eye was then injected into the anterior chamber of the left eye of another rabbit (Rabbit 94). After ten days the rabbit was necropsied, and the organism was recovered from the iris of the uninjected right eye, thus showing that the organisms gained access to the blood-stream of the injected eye and collected in the other eye. There were hemorrhagic lesions found in other parts of the body which also yielded pure cultures of green-producing streptococci. The same organism was also recovered in cultures that were made of the blood of the heart.

The organisms most frequently obtained in the cultures from dental abscesses and granulomata were green-producing streptococci (in short chains and as diplococci, streptococcus viridans) and staphylococci. In watching these experiments we were convinced that the streptococcus viridans was the organism that produced the lesions in rabbits and that the staphylococcus was a harmless organism. The best proof of this assumption came from the culture made of the lesions produced in the animals by the inoculation of the mixed primary culture. In all instances the cultures made of hemorrhagic lesions around the muscles, the periosteum, the jaws, from the anterior chambers of the eyes, and of bits of infected iris tissue produced only streptococcus viridans. Staphylococci were not present.

Plate cultures of the organisms were made at the time the cultures were made in long tubes of liquid medium. On the plates large numbers of colonies of streptococci and a few colonies of staphylococci appeared. Attempts to produce iritis in rabbits with organisms grown on the plates were never successful, since the bacteria grown in this manner soon lose their peculiar infecting power for certain tissues; they retain it, however, when grown in tall tubes of medium.

Our experiments sustain Rosenow's contention that in order to retain a specific affinity the organisms must be grown under conditions of oxygen tension similar to those to which they are accustomed. In the tall tube the organisms usually develop near the bottom and gradually come to the top as they acquire the ability to grow in the presence of more oxygen. One reason why other experiments have failed to produce the organisms with selective affinity probably is owing to the fact that the organism responsible for the specific lesion succumbed to the air during the growth of the culture, or lost its affinity through acquiring ability to live under changed environment.

The largest hemorrhages in the iris of the rabbits in which iritis was produced occurred at the juncture of the iris and the ciliary body, where there is a change from highly vascularized tissue to relatively poorly vascularized tissue, with resulting diminution of available oxygen, and in consequence diminished resistance to invading organisms. Similar lesions were found in muscles of the legs, near the tendons, in the periosteum, and around the roots of the teeth. Whether oxygen tension is the chief factor in the selection of the tissue affected cannot be determined from these experiments, but they sustain the conclusion suggested in Rosenow's experiments with streptococci of muscular rheumatism and arthritis.

We may, therefore, conclude that iritis is produced by bacteria arising from foci of infection around the roots of tèeth and in the tonsils; that it is an inflammatory reaction brought about by the presence of bacteria in the tissue of the iris carried to the iris by the blood-stream from the foci of infection, and that such bacteria have the ability to grow and do grow in such environments. Iritis caused by bacterial infection seems to be an inflammation of muscle tissue at the place corresponding to the parts of muscles affected in rheumatic affections of the limbs and trunk. Organisms have repeatedly been recovered from muscular lesions of the legs and trunk, and when injected into animals, produced similar lesions. In numerous instances the muscles and parts of muscles affected in the animal correspond to the muscles and parts of muscles affected in the host from which the organisms were obtained. That there is a close similarity between the lesions of the leg and the trunk muscles in rheumatism, and the lesion of the iris in iritis has been demonstrated time and again in the cases here reported. That they may have a common source is suggested by the fact that they can be produced in the rabbit by the same culture at the same time, almost to the total exclusion of other types of lesions or similar types of lesions in other than muscle tissue.

Therefore we may conclude that iritis of focal infection origin is a myositis caused by an organism that at some period of its growth may cause iritis, and at other periods inflammation of some other muscle. We may further conclude that this affinity for iris tissue becomes a function of the organism spontaneously, or may be acquired by growing on iris tissue; that the affinity for the iris is easily lost by the organism when grown in different environments, and that it will change its affinity for special structural tissue or even lose its virulence to a marked extent.

As the bacteria around the teeth and tonsils are constantly undergoing changes of environment, they suffer a change of function and a change of virulence. There is also a change in the resistance of the body to bacterial invasion, so that in the human body a constant warfare is going on between bacteria and the body tissues and fluids. Iritis occurs as a localized seat of this warfare within the eye, and is in all possible respects similar to reactions brought about in other parts of the body by the presence of the same bacteria at different times of the life cycle of the organism.

REFERENCES.

1. Benedict, W. L.: Value of Dental Examination in the Treatment of Ocular Disorders, Amer. Jour. Ophth., 1920, iii, 860–865.
2. Brown, E. V. L., and Irons, E. E.: The Etiology of Iritis, Trans. Amer. Ophth. Soc., 1915–1916, xiv, pt. 2, 495–517.
3. Irons, E. E., Brown, E. V. L., and Nadler, W. H.: The Localization of Streptococci in the Eye. A Study of Experimental Iridocyclitis in Rabbits, Jour. Infect. Dis., 1916, xviii, 315–334.
4. Lang, W.: The Influence of Chronic Sepsis upon Eye Disease, Lancet, 1913, i, 1368–1370.
5. Levy, J. M., Steinbugle, W. F. C., and Pease, M. C.: Investigations as to Frequency of Metastatic Eye Infections from Primary Dental Foci. Preliminary Report, Jour. Amer. Med. Asso., 1917, lxix, 194–198.
6. Lewis, F. P.: Discussion, Jour. Amer. Med. Asso., 1919, lxxiii, 1132.
7. Rosenow, E. C.: The Etiology of Acute Rheumatism, Articular and Muscular, Jour. Infect. Dis., 1914, xiv, 61–80.
8. Rosenow, E. C.: Iritis and Other Ocular Lesions on Intravenous Injection of Streptococci, Jour. Infect. Dis., 1915, xvii 403–408.
9. Rosenow, E. C.: Studies on Elective Localization: Focal Infection with Special Reference to Oral Sepsis, Jour. Dent. Res., 1919, i, 205–267.

SUGGESTIONS FOR A UNIFORM METHOD OF ESTIMATING LOSS OF VISUAL EFFICIENCY FOLLOWING INDUSTRIAL EYE INJURIES.*

NELSON M. BLACK, M.D.,
Milwaukee, Wisconsin.

The work involved as the result of the appointment as chairman of the Committee of the Section on Ophthalmology of the American Medical Association, to report on "Compensation for the Loss of Vision in Industrial Eye Accidents" suggested the above title as a subject for an entrance thesis for the American Ophthalmological Society.

As stated in the title, the paper is in the form of suggestions. If they are properly coördinated, if they are grounded on a sufficiently scientific basis and can be authoritatively supported by this Society, they may assist in bringing order out of the chaotic state now existing.

The suggestions are as follows:

I. That the *economic* loss of the essential physical, physiologic, and psychologic functions of *both eyes*, which combined constitute standard (normal) vision, be considered as 100 per cent. loss in efficiency, entitling the individual to 100 per cent. compensation.

II. That the *economic* loss of the above-mentioned functions of *one eye* be considered as 50 per cent. loss in efficiency, entitling the individual to 50 per cent. compensation.

III. That the enucleation of one eye be considered as 60 per cent. loss in efficiency, entitling the individual to 60 per cent. compensation.

IV. That compensation should not be computed until all

* Candidate's thesis accepted for membership by the Committee on Theses.

adequate and reasonable operations and treatment known to medical science shall have been attempted to correct the defect.

V. That the above estimates for compensation for eye accidents do not take into account any cosmetic defect which may result, which must be an additional compensation to be adjusted by the Industrial Commission or the insurance companies concerned.

VI. That deviations from the average normal in the following essential functions of the eye be the basis for estimating compensation for industrial eye injuries, unless it can be established that such defects existed before the injury.

	COMPENSATION	
	Distance	Near
	Per cent.	Per cent.
Function A: Central visual acuity for distance for one eye in occupation in which the working distance is greater than arm's length. Economic loss of which.	25	..
Function B: Central visual acuity for near for one eye in occupation in which the working distance is within arm's length. Economic loss of which....	..	25
Function C: Binocular single vision. Economic loss of which....................................	10	10
Function D: Depth perception. Economic loss of which..	5	5
Function E: Field of vision for one eye. Economic loss of which................................	10	10
Economic loss of the above for one eye.............	50	50
Economic loss of the above for both eyes	100	

VII. That visual acuity for distance be determined at 20 feet, using any test conforming to the Snellen standard.

That vision 20/20 = Standard or normal vision for distance.

That vision 20/220 = Economic loss of vision or industrial blindness for distance.

That visual acuity for near be determined at 14 inches, using any test conforming to the Snellen standard.

That vision 14/14 = Standard or normal vision for near.

That vision 14/154 = Economic loss of vision or Industrial blindness for near.

VIII. That this Society use its utmost endeavor to bring to the attention of industrial corporations and labor organizations the necessity for, and convince them of the value of, visual tests as an essential part of the physical examination of applicants for employment.

The following reasons are given for the selection of the above standards, together with the arguments in their favor:

It will be noted that distance vision is not used as a constant primary factor in estimating compensation for eye injuries.

It is the opinion of the writer that it is entirely wrong to attempt to estimate compensation for an injured eye on central visual acuity for distance except in occupations in which the working distance is greater than arm's length. By far the largest number of industrial injuries occur in occupations in which the working distance is within arm's length; furthermore, it is well known that, as a result of an injury, an eye may have a corneal scar, a partial traumatic cataract, or the vitreous body be filled with opacities, and the eye have fair distance vision, but be absolutely incapacitated for close work. In such cases, if compensation is based on the distance vision, the individual is not being paid the amount he should receive for the loss he has sustained.

It is proposed, therefore, that visual acuity for near be the basis for estimating compensation in occupations in which the working distance is at or within arm's length, that in those occupations in which the working distance is greater than arm's length visual acuity for distance be the basis for estimating compensation.

Standard or 100 Per Cent. Vision for Distance.—Usage has already established the unit for standard or normal vision based on the five-minute (5′) angle or V. $= \frac{20}{20} = 100$ per cent. visual acuity.

Industrial Blindness for Distance.—Reasons for the adoption of 20/220 as the unit to represent economic loss of distance vision or industrial blindness for distance.

Replies received in answer to a questionnaire sent to the Industrial Commissions throughout the United States gave from "ability to count fingers at six feet" as the minimum, to 20/100 as the maximum for industrial blindness. The intermediate values given being 5/200, 20/320, 20/220, and 20/200. V. $= 20/200$ was given in the majority of the replies.

The determination of the unit to represent industrial blindness must of necessity at the present time be more or less empirical and rather arbitrarily chosen.

Computing the average of the various units which have been used throughout the United States to represent industrial blindness indicates that a character or letter subtending an angle of between 50 and 60 minutes at 20 feet is in general use.

Therefore it is suggested that 20/220 represent the unit of economic loss of vision for distance, as at 20 feet the angle subtended by the character or letter on test charts for such vision is 55 minutes, or the mean between 50 and 60 minutes —a further reason being the ease with which this unit lends itself to the computing of the percentage of vision.

Table for Visual Acuity in Per Cent. for Substandard Distance Vision.—The determination and adoption of a table for estimating in per cent. the visual acuity for distance in case of injury to one eye.

It is suggested that such a table be based upon the increase in the linear dimensions of the letters or characters used in testing vision at 20 feet, which subtend a five-minute (5′) angle, and whose component parts subtend a one-minute (1′) angle. Such a table was prepared from the formula worked out by Mr. Arthur J. Sweet, consulting engineer of Milwaukee, Wisconsin, as follows: V. = 20/20, representing standard or normal vision, and V. = 20/220, representing industrial blindness.

The percentage of visual efficiency is obtained by dividing the linear dimensions of the letter perceived at 20 feet by the constant factor .07 inch (approx.) (which is the length in inches of one minute (1′) of the circumference of a circle having a radius of 20 feet) to determine the increased size of the test-object in minutes. From the quotient thus obtained subtract 5′, or the minutes actually subtended at the retina by a 20/20 test-object, thus giving in minutes the increase in size of the angle required for the vision of the defective eye. Industrial blindness being considered as 20/220, each minute increase in size of the angle represents 2 per cent. loss in acuity, so multiply the increase in size in minutes of the visual angle of the defective eye by two, giving the loss of vision in per cent. This, subtracted from 100 per cent., gives the visual acuity in per cent.

Example.—The cord subtending a 5′ angle at 20 feet = 0.3491 inch. 0.3491 divided by .07 = 4.99, or approximately 5, subtracting 5′ = 0 × 2 = 0, 100 − 0 = 100 per cent., or standard vision.

The cord subtending a 5′ angle at 220 feet = 3.85 inch. 3.85 divided by .07 = 55′ − 5′ = 50′ × 2 = 100 per cent. 100 per cent. − 100 per cent. = 0 per cent., or industrial blindness.

TABLE A.—VISUAL ACUITY IN PER CENT. FOR SUBSTANDARD DISTANCE VISION.

Vision	Visual Acuity	Vision	Visual Acuity
20/20	100 Per Cent.	20/120	50 Per Cent.
20/30	95 "	20/130	45 "
20/40	90 "	20/140	40 "
20/50	85 "	20/150	35 "
20/60	80 "	20/160	30
20/70	75 "	20/170	25 "
20/80	70 "	20/180	20
20/90	65 "	20/190	15 "
20/100	60 "	20/200	10
20/110	55 "	20/220	0 "

The determination and adoption of a table for estimating the per cent. of visual acuity for the distance of the combined vision of the two eyes, binocular vision, depth perception, and field of vision remaining unaffected.

Such a table must to a large extent be arbitrarily determined on the basis of the per cent. of visual acuity existing in a case of vision reduced to industrial blindness 0 per cent. (20/220) in one eye, and with 100 per cent. (20/20) vision in the other. An individual with 50 per cent. distance vision in each eye would have no better than 50 per cent. acuity. According to the usual method of estimating compensation now in vogue, if the central vision for distance in one eye is reduced to 20/200 − 20/220, that of the other being 100 per cent., the compensation is estimated at from 50 to 90 per cent. That this amount of compensation is too high must be manifestly apparent, for the individual has not lost that amount of vision. Any one who will make the trial of reducing his distance vision in one eye to below that considered as industrial blindness, the other being 100 per cent., and compare the result with that vision reduced to 50 per cent. in each eye, will quickly decide in favor of the former.

As to the probable loss of acuity with central vision reduced to industrial blindness in one eye (20/220), and 100 per cent. vision in the fellow, the other functions being normal, opinions vary between 10 and 25 per cent. loss (90 − 75 per cent. acuity).

It is suggested that a basis for a table to show per cent. of central visual acuity for the combined vision of the two eyes be V. = 100 + V. = 0 = 75 per cent. acuity.

The following table is made up on this basis. The horizontal column represents the vision of the injured eye. The vertical column represents the vision of uninjured eye. The per cent. of visual acuity of the combined vision for distance is found at the intersection of the horizontal and vertical columns.

TABLE FOR DETERMINING PER CENT. OF CENTRAL VISUAL ACUITY FOR DISTANCE OF BOTH EYES.

(Having obtained visual acuity for each eye separately for distance, read intersection of horizontal and vertical columns—the horizontal column representing the visual acuity of the injured eye for distance, the vertical that of a fellow eye. It is understood that visual acuity means the best vision that may ɔe obtained by the correction of any existing errors of refraction.)

VISION—PER CENT. ACUITY	$\frac{20}{20}$ 100 Per Cent.	$\frac{20}{40}$ 90 Per Cent.	$\frac{20}{60}$ 80 Per Cent.	$\frac{20}{80}$ 70 Per Cent.	$\frac{20}{100}$ 60 Per Cent.	$\frac{20}{120}$ 50 Per Cent.	$\frac{20}{140}$ 40 Per Cent.	$\frac{20}{160}$ 30 Per Cent.	$\frac{20}{180}$ 20 Per Cent.	$\frac{20}{200}$ 10 Per Cent.	$\frac{20}{220}$ 0 Per Cent.
20/20 = 100	100	97.5	95	92.5	90	87.5	85	82.5	80	77.5	75
20/40 = 90	97.5	90	87.5	85	82.5	80	77 5	75	72.5	70	67.5
20/60 = 80	95	87.5	80	77.5	75	72.5	70	67.5	65	62.5	60
20/80 = 70	92.5	85	77.5	70	67.5	65	62.5	60	57.5	55	52 5
20/100 = 60	90	82.5	75	67.5	60	57.5	55	52 5	50	47.5	45
20/120 = 50	87.5	80	72.5	65	57.5	50	47.5	45	42.5	40	37.5
20/140 = 40	85	77.5	70	62.5	55	47.5	40	37.5	35	32.5	30
20/160 = 30	82 5	75	67.5	60	52.5	45	37.5	30	27.5	25	22 5
20/180 = 20	80	72.5	65	57.5	50	42.5	35	27.5	20	17.5	15
20/200 = 10	77.5	70	62.5	55	47.5	40	32.5	25	17.5	10	7.5
20/220 = 0	75	67.5	60	52.5	45	37.5	30	22.5	15	7 5	0

Standard or 100 Per Cent. Vision for Near.—The determination and adoption of a unit to represent standard or normal vision for near.

It is suggested that standard or normal vision for the near be assumed when the eye is able to distinguish objects, or read type, that subtend a 5′ angle at 14 inches, the component parts of the character subtending a 1′ angle.

It is further suggested the standard or normal vision for near be represented by the fraction N. V. (Near Vision) = 14/14.

It is further suggested that as an adjunct to the ordinary test-card with printed matter for the near test, that test-cards be prepared for the various distances, from the characters selected by the Ophthalmic Section of the American Medical Association as the best so far devised for the illiterate test-objects. Such a test should, at least, be used to check the acuity for near found with the printed card. Further, that each size of print or character be upon separate cards, so there will be no chance for comparison, as would be the case if all the different sizes were printed on one card.

24

The reason for the above suggestions is that the average workingman is not, as a rule, concerned with letters or printed matter in his near work, but has to distinguish the form and shape of the material with which he is concerned.

Industrial Blindness for Near.—The adoption of a unit to represent loss of economic near vision or industrial blindness for the near.

Inasmuch as the angle subtended by the test-object selected for industrial blindness for distance is 11 times greater at 20 feet than that for V. = 100 per cent., it is suggested that the same ratio be used for industrial blindness for near, *i. e.*, N. V. 14/14 = 100 per cent.; N. V. 14/154 = 0 per cent.

Table for Visual Acuity in Per Cent. for Standard Near Vision—The Determination and Adoption of a Table for Estimating in Per Cent. the Visual Acuity for Near in Case of Injury to One Eye.—It is suggested that such a table be based upon the increase in the linear dimensions of the letters or characters used in testing vision at 14 inches which subtend a five-minute (5′) angle, and whose component parts subtend a one-minute (1′) angle, using the same formula used for estimating acuity for distance.

N. V. = 14/14, representing standard or normal vision for near, and N. V. 14/154, for industrial blindness.

P = percentage of visual acuity.

C = five-minute angle (5′) at retina.

X = length of cord subtending five-minute (5′) angle of character or letter perceived.

0.00407 = length of cord in inches subtending one-minute (1′) angle at 14 inches distance, or constant factor.

2 = per cent. loss in visual acuity for each one-minute (1′) increase in size of letter perceived.

Near Vision 14/14 equals 100 per cent. acuity; N. V. 14/154 = industrial blindness for near.

Formula $P = \left(\dfrac{X}{0.00407}\right) - C) \times 2$. 100 per cent. − P = Visual acuity for near.

Example:—When near vision = 14/70, $P = \left(\dfrac{0.10178 - 5}{0.00407}\right) \times 2$.

P = 40 per cent.

100 per cent. − 40 per cent. = 60 per cent. Visual acuity for one eye for near with vision 14/70.

TABLE C.—VISUAL ACUITY IN PER CENT. FOR SUBSTANDARD
NEAR VISION.

VISION	VISUAL ACUITY		VISION	VISUAL ACUITY	
14/14 =	100 Per Cent.		14/84	= 50 Per Cent.	
14/21 =	95	"	14/91	= 45	"
14/28 =	90	"	14/98	= 40	"
14/35 =	85	"	14/105	= 35	"
14/42 =	80	"	14/112	= 30	"
14/49 =	75	"	14/119	= 25	"
14/56 =	70	"	14/126	= 20	"
14/63 =	65	"	14/133	= 15	"
14/70 =	60	"	14/140	= 10	"
14/77 =	55	"	14/154	= 0 industrial blindness.	

The determination and adoption of a table for estimating the per cent. of visual acuity for near of the combined vision of the two eyes; binocular vision, depth perception, and field of vision remaining unaffected.

It is suggested that such a table be made up in the same ratio as that for distance vision, *i. e.*: N. V. = 100 per cent. + N. V. = 0 = 75 per cent. acuity.

The following table is made up on this basis—the horizontal column representing the vision of the injured eye, the vertical column the vision of the uninjured eye. The visual acuity of the combined vision for near is found at the intersection of the horizontal and vertical columns.

Binocular Single Vision.—The determination and adoption of a unit representing the value of binocular single vision: Function B.

With diplopia resulting from an injury to the eyes or head, the individual cannot use the two eyes in conjunction, but must depend on monocular vision, although he may be able to use the two eyes alternately. According to Table D, he would be entitled to 25 per cent. loss providing the acuity of the fixing eye were 20/20; to this must be added the loss of function C (binocular single vision) and function D (depth perception).

Binocular single vision is of comparative minor importance in the economy of the visual act, however its loss must be compensated; therefore, it is suggested that B.S.V. be given the value of 10 or 10 per cent.

TABLE D.—TABLE FOR DETERMINING PER CENT. OF CENTRAL VISUAL ACUITY FOR NEAR OF BOTH EYES.

(Having obtained visual acuity for each eye separately for near, read intersection of horizontal and vertical columns—the horizontal column representing the visual acuity for near of the injured eye, the vertical that of the fellow-eye. It is understood that visual acuity means the best vision that may be obtained by the correction of any existing errors of refraction or presbyopia that may exist.)

VISION—PER CENT. ACUITY	$\frac{14}{14}$ 100 Per Cent	$\frac{14}{28}$ 90 Per Cent.	$\frac{14}{42}$ 80 Per Cent.	$\frac{14}{56}$ 70 Per Cent.	$\frac{14}{70}$ 60 Per Cent	$\frac{14}{84}$ 50 Per Cent.	$\frac{14}{95}$ 40 Per Cent.	$\frac{14}{112}$ 30 Per Cent.	$\frac{14}{126}$ 20 Per Cent.	$\frac{14}{140}$ 10 Per Cent.	$\frac{14}{154}$ 0 Per Cent.
14/14 = 100	100	97.5	95	92.5	90	87.5	85	82.5	80	77 5	75
14/28 = 90	97 5	90	87.5	85	82.5	80	77.5	75	72.5	70	67 5
14/42 = 80	95	87.5	80	77.5	75	72.5	70	67 5	65	62.5	60
14/56 = 70	92.5	85	77 5	70	67.5	65	62 5	60	57.5	55	52 5
14/70 = 60	90	82.5	75	67.5	60	57.5	55	52.5	50	47.5	45
14/84 = 50	87.5	80	72 5	65	57 5	50	47.5	45	42.5	40	37 5
14/98 = 40	85	77.5	70	62.5	55	47 5	40	37.5	35	32.5	30
14/112 = 30	82 5	75	67.5	60	52.5	45	37.5	30	27.5	25	22 5
14/126 = 20	80	72.5	65	57.5	50	42 5	35	27.5	20	17.5	15
14/140 = 10	77 5	70	62.5	55	47.5	40	32 5	25	17 5	10	7.5
14/154 = 0	75	67.5	60	52.5	45	37.5	30	22.5	15	7.5	0

The character and amount of diplopia are only to be considered a factor in compensation when the defect may be corrected by prisms or operation, as compensation should not be estimated until all adequate and reasonable operations and treatment known to medical science have been attempted to correct the defect.

Depth Perception.—The determination and adoption of a unit representing the value of depth perception: Function D.

"Agreeing with the views of other investigators, Pfalz reports (Ophth. Klinik, 1898) that when the refraction was equal in both eyes and there was no squint, a good estimation of depth was present provided the vision of one eye was 1/10 or more, that of the other eye being normal."

"Axenfeld (Tenth International Congress, 1904) considers that, with a unilateral reduction of the visual acuity to not less than 1/6 in one eye, good binocular vision can be assumed without special testing.''

It is the opinion of the writer that depth perception persists in individuals who have possessed the function before one eye accident, when the difference in acuity between the two eyes is even greater. A confrère who has uncorrected vision in either eye of less than 5/200 (with correction 20/20) has excellent depth perception, without glasses, also with one eye corrected and the other uncorrected. In the above instance there is considerably over 1/10 difference in the acuity of the two eyes.

Therefore it is suggested that the value of 5 or 5 per cent. be given this function as its loss, excepting in case of diplopia, becomes practically apparent only when the vision in one eye is reduced below that considered in this paper as industrial blindness; further, as the individual becomes adapted to the new environment, ability to determine the third dimension is fairly well reëstablished.

Field of Vision.—The determination of a table representing the loss in visual efficiency for various degrees of contraction and for loss of the field of vision.

The loss in visual efficiency from contraction of the fields must be determined empirically, and the per cent. of loss must, at least at the present time, be discretionary. It cannot be associated in estimating compensation with acuity of vision for distance or near except when central acuity is lost, as in absolute central scotoma, but must be an additional factor and should not be added if it will increase the total percentage of loss above 100 per cent.

The great variation in the functional activity of the different portions of the retina serves as a basis of a table for estimating per cent. of loss for contraction of the fields. Central vision or qualitative vision is infinitely superior to peripheral in the perception of fine detail and optical perfection of the image; peripheral vision, or quantitative

vision, is superior in the perception of movement and the
ability to see in subdued light.

The change from quantitative vision to qualitative occurs
quite abruptly near the borders of the fovea.   According to
Dor (Arch. f. Ophth., xix), "a spot 5′ eccentric from the

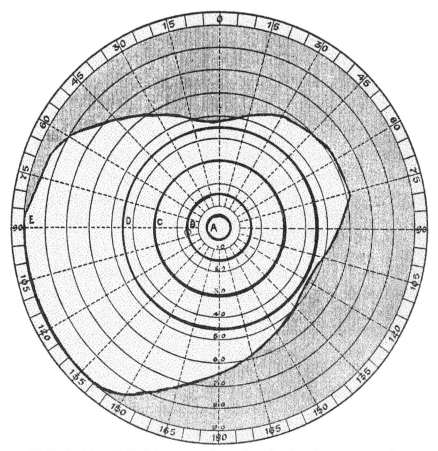

Field of vision divided into zones for estimating loss for compensation.

macula has an acuity of only 1/4, and one 15′ eccentric,
that of only 1/30."

Thus the contraction of the visual fields of both eyes to
15′ or even 5′ would not necessarily effect central visual
acuity.   If contracted to 5′ in one eye there would be prae-

tically no loss in efficiency from an industrial standpoint, as the overlapping of the field of the fellow-eye, if normal, would furnish a functionally active field up to practically 60′ from the point of fixation.

Therefore it is suggested that concentric contraction of the field of vision for one eye to 5′, or practically loss of the field, that of the opposite eye being normal, be rated as 10 per cent. loss in efficiency.

In estimating the loss in efficiency for concentric contraction of both visual fields, it is suggested that the fields be divided into 5 zones—*i. e.*, Zone A, extending from the fixation-point outward to 5′; Zone B, from that point outward to 15′; Zone C, outward to 30′; Zone D, outward to 45′; Zone E, outward to the limit of the field.

It is suggested that the loss in efficiency be as follows, for concentric contraction of the fields of both eyes to:

$$45' = 12\tfrac{1}{2} \text{ per cent. loss in efficiency.}$$
$$30' = 25 \quad \text{`` `` `` `` ``}$$
$$15' = 50 \quad \text{`` `` `` `` ``}$$
$$5' = 100 \quad \text{`` `` `` `` ``}$$

Homonymous hemianopsia, lateral, superior, or inferior, extending to Zone A, or

To 15′ from fixation point = 12½ per cent. loss in efficiency.
" 10′ " " " = 25 " " " " "
" 5′ " " " = 50 " " " " "
Bitemporal hemianopsia = 15 " " " " "
Binasal " = 25 " " " " "

The determination and adoption of a table of compensation for loss of visual efficiency of the remaining eye, the other being absent or economically blind from an industrial injury.

The suggested compensation for economic loss of vision of both eyes is 100 per cent. That for one eye 50 per cent. A one-eyed man or one with an industrially blind eye would, therefore, be entitled to 50 per cent. compensation for economic loss of vision of his remaining eye. The 50 per cent. compensation for economic loss of vision of the first eye does not indicate he has lost 50 per cent. of his visual efficiency. In the majority of instances the individual can, after an interval, return to his former occupation without material loss to his earning power. An injury to his remaining eye, reducing vision, would be a much more serious affair and should, therefore, receive a larger compensation than for injury to the first eye, but should not exceed 100 per cent. for the two eyes.

Individuals with economic loss of vision in one eye the result of disease (not of industrial origin), or with congenital or acquired amblyopia, should not be classed under this heading.

Such a ruling would make it almost imperative that the visual acuity for distance and near, of all employees, be recorded (and retested at least once a year), as this would be the only means of determining the acuity of vision before an injury.

It is suggested that compensation for loss of visual efficiency in one-eyed individuals from industrial injuries be based upon industrial blindness having been reached when visual acuity for distance (in greater than arm-length occupation) and near (in less than arm-length occupation) is reduced to 20/180 and 14/126 respectively, *i. e.*, to 20 per cent. visual acuity. This proposal is absolutely arbitrary, but its adoption is suggested until experience has given us an empirical factor or unit to work upon.

Tests of Visual Efficiency as Part of the Physical Examination of Employees.—The necessity for the physical examination of individuals, male or female, applying for positions in any manufacturing establishments, will be apparent upon a little thought. For instance, no manufacturer, factory superintendent, or foreman would accept or install a machine without inspecting it to see if it were complete in every detail and in good working order. Every employee is a part of the whole working machine of the factory, and any defect in any one part affects the whole. For example, a person with one-fourth, one-third, or even one-half of standard vision cannot be considered as competent a workman as one with standard vision. Again, one may have standard vision according to the test, but may have far-sighted or astigmatic eyes. The use of the eyes for detail work for long periods under such conditions causes eye-strain, which results in pain and discomfort in the eyes and in headaches, and thus interferes with the efficiency of the individual.

TABLE E.—TABLE OF COMPENSATION FOR REDUCED VISUAL EFFICIENCY FOR ONE-EYED INDIVIDUALS.

Distance Vision	Acuity	Compensation	Near Vision	Acuity
20/20	100 per cent.	0 per cent.	14/14	100 per cent.
20/30	95 "	12.5 "	14/21	95 "
20/40	90 "	15 "	14/28	90 "
20/50	85 "	17.5 "	14/35	85 "
20/60	80 "	20 "	14/42	80 "
20/70	75 "	22.5 "	14/49	75 "
20/80	70 "	25 "	14/56	70 "
20/90	65 "	27.5 "	14/63	65 "
20/100	60 "	30 "	14/70	60 "
20/110	55 "	32.5 "	14/77	55 "
20/120	50 "	35 "	14/84	50 "
20/130	45 "	37.5 "	14/91	45 "
20/140	40 "	40 "	14/98	40 "
20/150	35 "	42.5 "	14/105	35 "
20/160	30 "	45 "	14/112	30 "
20/170	25 "	47.5 "	14/119	25 "
20/180	20 "	50 "	14/126	20 "

In a very large proportion of the cases of poor sight, properly fitted glasses will correct the vision, and if a rule existed requiring physical examination, as suggested above, men with poor vision would find out their difficulty when applying for a position, and would, if possible, have their sight improved by glasses. This would prevent many accidents, as well as relieve the individual from eye-strain and headaches, and also enable him to do his work much better and more easily.   In many cases the glasses would be a protection against eye injuries.   Another factor which should be kept in mind while speaking of eye examinations for applicants for a position is the payment of indemnity for loss of vision in case of accident to the eye.   If there were a record of the man's vision made at the time he was employed, and through an accident he lost one-half or all the vision of an eye, the basis of settlement would at once be determined without the man's having to pay a lawyer to fight his employers and try to prove he had perfect vision before the accident.

Further, poor vision or inability to see well may be a factor in causing general accidents, because a man with poor vision cannot see the details of his work or the parts of the machine with which he is working sufficiently well to protect himself against injury.   Again, his vision may be so poor that he cannot see to get about the shop without running into objects or machinery in motion which might cause an injury, especially if the general lighting is poor.   It may be said, of course, that such a man should not be employed in such a place.   That is true enough, and such would not be the case if every man who applies for a job had to submit to a physical and visual examination as one must before enlisting in the army or navy, or when applying for a position in railroad or street-car service.   With a knowledge of the visual ability of an applicant he can be placed in a position where visual defects will be less of a handicap to himself and less of a menace to fellow employees, on the one hand, and be informed of his visual shortcomings and directed as to means of obtaining relief, on the other.

A letter of inquiry to Dr. Harry E. Mock, of Chicago, Illinois, relative to physical examinations in industrial corporations, elicited the following illuminating reply:

"To take up your questions as you ask them:

"First: Figures are not available as to the number of industrial corporations having physical examinations.   Many corporations have reported that they have, but on investigation one finds their physical examination is a mere inspection by a doctor and ofttimes by a nurse. From my studies of the various systems in vogue in other plants, and from the reports of Dr. Clarence Selby, Toledo, Ohio, who investigated industrial hygiene for the U. S. P. H., we have estimated that approximately 150 representative industrial corporations in this country really have an adequate system of physical examination of employees.

"Second: Approximately an equal number of industries require determination of visual acuity.

"Third: Unions object to the physical examination of applicants for work on the ground that employees often use this as a subterfuge for rejecting labor leaders, or so-called undesirables in the labor ranks, for employment. They object to the examination of employees on the ground that many industries discharge employees who are found to have physical defects, and that these men are unable to secure employment elsewhere because of this discharge. Also they claim that the doctor will sometimes find some alleged physical defect, and recommend the work as being too hard for that individual, when no defect is present, and the only desire of the management is to find some excuse to discharge a union man. These are not specific charges, but are conditions insinuated by the unions.

"The real facts of the case are, that some large industries have rejected as high as 15 or 20 per cent. of the applicants examined for work. This means that these industries are picking only the physically fit, and are not taking their share of the burden by selecting suitable occupations for the slightly handicapped worker, occupations in which the handicapped man can be 100 per cent. efficient if proper selection of the job is made. In these industries, where the best form of industrial medicine and surgery is practised, the percentage of applicants rejected for work ranges between 1 and 3 per cent. These medical departments reject an applicant only when he has some condition which makes his presence in the plant dangerous for himself, his fellow-workers, or for property. All other applicants who have defects are considered and placed according to this formula— physical qualifications plus occupational qualifications equals the job.

"Fortunately, a great many industries are yearly obtaining this broader vision and are utilizing physical examinations, including examination of vision, for the purpose of scientific placement of men on jobs. They realize that it is an efficiency measure par excellence. Naturally, labor unions are gaining a better viewpoint regarding physical examinations, and the objections formerly heard are gradually being wiped out. Mr. Gompers has assured me that if industries would adopt physical examinations from the broad humanitarian standpoint above outlined, labor unions would be absolutely in favor of this procedure.

"Fourth: All I have said relative to physical examinations applies to the examination of vision."

It is appreciated that the suggestions herein contained by no means cover all the essential factors in industrial compensation for eye injuries. For the most they have not a solid scientific foundation, but are arbitrarily selected standards. It is, however, the hope of the writer that they may be of assistance in solving this complicated and very important question.

THE COMPENSATION PROBLEM IN OPHTHAL-MOLOGY.*

ERASTUS EUGENE HOLT, JR., A.B., M.D.,
Portland, Me.

1. In the Workmen's Compensation Act of the Legislature of Maine, passed at the session of 1919, provision is made for the loss of an eye as follows: "For the loss of an eye, or the reduction of sight of an eye with glasses to 0.1 of the normal vision, three-fifths the average weekly wages during one hundred weeks."

2. If every injury or disease caused the loss of an eye, or the reduction of the sight of an eye with glasses to 0.1 of the normal vision, it would be a simple matter to determine the compensation according to this law. However, in consequence of injury or disease, the three indispensable functions of vision, namely, central vision, field of vision, and muscular functions, may sustain a variety of losses. To provide for the adjustment of these losses a blanket clause is given to cover them with reference to the schedule in the compensation act, as follows: "In all cases in this class where the usefulness of a member or any physical function thereof is permanently impaired the compensation shall bear such relation to the amount stated in the above schedule as the incapacity shall bear to the injury named in the schedule and the commission shall determine the extent of the incapacity."

3. The law makes reference only to sight, the first indispensable part of vision. If there is a permanent partial loss of it, that is a loss between 0.1 and 0.7, the compensation for this permanent partial loss of central sight shall bear such

* Candidate's thesis accepted for membership by the Committee on Theses.

381

relation to the amount named in the schedule as the incapacity shall bear to the incapacity caused by the injury named in the schedule. It also means, if we interpret the text correctly, that if an injury or disease caused a permanent loss in the second indispensable part of vision, namely, in the field of vision, or in the third indispensable part of vision, namely, in the muscular functions of an eye, the compensation shall also bear such relations to the amount named in the schedule as the incapacity shall bear to the incapacity caused by the injury named in the schedule.

4. The Workmen's Compensation Act, from which quotations have been made, being one of the most recent laws passed by a legislature, is undoubtedly a composite of those heretofore enacted in other states, and must therefore fairly represent the status of the compensation laws of the United States. It provides for compensations for disabilities equivalent to those named in the schedule and for partial disabilities ("the usefulness of a member or any physical function thereof"), but it does not provide any method by which the disability is to be determined. It simply states that the commission shall determine the incapacity.

5. It is obvious that the commission must depend upon the medical examiner for information regarding disabilities equivalent to those named in the schedule and partial disabilities ("the usefulness of a member or any physical function thereof"), as to whether they are permanently impaired and the relationship their impairment bears to the disability caused by an injury named in the schedule. This throws the responsibility for the determination of a compensation upon the medical examiner, the specialist who examines the eyes and makes his report to the commission. After an ophthalmologist makes an examination of the three indispensable parts of vision—central vision, field of vision, and muscular functions of the eyes—he has had no method by which he could demonstrate mathematically how any permanent loss

in these functions caused a loss in the earning ability of the employee in the vocation he followed. The ophthalmologist, therefore, has had no method by which he could determine in a logical manner the relationship between the loss of functions and the disabilities named in the schedule; so that the commission or another medical examiner could readily understand just how the determination was made. As the actual value of the weekly compensation, and its total amount, has to be determined by the natural science method, it is self-evident that in order to determine every part of it in a logical manner this self-same method must be used.

6. We find the value of a compensation under this Act is determined by mathematics. For this purpose we must first determine, as the law provides, what the average weekly wages of the employee have been for the previous year. We find this Act limits the weekly wages to be not less than $10 per week nor more than $25 per week. For an example, we will assume that the employee has lost the left eye and was earning $25 per week. We therefore have 25 for the factor of the multiplicand and 3/5 for the factor of the multiplier in the natural science formula to obtain a product as follows: $25 \times 3/5$ = weekly compensation to be paid the employee. Multiplying, we obtain 15. Therefore, the weekly compensation for the loss of the left eye of this employee is $15.

7. In order to obtain the total amount this employee will receive for the loss of his left eye we must again use mathematics and make 15 the factor of the multiplicand and 100 for the factor of the multiplier in the natural science formula to obtain a product, as follows: 15×100 = the total compensation. Multiplying, we obtain 1500. Therefore, the total compensation to be paid the employee for the loss of his left eye is $1500. It will thus be seen that in order to obtain the value of the weekly and the total compensation for this employee it was necessary to employ the natural science

formula of multiplicand and multiplier to obtain a product. Mathematicians tell us there is no other way to obtain these values. If this is true as regards a part of a compensation, it must be true as regards the whole of it if the problem is to be solved by mathematics in a scientific manner.

8. In our example the employee was earning $25 per week. This was his capacity to earn, or his power to earn, or his earning ability. It makes no difference which term is used to express it, so long as it definitely conveys the fact that whatever an employee may receive for his services depends entirely upon his earning ability.* This is so self-evident that it should seem apparent to any one, but that it has not been so viewed is apparent to any one who has studied the meager literature upon the subject.

9. This fact is stated very clearly in a recent well-prepared paper by Colonel C. W. Belton, Medical Adviser of the Board of Pension Commissioners for Canada,[5] after he had studied all available methods, as follows: "As far as could be learned, there was no basic principle from which might be deduced in manner more or less logical an award for any given damage. Yet it was fairly apparent that the effect of the damage on the earning power was in some way concerned with the assessment." As regards the status of his own government, he says: "Although the present regulations make no reference to earning power, there is no reason to believe that this has been set aside. In fact, certain clauses may be taken to confirm it. These clauses are important in other respects as well, and should be carefully considered."

10. Thus it will be seen from these two quotations that Colonel Belton approaches the solution of the compensation

---

* This term should be preferred when it refers to a human being, because a machine has a capacity to earn, or an earning power, when directed and controlled by a human being, while a human being directs and controls himself in order to have an earning ability. Therefore, ability implies an intellectuality which a machine doesn't have and which is not expressed in the word capacity or power.

problem with an open mind, which enables him to discern that "there was no basic principle from which might be deduced in manner more or less logical an award for any given damage," yet that "it was fairly apparent that the effect of the damage on the earning power was in some way concerned with the assessment," and finally as regards his own government he observes that "although the present regulations make no reference to earning power, there is no reason to believe that this has been set aside. In fact, certain clauses may be taken to confirm it" which he regards as important in other respects and which should be carefully considered.

11. These observations of Colonel Belton are of great importance because they come from one high in an official position, seeking the truth about the status of the solution of the compensation problem. I am persuaded by them in the belief that it is a duty I owe to the medical profession to do whatever I can to bring into practice a logical method of solving this problem, namely, the natural science method, having had instruction in its solution by this method since childhood from my father, who has made the solution of this problem a life-long study.

12. A Workmen's Compensation Act is designed primarily to reimburse in an equitable manner the employee for a certain loss he has sustained in his earning ability from injury or disease. The parties primarily concerned in the transaction are the employee and the employer, although the cost is eventually borne by the public which, of course, includes both the employee and employer. A law which requires all the people to contribute to the expense of its administration should certainly have a "basic principle from which might be deduced in manner more or less logical an award for any given damage." This certainly can be accomplished by determining the loss to the earning ability of the employee through the use of the natural science method.

13. The fact stated in a previous paragraph (¶8) that the

25

wages an employee receives for his services depend entirely upon his ability to earn, brings to view another fact that a loss in wages from injury or disease is due to a loss in the earning ability of that employee. In order to determine in a logical way what this loss is we must employ mathematics, the same as we would employ mathematics to determine the loss from anything else in the world. We have already shown in ¶6 and ¶7 how the weekly and the total compensation for the loss of the left eye of an employee were determined by the natural science method. Therefore, we must employ it to determine the true value of the earning ability of an employee and thereby any loss that may occur to it. In order to do this we must find an indispensable part of the earning ability of an employee to represent the factor of the multiplicand and another indispensable part to represent the factor of the multiplier to obtain a product. It is a law in mathematics, self-evident to any one who can comprehend a mathematical problem, that we must have at least these two factors to solve any problem.

14. The natural science method comprises an analysis of anything by which its indispensable parts are determined so that these can be used as factors in its formula of multiplicand and multiplier to obtain a product which represents the value of the thing analyzed. By this analysis it is self-evident that the first indispensable part of the earning ability of an employee is the functions of the body, for without them he would have no earning ability. For economic purposes the functions of the body would include the training of both the mind and the body. This complex quantity may be termed the functional ability of the employee, and for convenience may be represented by F as a symbol of the factor of the multiplicand. The other indispensable part of the earning ability to represent the factor of the multiplier is the ability of the employee to compete in the labor market. This may be termed the competing ability

of the employee. It may be defined as that part of his earning ability which enables him to secure an occupation, or to establish one for himself, and then to perform the duties thereof successfully enough to have an earning ability of economic value. It may be represented by C as a symbol for the factor of the multiplier. With E for the symbol of the earning ability of the employee we have for the equation as follows: (1) F C = E, the statement of the earning ability of an employee in the natural science formula for the purpose of determining its status on the basis of 1, that is to say, if all the functions of the body are normal and therefore equal to 1, then the coefficient of F, the functional ability of the employee, is equal to 1. This would be true of C, the competing ability of the employee, for his ability to compete in the labor market depends upon the functional ability of the body, for without the functional ability of the body there would be no competing ability of the employee. Hence, in such a case, the coefficient of C, the competing ability, would be 1, and if the coefficient of each of the factors of the multiplicand and multiplier is 1, the product E, the earning ability of the employee, must be equal to 1 or normal, for that employee.

15. In demonstrating in a logical manner how a compensation is assessed by the natural science method, we must have a standard of measurement for the proportionate part that each function of the body bears to the functional ability of the whole body, that is, for the loss of an eye the standard of measurement has been determined to be .18 of the functional ability of the whole body.[10] Hence by the natural science method as worked out in physical economics, the loss of the functions of an eye would be stated as follows: By subtracting .18 from 1, we have .82 for the coefficient of F, the functional ability of the whole body (.82F). As C, the competing ability of a person (as per ¶14), depends upon the same identical functions of the body for its existence, it

must have at first the same coefficient .82C. Hence, we have .82F .82C = E, the statement of the earning ability of an employee in the natural science formula for the loss of the functions of one eye for economic purposes. In the solution of this statement, if the medical examiner determines from all the conditions and circumstances surrounding this employee in the vocation he follows that the damage to C, the competing ability, is similar in amount to the loss to F, the functional ability, the remaining earning ability of the employee would be the product of these two factors. Hence, multiplying, we have E = .6724, and the loss is .3276, or 32.76 per cent.; 32.76 per cent. of $25, the weekly wages of the employee, is $8.19. This is the logical weekly compensation according to the determination of the medical examiner upon whose report the values in this problem must always depend. If another medical examiner is called to make an examination and report according to the natural science method as worked out in physical economics, and the report should differ from that of the first medical examiner, the commission can see at once why it differs, and knowing the method by which the percentage of loss to the earning ability is determined, they can thereby better judge which medical examiner is nearer the exact existing condition of the damage to the competing ability of the employee in the vocation he follows, and whether it is necessary to call in another medical examiner in order to determine the loss to the earning ability of the employee in a just and equitable manner.

16. For instance, if the medical examiner had determined that a machinist, aged thirty, had permanently lost one-half the central sight of the left eye, the field of vision and muscular functions of this eye being normal, with all three functions of the right eye normal, he could not report that this disability was equal to one-half the disability named in the schedule. This would be no more equitable than to

establish a standard that the compensation for the loss of the sight of the left eye should be equal to one-half the compensation given for the loss of sight in both eyes. In the case of the machinist, the loss would be one-half of .18, the standard of measurement for the loss of one eye, or .09. This we subtract from 1, the normal coefficient, and we have .91 for the coefficient of F, the functional ability of the body (.91F). As C, the competing ability of the machinist, depends upon the same identical functions of the body for its existence (¶14), it also must have the same coefficient (.91C), and we have as follows: .91F .91C = E, the statement of the earning ability of the machinist after the loss of one-half the sight of the left eye. Although the loss of one-half the sight of the left eye of the machinist is a severe loss to the eye itself, its proportionate loss to F, the functional ability of the whole body, is a slight loss, especially when the field of vision and muscular functions are normal. Hence, the medical examiner reported according to Physical Economies as follows: Loss to F = .09; Damage to C, 5° slight.* With these we find in Computation Table No. 3 that the loss to E = 11.92 per cent. The "damage to C, 5° Slight," represents that the medical examiner determined that the loss of sight to the machinist was slight and of the 5° slight, that is, it was next to a severe loss of vision in the vocation of a machinist. It will be seen that it was only necessary for the medical examiner to report the loss to F, the functional ability, and the degree of damage to C, the competing ability of the machinist, which he determined upon in order for the commission to quickly find by Table 3 the exact loss to the earning ability of the machinist for the loss of one-half of the vision in the left eye.

17. A comprehensive view of the natural science method is necessary in order to use it successfully in the determina-

---

* This statement in the formula would be as follows: .91F .91C ⅓ = E. Hence E = .8808, and the loss is .1192, or 11.92 per cent.

tion of damages to the functions of the eyes, or any other part of the body, from injury or disease, and thereby the loss to the earning ability upon which a compensation must always be based if we are to employ the only "basic principle" known by which "might be deduced in manner more or less logical an award for any given damage." For this purpose reference must be made first to the analysis of the body, by which it is resolved into its indispensable parts so that these parts may be used as factors in the multiplicand (¶14) as readily as though there were but one factor; second, to the standard of measurement by which any loss to the functions of the eyes may be determined; and third, to the method of grading the damage to the competing ability and thereby the loss to the earning ability of an employee in any vocation.

18. With this working knowledge of the natural science method as elucidated in the papers to which reference has been made, the medical examiner first determines the status of the functions of the eyes by an examination with instruments and methods of precision and thereby any loss in those functions. Remembering that the total loss to the functional ability of the whole body for the loss of the functions of one eye is .18, he determines whether the loss found, for instance, in one eye, is a slight loss, and if so, it is one-sixth of .18 or .03; whether it is a severe loss, and if so, it is one-half of .18 or .09; whether it is a nearly total loss, and if so, it is five-sixths of .18 or .15; and finally, whether it is a total loss, and if so, it is .18 of the functional ability of the whole body. The medical examiner makes his report in accordance with these determinations, as per example of the machinist in ¶16. With this report of the medical examiner the commission can quickly find by Table 3 the loss to the earning ability of the machinist to be 11.92 per cent.

19. With reference to the determination of the damage to C, the competing ability of an employee, from the loss to F, the functional ability, it must be kept constantly in view

that there can be only 100 per cent. damage to it; that this 100 per cent. damage is divided into three groups and for convenience named slight damage, of which there are designated five degrees; severe damage, of which there are six degrees; and nearly total damage, of which there are five degrees—making 16 degrees into which the 100 per cent. damage to C, the competing ability, is divided. This division of the 100 per cent. damage to the competing ability facilitates the work of the medical examiner in that he can readily determine whether the loss to F, the functional ability, damages C, the competing ability of an employee to a slight degree, or to a nearly total degree. If he determines from all the conditions and circumstances under which the employee will work, that he has sustained neither of these degrees of damage, then the damage to his competing ability inevitably comes between the two, which is severe, or it is a total damage which would be apparent without any comparison. When the medical examiner determines to which group the damage to the competing ability comes under, he then by the same logical process by which this was ascertained determines which degree of the group gives the loss to E, the earning ability of the employee, in accordance with the loss to the functional ability and the resulting damage to the competing ability of the employee in the vocation followed.

20. With a working knowledge of the "basic principle" as elucidated in the papers to which reference has been made, and mindful of the indisputable mathematical laws among which is the fact that the loss, or damage, to anything in this world can never be more than 100 per cent., a medical examiner may approach the solution of the compensation problem in ophthalmology with an assurance that his reports will obviate the criticism of Colonel Belton, for they will be made upon the "basic principle" of the natural science method from which may be "deduced in manner more or less logical an award for any given damage."

REFERENCES.   .

1. Vital Statistics, by William Farr, M.D., D.C.L., C.B., F.R.S.
2. Visual Economics, by H. Magnus, M.D., Breslau, Germany, translated with amendations by H. V. Würdemann, M.D., Seattle, Washington.
3. Bureau of Pensions, Department of the Interior, United States.
4. Bureau of War Risk Insurance, Department of the Interior, United States.
5. Pensions for the Disabled Soldiers, Canadian Expeditionary Forces, Colonel C. W. Belton, Medical Adviser to the Board of Pension Commissioners for Canada.
6. Estimation of the Amount of Injury to the Business Capacity of the Individual from Partial or Complete Loss of Vision. H. F. Hansell, M.D., Philadelphia.
7. The Computation of Compensation for Ocular Injuries, Major H. S. Gradle, M.R.C., U.S.A., Chicago.
8. Indemnities Following Injuries to the Eyes. How Shall we Determine Them? V. A. Chapman, M.D., Milwaukee, Wisconsin.
9. A Method of Computation for Ocular Injuries, Applicable to the New York State Workmen's Compensation Law, A. C. Snell, M.D., Rochester, New York.
10. Physical Economics, E. E. Holt, M.D., Portland, Maine.
Transactions Amer. Assn., U. S. Pension Exam. Surgeons, 1904. Transactions, Section of Ophthalmology, Amer. Med. Assn., 1906. Transactions Amer. Ophth. Soc., 1909 and 1920. Transactions Amer. Otol. Soc., 1912. Transactions Amer. Acad. of Ophth. and Oto-Laryn., 1914. Visual Economics, in Amer. Encyclo. of Ophth., 1921.

INDEX.

393

Lightning Source UK Ltd.
Milton Keynes UK
UKHW021524090219
336936UK00007B/780/P